Vagueness in Psychiatry

International Perspectives in Philosophy and Psychiatry

Series editors: Bill (K.W.M.) Fulford, Lisa Bortolotti, Matthew Broome, Katherine Morris, John Z. Sadler, and Giovanni Stanghellini

Vagueness in Psychiatry

Edited by

Geert Keil

Lara Keuck

Rico Hauswald

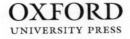

OXFORD

UNIVERSITY PRESS

OXFORD

UNIVERSITY PRESS

Great Clarendon Street, Oxford, OX2 6DP,
United Kingdom

Oxford University Press is a department of the University of Oxford.
It furthers the University's objective of excellence in research, scholarship,
and education by publishing worldwide. Oxford is a registered trade mark of
Oxford University Press in the UK and in certain other countries

Published in the United States of America by Oxford University Press
198 Madison Avenue, New York, NY 10016, United States of America

British Library Cataloguing in Publication Data
Data available

Library of Congress Control Number: 2016950024

ISBN 978-0-19-872237-3

Printed in Great Britain by
Ashford Colour Press Ltd, Gosport, Hampshire

Contents

List of contributors

John H. Blume
Cornell Law School,
NY, USA

Lisa Bortolotti
Department of Philosophy,
University of Birmingham, UK

Matthew Broome
Department of Psychiatry,
University of Oxford, UK

Allen Frances
Duke University School of Medicine,
Durham, NC, USA

Rico Hauswald
Department of Philosophy,
Dresden University of Technology,
Germany

Hanfried Helmchen
Department of Psychiatry
and Psychotherapy,
Charité Universitätsmedizin Berlin,
Germany

Amelia C. Hritz
Department of Human Development
and Law School,
Cornell University,
NY, USA

Peter Hucklenbroich
Institute for Ethics, History
and Theory of Medicine,
University of Münster,
Germany

Sheri L. Johnson
Cornell Law School, NY, USA

Geert Keil
Department of Philosophy,
Humboldt University of Berlin,
Germany

Lara Keuck
Department of History,
Humboldt University of Berlin,
Germany

Hans-Ludwig Kröber
Institute of Forensic Psychiatry,
Charité Universitätsmedizin Berlin,
Germany

Orly Lewis
Department of Classics,
Humboldt University of Berlin,
Germany

Matteo Mameli
Department of Philosophy,
King's College London,
UK

Richard J. McNally
Department of Psychology,
Harvard University,
Cambridge, MA, USA

Dan J. Stein
Department of Psychiatry &
Mental Health,
University of Cape Town,
South Africa

Ralf Stoecker
Department of Philosophy,
University of Bielefeld,
Germany

Ema Sullivan-Bissett
Department of Philosophy,
University of Birmingham,
UK

Tim Thornton
School of Nursing,
University of Central Lancashire,
UK

Chiara Thumiger
Department of Classics and
Ancient History, University
of Warwick, UK

Philip van der Eijk
Department of Classics,
Humboldt University of Berlin,
Germany

Peter Zachar
Department of Psychology,
Auburn University Montgomery,
Montgomery, AL, USA

Part I

Overview of vagueness in psychiatry

Chapter 1

Vagueness in psychiatry:
An overview

Geert Keil, Lara Keuck, and Rico Hauswald

1 Introduction

Many philosophers of psychiatry agree that in psychiatry there is no sharp boundary between the normal and the pathological. Although clear cases abound, it is often indeterminate whether a particular condition does or does not qualify as a mental disorder. For example, many disorders and diseases come in degrees. Definitions of 'subthreshold disorders' and of the 'prodromal stages' of diseases are notoriously contentious. Medical classification systems and diagnostic manuals may define thresholds, but such definitions are often stipulative and do not claim to carve nature at its joints.

Philosophers and linguists call concepts that lack sharp boundaries 'vague'. 'Vagueness' is a term of art that denotes a semantic property of linguistic expressions. Vague terms admit of borderline cases because they draw no sharp distinction between their extension and their anti-extension, that is, between the phenomena they apply to and those they do not apply to. Arguably, the concepts of mental health, disease, and disorder[1] are vague in this sense.

While blurred boundaries between the normal and the pathological are a recurrent theme in almost every publication concerned with the classification of mental disorders, systematic approaches that take into account the philosophical discussions about vagueness are rare.[2] Usually the indeterminacy of nosological categories is invoked either as an argument against essentialist definitions or 'reifications' of diseases (see Bolton 2008) or as being heuristically

---

[1] We are well aware of the difficulties that arise from attempts at adequately naming our object of inquiry. The terms 'mental disease', 'psychiatric disease', 'mental disorder', and 'mental illness' have no standard meanings and often connote different things, depending on the context of their use. In this introduction we do not reflect on these differences, but several of the chapters in this book do.

[2] A notable exception is Sadegh-Zadeh's *Handbook of Analytic Philosophy of Medicine*, which contains a discussion of the vagueness of medical language (Sadegh-Zadeh 2012, 37–47).

useful for reasoning about, and refining, diagnostic classifications (see Kendler and Parnas 2012). In the literature, the following issues dominate discussions about the fundamentals of psychiatric nosology:

- Categorical versus dimensional approaches in current psychiatric classification systems: Should diagnostic manuals move away from binary categorizations (e.g. affected vs not affected)?[3] If so, how should non-categorical approaches be represented in the manuals and implemented in medical, administrative, and juridical practice?[4]

- Principles of psychiatric classification, particularly with respect to questions like these: Are mental disorders natural kinds with sharp boundaries, are they instead simply arbitrary or pragmatic conventions, or is this opposition artificial?[5] Does the concept of disease itself (as opposed to particular disease concepts) correspond to a natural kind, or is it a Roschian prototype concept? Or does it have a family resemblance structure?[6]

- Prodromal phases and subthreshold disorders, especially in the case of controversial states at the boundary between health and disease.[7]

- The problem of overdiagnosis in psychiatry: responding to the recent revision of the *Diagnostic and Statistical Manual of Mental Disorders* (*DSM*; APA 2013), a number of psychiatrists have warned against the trend of shifting the admittedly vague borderline between the normal and the pathological by lowering the thresholds for certain diagnostic criteria.[8]

Although conceptual problems surrounding the fuzziness in the classifications of mental disorders feature prominently in all of these debates, there have been

---

[3] See, for example, the books edited by Widiger et al. (2006), Helzer et al. (2008), and Zachar and Ellis (2012).

[4] The new Research Domain Criteria (RDoC) introduced by the National Institute of Mental Health (NIMH) are already in use and an example of a new, multidimensional taxonomy of mental disorders that doesn't rely on disease constructs as we know them; see the papers by Hyman (2010) and Tabb (2015) and the influential NIMH director's blog entry (Insel 2013).

[5] See the special issue titled *Classification and Explanation in Psychiatry*, edited by Bortolotti and Malatesti (2010), and book chapters by Cooper (ch. 2 in Cooper 2005), Zachar (2008), and Samuels (2009).

[6] See the journal articles by D'Amico (1995), Lilienfeld and Marino (1995), and Sadegh-Zadeh (2008).

[7] See the books by Horwitz and Wakefield (2007; 2012), the book chapter by Broome et al. (2011), or the special issue titled *Mild Cognitive Impairment*, edited by Hughes (2006).

[8] See e.g. Frances (2013) and Paris (2015). For an overview of debates that the *DSM-5* sparked within the philosophy of psychiatry, see also Demazeux and Singy (2015).

no systematic efforts to draw these lines of inquiry together and explore their connections to philosophical debates on vagueness. This is true not only for psychiatry, but also for the philosophy of medicine in general. As Djulbegovic, Hozo, and Greenland (2011, 329) observed, 'despite its importance and its roots dating back to the ancient Sorites paradox, little work has been done on examining the role of vagueness in medicine'.

The present book aims to address this lacuna and, moreover, to discuss the particular consequences of dealing with vagueness in psychiatry. A number of chapters apply philosophical and linguistic insights on vagueness and demarcation problems to psychiatric theory and practice. Philosophical terms of art such as 'soritical vagueness' or 'combinatorial vagueness' may be unfamiliar to many clinical psychiatrists. One of the aims of the book is to demonstrate that philosophical distinctions and clarifications can provide useful tools for elucidating problems of psychiatric nosology and classification. Conversely, philosophical treatments of vagueness have hitherto displayed little concern for socially or otherwise *relevant* demarcation problems. Although psychiatric classifications seem to provide paradigmatic examples of vague concepts and categories, the philosophical debates on vagueness have largely focused on heaps, bald heads, colours, clouds, or mountains, all of which have few or no implications for real-life problems. In the literature on vagueness there is only one field that can point to a tradition of collaboration between philosophers and non-philosophers and that emphasizes real-world demarcation problems, namely the field of vagueness *in law* (see Endicott 2000; Poscher and Keil 2016). The present book aims at establishing a second such field.

The book examines the sources, kinds, and consequences of the fuzziness of psychiatric classification, proposes some remedies, and discusses the pros and cons of gradualist approaches to health and disease. The 13 chapters explore the field from different perspectives, including theoretical philosophy, philosophy of psychiatry, and forensic psychiatry. They draw on examples and experiences from the clinic, the courtroom, and everyday life in current and past cultures and discuss them in the light of philosophical accounts of vagueness, disease entities, and psychiatric classification.

2 What is vagueness?

The adjective 'vague' has both an ordinary and a technical meaning. In ordinary language, the word is mostly used pejoratively: vague hints, vague promises, or vague announcements are airy and nebulous, in the sense that the speaker is deliberately less specific than is contextually appropriate. By speaking vaguely, one can hide intentions and withhold information. In linguistics and philosophy, by contrast, 'vague' is a technical term. Vagueness is a semantic property of linguistic expressions. Vague terms draw no sharp boundary between their extension and their anti-extension. They tolerate marginal changes, admit of borderline cases, and give rise to the paradox of the heap—that is, the paradox that you can 'prove', by a series of incremental arguments (if 1,000 grains of sand make up a heap, then so do 999 grains, as do 998, etc.), that a single grain of sand makes up a heap. Soritical reasoning from impeccable premises to absurd conclusions is certainly fallacious, but it has proved notoriously hard to pinpoint the fallacy. The sorites paradox can be traced back to the ancient philosopher Eubulides of Miletus, who used the examples 'heap' (Greek *sōros*) and 'bald man'. Vague predicates are the logician's nightmare because they challenge *bivalence*, the logical principle that every sentence or proposition is either true or false.

Over the past two decades, vagueness has become one of the hottest topics in the philosophy of language. There is a vast literature that discusses the semantic, pragmatic, logical, and metaphysical aspects of the phenomenon.[9] In the philosophy of language, vagueness has been recognized as a challenge to the project of developing a systematic theory of meaning. The vagueness of countless ordinary predicates is an undeniable trait of natural languages. Semantic theories that deny this trait or do not take it seriously are descriptively inadequate. In order to solve the sorites paradox without denying the phenomenon, philosophers have developed a number of *theories* of vagueness that are largely unknown outside academic philosophy, the most important ones being supervaluationism, contextualism, epistemicism, many-valued logic and degree theories, and incoherentist or nihilistic theories.[10]

The point of departure of this book, however, is not a particular *theory* of vagueness, but the *phenomenon* of vagueness and its implications for demarcation problems in psychiatry. Recent philosophical discussions on vagueness in semantics, logic, and metaphysics have become sophisticated and sometimes arcane, and the aim of this book is not to make a major contribution to the refinement of theories of vagueness. Progress on this front can be made without examples from medicine, psychiatry, or law. And, conversely, not all ramifications of the competing theories of vagueness are relevant to phenomena of vagueness and indeterminacy in psychiatry. For our present purposes, however, we have selected four topics from the multifaceted philosophical discussion that do have implications for demarcation problems in psychiatry: (1) the

---

[9] For an overview, see Williamson (1994); Pinkal (1995); Keefe and Smith (1997); Keefe (2000); Sorensen (2001); Graff and Williamson (2002); Shapiro (2006); Hyde (2008); Ronzitti (2011); Raffman (2014); Hyde (2014); Sorensen (2016).

[10] For an overview, see Keefe (2000) and Sorensen (2016).

clarification that vagueness is not a consequence of an epistemic deficiency; (2) the debate on whether all vagueness is representational; (3) the distinction between vagueness and other indeterminacy phenomena; and (4) the discussion about the potential value of vagueness.

2.1 Vagueness versus epistemic uncertainty

While vagueness may manifest itself in a speaker's uncertainty about what to say, it is not a result of that speaker's ignorance of empirical facts. Hence the uncertainty cannot be remedied by accessing further information:

> To say that an expression is vague . . . is . . . to say that there are cases (actual or possible) in which one just does not know whether to apply the expression or to withhold it, and one's not knowing is not due to ignorance of the facts. (Grice 1989, 177)

> [V]agueness is taken as a semantic property of expressions which is independent of the speaker's ignorance of facts. The indeterminacy is due to an aspect of the meaning of the term rather than to our current state of knowledge. (Gullvåg and Næss 1996, 1417; see Alston 1967, 218)

> No amount of conceptual analysis or empirical investigation can settle whether a 1.8-meter man is tall. Borderline cases are inquiry resistant. (Sorensen 2016, section 1)

The word 'heap' is vague precisely because a speaker may know the exact number of grains and still wonder whether the collection comprises a heap or not. The vagueness of a linguistic expression not only raises the practical problem of *where* to draw the line, but also the *conceptual* problem that, wherever the line is drawn, it will yield borderline cases. Demarcations that work with numerical values (50 grains of sand, wavelengths $\geq$ 600 nm, symptoms lasting for 14 days or more) may circumvent this problem, but, if the concept in question is semantically vague, then such precisifications are arbitrary and underdetermined by empirical data. There simply is no matter-of-fact answer to the question of how many grains a heap must have or at precisely which wavelength light begins to look red.

Now, 'many psychiatrists and psychologists believe that much of the vagueness in psychiatry is epistemic. Their hope is that yet to be discovered information involving biomarkers, endophenotypes, and underlying mechanisms will lead to increased diagnostic clarity' (Zachar and McNally, Chapter 9.1). In the same vein, Hucklenbroich argues that vagueness in psychiatry merely indicates the scientifically immature status of this branch of medicine (Chapter 4). Epistemic deficits, however, must be distinguished from conceptual challenges. While a lack of knowledge poses an additional obstacle to clear-cut psychiatric diagnoses and classifications, semantic vagueness by its very nature cannot be eliminated through scientific discoveries. If medical classifications and diagnostic categories are fuzzy due to semantic vagueness, then scientific progress will not remove this fuzziness. If 'disease' is an essentially vague notion, then it behaves semantically very much like 'heap': a clinician confronted with mild symptoms of prodromal forms may know the exact medical condition of that patient and still wonder whether the condition should qualify as a disease or not.

2.2 Is all vagueness representational?

In a seminal paper from 1923 Bertrand Russell argued that all vagueness is linguistic, or at least representational:

> [V]agueness and precision alike are characteristics which can only belong to a representation, of which language is an example. They have to do with the relation between a representation and that which it represents. Apart from representation . . . there can be no such thing as vagueness or precision; things are what they are, and there is an end of it. Nothing is more or less what it is, or to a certain extent possessed of the properties which it possesses. (Russell 1923, 85)

Michael Dummett and David Lewis concur: '[T]he notion that things might actually *be* vague, as well as being vaguely described, is not properly intelligible' (Dummett 1975, 111). 'The only intelligible account of vagueness locates it in our thought and language' (Lewis 1986, 212). Every now and then, however, it has been suggested that, in addition to semantic or representational vagueness, there might be an 'ontological' or 'metaphysical' kind of vagueness. Since the last decades of the twentieth century, a growing minority of philosophers have suggested that the idea of vagueness in the world—vagueness *in rebus*—is not absurd.[11]

On a closer look, it seems that Russell's unintelligibility objection does not go very deep. It does little more than remind us of a linguistic fact about the established use or meaning of the term 'vague'. The word has such heavy semantic connotations that it sounds odd to apply it to non-linguistic items. The question is whether this oddity reflects some deeper mismatch. So let us change the wording: plausibly, physical objects cannot be vague in exactly the same sense in which linguistic expressions can be, but few would deny that mountains, clouds, or forests can have 'fuzzy', 'blurry', or 'unsharp' boundaries, both spatially and temporally. These adjectives apply to both representational and non-representational items. As soon as we change the wording from 'vague' to 'blurred' and its cognates, the impression of categorical absurdity vanishes.

A pivotal question in the debate on ontic vagueness is how the vagueness of linguistic expressions and the fuzziness of spatio-temporal boundaries *relate* to each other. One suggestion is that psychiatric concepts and classifications are

---

[11] For an overview, see Keil (2013). The present section draws on this article.

vague *because* the reality that they aim to capture is continuous rather than discrete. Let us call *gradualism* about health and disease the view that (many) diseases and disorders come in degrees and that there is no natural lower threshold that demarcates health from disease. Gradualism is not a claim about language, but about the underlying reality. It relates to a highly general principle in natural philosophy: the *principle of continuity*, which philosophers since antiquity have expressed through the dictum *natura non facit saltus* (nature makes no leaps). A prominent representative of this principle is Leibniz, who argued that all differences and transitions in nature are gradual. The principle of continuity has both static and dynamic readings, both of which are relevant to medical nosology: gradualism may hold for synchronic *differences* between states, or for *changes* from one state to another, or for both.

Imagine by contrast a 'Lego world' where all objects have simple, static, geometric forms with sharp edges: a universe that consists of just Lego bricks and the void. In such a world, predicates like 'flat' or 'cubic' or 'red' are still *intensionally* vague, in other words their linguistic meanings are such that they do not rule out the *possibility* of borderline cases, but, as long as their *extensions* are clear-cut—that is, as long as borderline cases do not actually occur—no non-philosopher will care.

On a closer look, it seems ill-advised to press the question of what the ultimate source of vagueness is, whether it be our representations or the things themselves, our language or the world. The relationship is dialectical because natural languages did not evolve in a Lego world. An analogy might be helpful to illustrate the dialectics at work. Think of language as a tool: sugar tongs are perfect tools for gripping sugar cubes. But if you try and fail to grip powdered sugar with sugar tongs, then who is to blame, the sugar or the tongs? This rhetorical question brings us back to the discussion about dimensional versus categorical approaches to psychiatric classification. Binary categories work well in clear-cut cases of severe illness and good health, but they cannot adequately capture mild or controversial forms of putative mental disorders. Again, we may ask: Who is to blame, the phenomena or the classifications? The sugar tongs analogy, however, suggests that this is not a good question to ask. We may say that the presence of natural continuities *makes* crisp classifications an inapt tool, but only in a non-causal sense of 'making'. The mismatch between a tool and the reality to be gripped can be described from either side.

2.3 Degree vagueness and other indeterminacy phenomena

Philosophers usually distinguish between *degree* (or *soritical*) vagueness and *combinatory* vagueness (Alston 1967, 219). Degree-vague concepts do not draw a sharp line in a single dimension. Combinatory vague concepts, on the other hand, comprise a cluster of independent dimensions, and these dimensions are such that, in some of their combinations, it is indeterminate whether or not the concept applies. The concept 'heap' is degree-vague because it does not draw a sharp line in a single underlying dimension, that is, in the number of grains. Alston's example of a combinatory vague concept is 'religion': religions are characterized by a number of features such as a belief in gods, regarding certain objects as sacred, ritual acts, a moral code, characteristic feelings, a world view, and a social organization bound together by these characteristics (Alston 1967, 219). The term 'religion' is combinatory vague because there is no fact of the matter as to how many of these characteristics, and which of them, must be present in order for the term to apply. It is clear, for example, that the presence of rituals is neither necessary nor sufficient for something to be a religion. But the presence of all the characteristics is not necessary either. In Buddhism there is no belief in gods, yet Buddhism still counts as a religion. Where to draw the line is not completely determinate, and borderline cases exist where it is not clear whether the phenomena constitute a religion or not (see Chapter 5.4).

These two main forms of vagueness need to be distinguished from other semantic forms of indeterminacy, such as *ambiguity* and *generality*, as well as from non-semantic forms of indeterminacy, such as natural *continuity* and epistemic *uncertainty.*

While vagueness, as characterized above, is a term's propensity to allow for borderline cases, a term is *ambiguous* if it has more than one meaning. For example, 'bank' is ambiguous because it can mean either a 'financial institution' or the 'edge of a river'. 'Depression' is ambiguous between a number of technical meanings, for example in psychiatry, economics, geography, and meteorology. In addition, it has a non-technical meaning in ordinary language that is closely related to its psychiatric meaning. While a vague term has one fuzzy extension, an ambiguous term has two or more distinct extensions.

Generality is a property of terms that have a broad, underspecified extension. To say that a term or a description is general is to say that it would be possible to give a more detailed description by using more specific terms. For example, 'beverage' is general since it comprises beer, wine, soft drinks, and so on. The category of 'unspecified mental disorder' in the International Statistical Classification of Diseases and Related Health Problems (ICD) is general as well.

Continuity is a real-world trait that does not depend on semantics. For example, clouds consist of swarms of water droplets whose density gradually diminishes towards the periphery of the cloud. Unlike Lego bricks, clouds have no sharp edges. A *class* of phenomena may be said to be continuous if it has no 'realization gaps' (Pinkal 1995, 106). Such realization gaps exist between natural kinds such as gold, silver, and copper: the natural world encompasses a fixed number of chemical elements, but no median elements. By contrast, between the highest mountain and the smallest hillock some intermediate promontory can always be built or found somewhere. The movie about the Englishman who once went up a hill but came down a mountain plays on arbitrary classifications, but real-world continuities are not artefacts of representational systems. Linguistic conventions, such as requiring a mountain to be 1,000 feet high, do not refute natural continuities. Likewise, progressive dementia remains a continuous phenomenon even if psychiatrists have decided to distinguish between five or seven stages of it, and even if the phenomenon is not called 'dementia' any more, but rather 'major neurocognitive disorder'.[12]

While all these forms of indeterminacy are distinct phenomena in their own right, this does not imply that they can always be easily distinguished or are completely independent of each other. For example, even though there is no necessary connection between a word's vagueness and the absence of realization gaps, the use of vague expressions is arguably more appropriate or useful when describing a continuous domain of reality, while precise expressions are better suited for describing discrete phenomena. Also, it is sometimes difficult to distinguish the various forms of semantic indeterminacy, since there are contexts in which a term exhibits several forms at once, for example soritical vagueness, combinatory vagueness, and generality. In psychiatry, semantic indeterminacy of diagnostic categories is typically overlaid with epistemic *uncertainty*, and often it is arduous to disentangle both: Is it hard to secure the diagnosis because we do not know the exact condition of the patient, or because the diagnostic category is vaguely defined, or because of both?

These intricacies have consequences for the design of this book. Many chapters, while focussing on vagueness, will also touch on questions of ambiguity, generality, ontological continuity, and epistemic uncertainty in psychiatry and will explore the relationships that hold between these phenomena.

2.4 The value of vagueness

Philosophers disagree about whether vagueness is a vice or a virtue, that is, whether the pejorative connotations of the ordinary notion encroach upon the technical term of semantic vagueness or not. The ends of the spectrum are marked by Frege and the later Wittgenstein. Frege compares concepts to areas

---

[12] The clinical dementia rating (CDR) divides the disease process into five stages. The global deterioration scale for assessment of primary degenerative dementia (GDS) distinguishes seven stages. The *DSM-5* has substituted the term 'neurocognitive disorders' for 'dementia'.

on a plane and argues from this analogy that concepts without sharp boundaries do not deserve their name:

> We may express this metaphorically as follows: the concept must have a sharp bound-
> ary .... To a concept without sharp boundaries there would correspond an area that
> had not a sharp boundary-line all around, but in places just vaguely faded away into the
> background. This would not really be an area at all; and likewise a concept that is not
> sharply defined is wrongly termed a concept. (Frege 1952 [1903], 159 [§ 56])

Wittgenstein (1953, § 99) tentatively agrees with Frege that '[a]n indefinite
boundary is not really a boundary at all', but he objects that vague concepts are
often useful and that their benefits are due precisely to their vagueness:

> But is it senseless to say: 'Stand roughly there'? Suppose that I were standing with some-
> one in a city square and said that. As I say it I do not draw any kind of boundary, but
> perhaps point with my hand—as if I were indicating a particular *spot*. (Wittgenstein
> 1953, § 71)

> Is it even always an advantage to replace an indistinct picture by a sharp one? Isn't the
> indistinct one often exactly what we need? (Ibid.)

One of Wittgenstein's favourite examples is the term 'game'. It has no sharp
boundaries, nor are we able to come up with a precise definition because 'game'
is a cluster concept that exhibits combinatory vagueness.

> But this is not ignorance. We do not know the boundaries because none have been
> drawn. To repeat, we can draw a boundary—for a special purpose. Does it take that
> to make the concept usable? Not at all! (Except for that special purpose.) (Ibid., § 69)

We may stipulate some definition, but the resulting concept would no longer
be our ordinary concept of 'game'. Arbitrary boundaries always need a special
justification: 'It is unnatural to draw a conceptual boundary line where there is
not some special justification for it, where similarities would constantly draw us
across the arbitrarily drawn line' (Wittgenstein 1980, II, § 626). What is more, it
is often exactly the imprecision that makes the concept valuable in our communicative practices. The concept that results from imposing sharp boundaries on
our ordinary word 'game' may be more precise, but at the same time less useful
for everyday communicative purposes. Ordinary language and communication
have not evolved in a Lego or a Minecraft world. Nor has psychiatry. The vague
terms 'game', 'heap', 'mountain', 'dementia', and 'post-traumatic stress disorder'
are useful precisely because the areas of reality that their use partitions exhibit
continuous transitions rather than sharp cut-offs.

Incidentally, Frege was well aware of the tension between precision and usefulness. His remark that ill-defined concepts are not concepts at all pertains exclusively to his *Begriffsschrift*, devised as 'a formal language of pure thought modeled
on that of arithmetic', while he acknowledges that predicates in natural languages

are more flexible: 'The shortcomings stressed [here] are rooted in a certain soft-ness and instability of [ordinary] language, which nevertheless is necessary for its versatility and potential for development' (Frege 1972 [1882], 86). Frege goes on to compare ordinary language to the human hand by illustrating its 'adaptability to the most diverse tasks', while artificial 'tools for particular purposes . . . work with more accuracy than the hand can provide' (ibid.).

Medical classification systems are applied across multiple contexts: on the one hand they face demands for reliability, precision, and stability, and on the other they must be open to scientific developments as well as adaptable to spe-cific doctor–patient encounters. The chapters in this book illustrate that it is often difficult to decide when the vagueness of psychiatric language is a vice and when it is a virtue. A general answer that is valid in all contexts is not to be expected.

3 Demarcation problems in psychiatry

The two main kinds of vagueness distinguished above beset any demarcation between mental health and disease, as well as between various diseases or path-ological conditions. First, due to gradual transitions from normal to pathologi-cal states, the phenomena exhibit *degree vagueness*. For example, according to *DSM-IV* (APA 2000, 42), persons count as 'mentally retarded' if their intellec-tual functioning is 'significantly subaverage', that is, 'approximately 70 or below'. 'Significantly subaverage' and 'approximately' are of course vague notions. That is to say, the concept of 'mental retardation' draws no sharp boundary along the IQ spectrum but instead accounts for gradual transitions from 'healthy' to 'pathological' conditions. *DSM-IV* then distinguishes four degrees of severity of intellectual impairment (mild, moderate, severe, profound). Further adjectives that the manual uses in specifying the degrees, such as 'considerable', 'notice-able', 'typical', and 'significant', are soritically vague as well.

Second, the concepts of 'mental disease' and of 'health' and 'normality', against which pathological conditions are demarcated, exhibit *combinatory vagueness*. The same holds for many particular mental disorders that are polythetically defined—that is, defined according to a minimum number of features on a list. The *DSM* frequently uses the formulation 'few, if any, symptoms in excess of those required to make the diagnosis' to characterize 'mild' forms of disorders (e.g. APA 2013, 60), thus indicating the presence of combinatory vagueness. For major depressive disorder, *DSM-5* requires five out of nine symptoms. Post-traumatic stress disorder (PTSD) can be diagnosed if six symptoms from a list of 20 are present, so that people can be diagnosed with PTSD without sharing a single symptom (see Chapter 9).

It is one thing to observe that many contemporary psychiatric concepts exhibit some forms of vagueness, and another to evaluate this situation. While all of the contributors to this volume diagnose some kind of imprecision in the concepts and classifications they examine, their evaluations differ considerably. Some authors argue that the indeterminacy that seems to be ubiquitous in psychiatry is a sign of its currently underdeveloped status and should be eliminated or minimized as psychiatry develops into a true science (Chapter 4; see also Murphy 2006). Others advocate gradualist approaches, arguing either that the reality psychiatry deals with is not divided into well-defined natural kinds or that psychiatry is imbued with inherent epistemic uncertainty—or both. Those who favour gradualist approaches do not expect psychiatry's language to become ever more precise; instead they advise against misleading claims of precision. As Zachar and McNally put it with respect to PTSD:

> Once we stipulate criteria, we can ask how many new cases of PTSD can be expected to develop in the United States in a single year or how many people in the United States can be expected to have PTSD in their lifetime. Because the *DSM* specifies precise diagnostic thresholds, we expect PTSD to be crisp and countable in these ways, but expecting such questions to have definitive answers is a bit like expecting that we can discover how many grains of sand one needs in order to have a genuine heap. If one is educated about the nature of the vague concepts, such questions are misplaced. (Zachar and McNally, Chapter 9.8)

Other authors argue that dealing reasonably and responsibly with vagueness is an integral part of diagnostic reasoning and that gradualist approaches can even increase therapeutic opportunities. A gradualist understanding of health and disease might shift the psychiatrist's attention away from the disabilities of a patient and towards that patient's remaining abilities as entry points for therapeutic interventions (see Chapter 7).

Some chapters see the appropriateness of gradualist or non-gradualist approaches as an unresolved problem, or at least as an issue that needs to be evaluated case by case: some phenomena, such as progressive neurodegenerative diseases, may always require that ultimately arbitrary boundaries be drawn along a continuum. Other medical conditions may be more easily captured by clear-cut classifications or may present better targets for scientific progress to reveal genuine differences that warrant fine-grained distinctions. Finally, it is also possible that our knowledge of some psychiatric phenomena is so underdeveloped that any attempt to define them with precision is premature, and even the question of whether gradualist or non-gradualist approaches are ultimately appropriate must be postponed. Nevertheless, as Chapter 5 attempts to do, we can at least provide some terminology for comparing various kinds of vague and precise medical classifications and weigh their pros and cons in different circumstances.

Despite its fuzziness, the boundary between health and disease plays a crucial role in our social practices; and these practices have, in turn, effects on individuals, on public health, and on society as a whole. To be classified as mentally ill has considerable social, normative, legal, and economic consequences. Who receives medical treatment? Who pays for it? Who is eligible for disability benefits? Who is allowed to stay off work? Who can purchase life insurance? Who is subjected to compulsory hospitalization? Which defendant can plead 'diminished responsibility'? Controversial in all of these cases is the question of what degree of impairment should correspond to exactly what sort of exculpation, entitlement, or compensation. Furthermore, attempts to draw boundaries between the normal and the pathological intersect with *normative* considerations. Concepts like 'health', 'disease', 'disorder', and 'abnormal' are often considered to have an evaluative dimension, whatever that precisely means. Normative considerations play some role in many of the chapters and occupy centre stage in Chapter 3.

Given the immense social importance of demarcating mental health and disease, it comes as no surprise that the development of each new edition of the major classification systems of mental disorders, the *DSM* and the ICD, is accompanied by heated debates inside and outside psychiatry. For instance, the psychiatrist Allen Frances, former chairman of the task force that published *DSM-IV*, has forcefully argued that *DSM-5* will promote 'diagnostic inflation' in psychiatry 'by reducing thresholds for existing disorders and by introducing new high prevalence disorders at the boundary with normality' (Frances 2012). The debate surrounding *DSM-5*'s lowered diagnostic thresholds provides examples for many of the analyses presented in this book (see Chapter 8). Other chapters remind us that issues concerning gradualist approaches to health and mental illness are by no means confined to current regimes of classification.

4 Guide to contents

4.1 Health and disease as matters of degree

After the introductory Part I, Part II of the book encompasses historical and recent philosophical positions regarding the nature of demarcation problems in nosology. The authors discuss the pros and cons of gradualist approaches to health and disease and the relevance of philosophical discussions of vagueness to these debates. The chapters in this part analyse the reasons and sources of indeterminacy in medical classification and examine how different theories of disease may account for them. Considering the differences and similarities between general medicine and psychiatry, the authors debate why the blurred boundary between health and disease is especially challenging in psychiatry. This sets the stage for later chapters that analyse clinical, social, and legal issues in greater detail.

Chapter 2 looks back in history. Orly Lewis, Chiara Thumiger, and Philip van der Eijk introduce ancient medical ideas about 'balance' and 'imbalance' and relate them to modern notions of degree vagueness and combinatorial vagueness. Gradualist notions of (mental) health and disease can be traced back to antiquity. Aristotle held that health

> admits of degrees . . . for it does not consist in the same proportion in everyone, nor is it even always the same one proportion in the same person, but even when it is fading it remains up to a point, and differs in degree. (Nicomachean Ethics, 10.3, 1173ª24; for discussion, see Chapter 2.2)

Ancient Greek and Roman physicians, most prominently Galen, followed this track. These ideas resonate with issues raised in almost all of the remaining chapters. Another characteristic of Graeco-Roman medicine that the chapter highlights is the fundamental consideration given to the body–mind continuum as an object of medical attention. It was impossible to discuss psychiatric matters in isolation, without paying heed to the health of the individual as a whole.

Chapter 3 discusses challenges to a crisp definition of 'disease' from a systematic perspective. Geert Keil and Ralf Stoecker argue that disease is a thick and vague cluster concept. As a cluster concept, it vacillates between biological malfunctioning, subjective suffering, and impaired ability for social interaction. As a thick concept, it has both descriptive and evaluative content. The soritical vagueness of the normal and the pathological, the combinatorial vagueness of the cluster concept, and the normativity of the thick concept have not yet been considered in combination. Using the example of major depressive disorder and discussing the *DSM-IV*'s bereavement exclusion criterion, the chapter explores how the definitional problems relate to one another. It draws conclusions for medical ethics on the basis of the observation that the various normative issues involved in receiving a psychiatric diagnosis hinge on different strands of the cluster concept 'disease'.

Chapter 4 focuses on disease from a biomedical perspective. Peter Hucklenbroich examines the notion of 'disease entities', which arose in the context of scientific developments in medicine in the nineteenth century. He argues that 'disease entity' has been and still is the most fundamental notion and theoretical tool of nosology. The chapter explains the distinction between tentatively proposed, clinically proven, and aetiopathogenetically defined disease entities and argues that disease entities are, by definition, distinct and mutually exclusive. Against this background, Hucklenbroich interprets vagueness and gradualism in present-day psychiatry as evidence of psychiatry's scientific immaturity. Psychiatry is not in need of gradations between health and disease in general, but rather of empirically sound and validated gradations that address the kind, stage, and severity of its nosological entities—including its provisional surrogates for proper disease entities.

Chapter 5 argues that discussions about the blurred boundaries and poor validity of current psychiatric classification draw on, and often confound, ontological, epistemic, and semantic aspects of indeterminacy. Rico Hauswald and Lara Keuck aim to clarify the terminology and interrelationship of these aspects. In contrast to Hucklenbroich's view that disease entities are mutually exclusive, the chapter argues that they can be either discrete or continuous, depending on whether realization gaps arise. Also, some disease classifications are more controversial than others. The chapter explains these differences by examining how the validity of a disease classification is assessed in various contexts of use and how it depends on the different (legitimate) interests and purposes of classifying. The epistemic aspect of uncertainty affects whether medical categories are defined vaguely or precisely. However, the chapter emphasizes that precise categories can be just as controversial as vague ones, thereby raising the question of how best to fit linguistic representations with the reality that medicine aims to classify and control.

4.2 Vagueness in psychiatric classification and diagnosis

The middle part of the book narrows the focus to psychiatric nosology. The authors approach the vagueness of psychiatric classification by drawing on contentious medical categories, such as PTSD or schizophrenia, and on the dilemmas of day-to-day diagnostic and therapeutic practice. Against this background, the chapters critically evaluate how current revisions of the ICD classification and *DSM* manual conceptualize mental disorders and how they are applied in various contexts. The authors also draft recommendations for future revisions of the DSM (Chapter 8) and put forward alternative accounts of how psychiatric diagnoses could be captured more appropriately (Chapters 6 and 9).

Chapter 6 provides a gestalt account of psychiatric diagnosis that is opposed to the current criteriological approaches taken in the *DSM* and the ICD. Tim Thornton shows that a central premise of criteriological approaches is the operationalization of isolated symptoms. This premise has been subject to criticism from phenomenologically oriented philosophers and psychiatrists. Following their lead, the chapter argues that abstract criteria, for instance those for schizophrenia as defined in psychiatric classifications, remain vague and fail to capture the precise connection between symptoms and skilled diagnostic judgements. By Thornton's alternative account, in an overall gestalt diagnostic judgement, the various criteria are abstractions from a whole that directly expresses the underlying psychopathological state of patients or clients. The chapter draws on philosophical theories from Polanyi and McDowell to explain how, for skilled clinicians, it is possible to recognize schizophrenia in a patient's psychopathological state, although this state might not be accessible and explicable through operationalized diagnostic criteria.

Chapter 7 approaches the question of fuzzy boundaries and tough decisions from a clinical perspective. Hanfried Helmchen explains how psychiatrists try to reduce medical uncertainty by stipulating strict definitions of clinical categories, by applying algorithms and methods of evidence-based medicine, and by operationalizing diagnoses. Helmchen stresses that clinical psychiatrists are well aware not only of the instrumental value but also of the limits of these means. The chapter provides an overview of the decisions psychiatrists have to make in reaching a diagnosis and of the ways in which regimes of standardization help or impede those decisions. Drawing on the example of subthreshold disorders, Helmchen discusses the pivotal importance of considering patients' individuality and of focusing not only on their diseases, but also on the remaining healthy portion of their personalities—especially in view of the unintended consequences of psychiatric diagnosis, such as the side effects of drug therapy and stigmatization.

Chapter 8 takes the harmful consequences and misuse of psychiatric diagnoses as a point of departure in reflecting on the roles that 'the normal', 'the not normal', and 'the in-between' play in psychiatric research, medical practice, and other fields where *DSM* classifications are used (e.g. for forensic purposes or for advisory opinions on special educational needs). Lara Keuck and Allen Frances argue that diagnostic inflation can be observed in two directions: in the pathologization of hitherto 'normal' behaviour; and in the pathologization of socially undesired 'not normal' behaviour. The chapter examines risk conditions, mild and prodromal disorders, and other states that are considered in-between the normal and the pathological. Keuck and Frances point out that these conditions exhibit not only vagueness, as described in Chapters 3, 5, and 9, but also ambiguity: in-between states represent conditions that do not (yet) count as disease, but they also signify the prodromal stages of mental disorders, thereby putting the emphasis on being not *yet* diseased. The chapter argues that the vagueness and ambiguity of in-between notions might be an adequate representation of the reality they try to capture; but they also serve as a gateway for disease-mongering and the misapplication of diagnostic labels. Against this background, the chapter formulates recommendations for future revisions of the *DSM*.

In Chapter 9 Peter Zachar and Richard J. McNally apply the notions of degree vagueness and combinatorial vagueness to characterize the conceptual structure of PTSD. There are clear cases of correct diagnosis and of false positives, but there is also a grey area between the two. PTSD is representative of how contemporary classificatory systems like the *DSM* portray many mental disorders. On the one hand, psychopathologists have developed precise diagnostic criteria for PTSD. On the other, concepts such as 'traumatic', 'severe', and 'impaired' generate borderline cases between subtraumatic and traumatic stressors. As in the sorites paradox, similar but successively milder traumatic events may produce PTSD symptoms. The boundary between normal and abnormal reactions is fuzzy as well. The chapter also discusses an alternative approach, according to which the various symptoms of PTSD are causally related mereological elements of PTSD.

4.3 Social, moral, and legal implications

Part IV is concerned with the social, moral, and legal implications that arise when being mentally ill is a matter of degree. Not surprisingly, the law is ill-equipped to respond to these challenges due to its binary logic. Still, the authors show that there are more and less reasonable ways of dealing with blurred boundaries—that is, of arriving at warranted decisions in hard cases.

Chapter 10 focuses on delusions and assessments of the extent to which an agent should be held responsible for actions that are motivated by delusional beliefs. Ema Sullivan-Bissett, Lisa Bortolotti, Matthew Broome, and Matteo Mameli maintain that there is no difference in kind between delusional and other epistemically faulty beliefs. Mere epistemic grounds that relate to the epistemic quality of the relevant belief-forming and belief-maintaining processes do not suffice to effectively demarcate pathological from non-pathological beliefs. Delusional beliefs, the authors argue, are continuous with other faulty beliefs. Since being diagnosed with a psychiatric disorder that features delusions is commonly associated with having reduced or no responsibility for delusion-based actions, the continuity thesis turns out to have significant moral and legal implications. On the basis of an analysis of three criminal cases, the authors conclude that the presence of delusions is rarely sufficient to determine whether agents are morally responsible and legally accountable for their criminal acts.

In Chapter 11 the forensic psychiatrist Hans-Ludwig Kröber discusses the difficulty of demarcating states that substantially diminish an agent's legal responsibility from states that do not. He argues that, although many impairments admit of degrees, there are categorical differences between some states, such as having schizophrenic delusions, and others, such as having only wishful illusions or a vivid imagination. He criticizes modern psychiatry for its use of 'mental disorder' as an umbrella term for various kinds of impaired functions on the grounds that this tends to mask important differences between patho-logical disorders, non-pathological disorders, and disorders that are similar to an illness. On the contrary, taking such differences into account is crucial when assessing a person's ability to act in accordance with an understanding of the wrongfulness of his or her actions. In the end, Kröber argues that this assessment is not possible only by psychiatric means, for it also involves normative questions, in particular the question of how much of the burden of presumed self-control and will power criminal law imposes upon a person.

In Chapter 12 the legal scholars John H. Blume, Sheri L. Johnson, and Amelia C. Hritz provide a detailed examination of so-called Atkins cases, that is, mentally disabled individuals who have committed capital murder. In *Atkins v Virginia* [2002], the US Supreme Court held that the execution of individuals with intellectual disabilities ran afoul of the constitution. It did so without specifying a precise IQ level or a definition of when someone counts as intellectu-ally disabled, permitting instead each state to establish its own criteria. Atkins cases constitute a paradigm for the troubling consequences of distinguishing between the normal and the pathological: the question of where to draw the line in a continuum turns literally into a matter of life and death. This brings the authors to articulate serious doubts about the fairness and morality of execut-ing someone who just barely falls on the 'wrong' side of the diagnostic line, but who is nevertheless disabled in every relevant respect.

Chapter 13 widens the focus by discussing the collaboration between medical and non-medical professionals in the prevention of conditions like substance use disorders or pathological gambling, both of which exhibit blurred bound-aries between normal and addicted behaviour. Drawing on the findings of cognitive–affective science about categorization, Dan Stein groups these condi-tions together as 'atypical disorders' and contrasts them with more typical ones. He then examines implications for individual and public healthcare, focusing on the ethics of collaboration between clinicians and representatives of the pharmaceutical, liquor, and gambling industries as well as on their ability to provide services or to conduct research on atypical disorders. He concludes that the liquor and gambling industries are particularly challenging for clinician-researchers and other stakeholders because they are associated with both social goods and social evils and have a spectrum of potential benefits and harms.

Acknowledgements

This book emerged from the research project 'Dealing Reasonably with Blurred Boundaries: Vagueness and Indeterminacy as a Challenge for Philosophy and

Law'. The project spanned four years and was supported by a research grant from the Volkswagen Foundation as part of the funding initiative 'Key Issues in the Humanities'. The main aims of the project were to identify and systematize phenomena of vagueness and indeterminacy in different fields of application, to examine their semantics, ontology, and epistemology, and to develop procedures of dealing reasonably with blurred boundaries.

We are indebted to Eric J. Engstrom, who translated Chapter 7 from the German and undertook the language editing of Chapters 1, 2, 3, 4, 5, 8, and 11. Eric's highly professional work was also funded by the Volkswagen Foundation. Gelareh Shahpar and Martin Klaus Günther assisted us with the preparation of the manuscript and with putting together the index. Lara Keuck would like to thank Katie Tabb, Maël Lemoine, and Steeves Demazeux for their always insightful discussions on the philosophy of psychiatry; she is also grateful to the Max Planck Institute for the History of Science and to the 'Society in Science—The Branco Weiss Fellowship', administered by the Federal Institute of Technology in Zurich, for supporting her work on this book. Finally, we wish to thank the anonymous reviewers for their helpful comments and suggestions, Manuela Tecusan for her meticulous copy-editing, and Oxford University Press and the series editors for including the book in the International Perspectives in Philosophy and Psychiatry series.

References

Alston, W. P. 1967. 'Vagueness'. In *Encyclopedia of Philosophy*, vol. **8**, edited by P. Edwards, pp. 218–21. New York, NY: Macmillan.

APA (American Psychiatric Association). 2000. *Diagnostic and Statistical Manual of Mental Disorders, Fourth Edition, Text Revision: DSM-IV TR*. Washington, DC: American Psychiatric Association.

APA (American Psychiatric Association). 2013. *Diagnostic and Statistical Manual of Mental Disorders, Fifth Edition: DSM-5*. Washington, DC: American Psychiatric Association.

Bolton, D. 2008. *What Is Mental Disorder? An Essay in Philosophy, Science and Values*. Oxford: Oxford University Press.

Bortolotti, L., and Malatesti, L. A. (eds.). 2010. *Classification and Explanation in Psychiatry: Philosophical Issues*. Special issue of the *European Journal of Analytic Philosophy* **6**.

Broome, M. et al. 2011. 'Neuroscience, continua and the prodromal phase of psychosis'. In *Vulnerability to Psychosis: From Neurosciences to Psychopathology*, edited by P. Fusar-Poli, S. Borgwardt, and P. K. McGuire, pp. 3–21. Hove: Psychology Press.

Cooper, R. 2005. *Classifying Madness: A Philosophical Examination of the Diagnostic and Statistical Manual of Mental Disorders*. Dordrecht: Springer.

D'Amico, R. 1995. 'Is disease a natural kind?'. *The Journal of Medicine and Philosophy* **20** (5): 551–69.

Demazeux, S., and Singy, P. (eds.). 2015. *The DSM-5 in Perspective: Philosophical Reflections on the Psychiatric Babel*. Dordrecht: Springer.

Djulbegovic, B., Hozo, I., and Greenland, S. 2011. 'Uncertainty in medicine'. In *Philosophy of Medicine*, edited by F. Gifford, pp. 299–356. Oxford: North Holland.

Dummett, M. 1975. 'Wang's paradox'. In *Vagueness: A Reader*, edited by R. Keefe and P. Smith, pp. 99–118. Cambridge, MA: MIT Press.

Endicott, T. 2000. *Vagueness in Law*. Oxford: Oxford University Press.

Frances, A. 2012. 'DSM 5 and diagnostic inflation: Reply to misleading comments from the task force'. Psychology Today. Posted 23 January 2012. https://www.psychologytoday. com/blog/dsm5-in-distress/201201/dsm-5-and-diagnostic-inflation (accessed 25 May 2016).

Frances, A. 2013. *Saving Normal: An Insider's Revolt against Out-of-Control Psychiatric Diagnosis, DSM-5, Big Pharma, and the Medicalization of Ordinary Life*. New York, NY: William Morrow.

Frege, G. 1952 [1903]. *The Fundamental Laws of Arithmetic II*, translated by P. T. Geach. In *Translations from the Philosophical Writings of Gottlob Frege*, edited by P. T. Geach, and M. Black, pp. 159–81 and 134–244. Oxford: Blackwell.

Frege, G. 1972 [1882]. 'On the scientific justification of the concept-script'. In *Conceptual Notation and Related Articles*, translated and edited by T. W. Bynum, pp. 83–9. Oxford: Clarendon.

Graff, D., and Williamson, T. (eds.). 2002. *Vagueness*. Aldershot: Ashgate.

Grice, H. P. 1989. *Studies in the Ways of Words*. Cambridge, MA: Harvard University Press.

Gullvåg, I., and Næss, A. 1996. 'Vagueness and ambiguity'. In *Sprachphilosophie—Philosophy of Language—La philosophie du langage: Ein internationales Handbuch zeitgenössischer Forschung*, vol. 2, edited by M. Dascal, D. Gerhardus, K. Lorenz, and G. Meggle, pp. 1407–17. Berlin: De Gruyter.

Helzer, J. E. et al. (eds.). 2008. *Dimensional Approaches in Diagnostic Classification: Refining the Research Agenda for DSM-V*. Arlington, VA: American Psychiatric Association.

Horwitz, A. V., and Wakefield, J. C. 2007. *The Loss of Sadness: How Psychiatry Transformed Normal Sorrow into Depressive Disorder*. Oxford: Oxford University Press.

Horwitz, A. V., and Wakefield, J. C. 2012. *All We Have to Fear: Psychiatry's Transformation of Natural Anxieties into Mental Disorders*. Oxford: Oxford University Press.

Hughes, J. C. (ed.). 2006. *Mild Cognitive Impairment*. Special issue of *Philosophy, Psychiatry, & Psychology* 13.

Hyde, D. 2008. *Vagueness, Logic and Ontology*. Aldershot: Ashgate.

Hyde, D. 2014. 'Sorites paradox'. In *The Stanford Encyclopedia of Philosophy*, edited by E. N. Zalta. http://plato.stanford.edu/archives/win2014/entries/sorites-paradox (accessed 25 May 2016).

Hyman, S. E. 2010. 'The diagnosis of mental disorders: The problem of reification'. *Annual Review of Clinical Psychology* 6: 155–79.

Insel, T. R. 2013. 'Transforming diagnosis'. Director's Blog, NIMH. http://www.nimh.nih. gov/about/director/2013/transforming-diagnosis.shtml (accessed 25 May 2016).

Keefe, R. 2000. *Theories of Vagueness*. Cambridge: Cambridge University Press.

Keefe, R., and Smith, P. (eds.). 1997. *Vagueness: A Reader*. Cambridge, MA: MIT Press.

Keil, G. 2013. 'Introduction: Vagueness and ontology'. *Metaphysica* 14: 149–64.

Kendler, K. S., and Parnas, J. (eds.). 2012. *Philosophical Issues in Psychiatry II: Nosology*. Oxford: Oxford University Press.

Lewis, D. 1986. *On the Plurality of Worlds*. Oxford: Blackwell.

Lilienfeld, S. O., and Marino, L. 1995. 'Mental disorder as a Roschian concept'. *Journal of Abnormal Psychology* **104** (3): 411–20.

Murphy, D. 2006. *Psychiatry in the Scientific Image*. Cambridge, MA: MIT Press.

Paris, J. 2015. *Overdiagnosis in Psychiatry: How Modern Psychiatry Lost Its Way While Creating a Diagnosis for Almost All of Life's Misfortunes*. Oxford: Oxford University Press.

Pinkal, M. 1995. *Logic and Lexicon: The Semantics of the Indefinite*. Dordrecht: Kluwer.

Poscher, G., and Keil, G. (eds.). 2016. *Vagueness and Law*. Oxford: Oxford University Press.

Raffman, D. 2014. *Unruly Words: A Study of Vague Language*. Oxford: Oxford University Press.

Ronzitti, G. (ed.). 2011. *Vagueness: A Guide*. Dordrecht: Springer.

Russell, B. 1923. 'Vagueness'. *Australasian Journal of Philosophy and Psychology* **1**: 84–92.

Sadegh-Zadeh, K. 2008. 'The prototype resemblance theory of disease'. *Journal of Medicine and Philosophy* **33** (2): 106–39.

Sadegh-Zadeh, K. 2012. *Handbook of Analytical Philosophy of Medicine*. Dordrecht: Springer.

Samuels, R. 2009. 'Delusions as a natural kind'. In *Psychiatry as Cognitive Neuroscience: Philosophical Perspectives*, edited by M. Broome and L. Bortolotti, pp. 49–79. Oxford: Oxford University Press.

Shapiro, S. 2006. *Vagueness in Context*. Oxford: Oxford University Press.

Sorensen, R. 2001. *Vagueness and Contradiction*. Oxford: Oxford University Press.

Sorensen, R. 2016. 'Vagueness'. In *The Stanford Encyclopedia of Philosophy*, edited by E. N. Zalta. http://plato.stanford.edu/archives/spr2016/entries/vagueness (accessed 25 May, 2016).

Tabb, K. 2015. 'Psychiatric progress and the assumption of diagnostic discrimination'. *Philosophy of Science* **82** (5): 1047–58.

Widiger, T. A. et al. (eds.). 2006. *Dimensional Models of Personality Disorders: Refining the Research Agenda for DSM-V*. Arlington, VA: American Psychiatric Association.

Williamson, T. 1994. *Vagueness*. London: Routledge.

Wittgenstein, L. 1953. *Philosophical Investigations*, translated by G. E. M. Anscombe. Oxford: Basil Blackwell.

Wittgenstein, L. 1980. *Bemerkungen über die Philosophie der Psychologie/Remarks on the Philosophy of Psychology*, edited by G. E. M. Anscombe and G. H. von Wright. Oxford: Blackwell.

Zachar, P. 2008. 'Real kinds but no true taxonomy: An essay in psychiatric systematics'. In *Philosophical Issues in Psychiatry: Explanation, Phenomenology, and Nosology*, edited by K. S. Kendler and J. Parnas, pp. 327–67. Baltimore, MD: Johns Hopkins University Press.

Zachar, P., and Ellis, R. D. (eds.). 2012. *Categorical versus Dimensional Models of Affect: A Seminar on the Theories of Panksepp and Russell*. Amsterdam: John Benjamins.

Part II

Health and disease as matters of degree

Chapter 2

Mental and physical gradualism in Graeco-Roman medicine

Orly Lewis, Chiara Thumiger, and
Philip van der Eijk

1 Introduction

The aim of this chapter is to explore how ancient medical ideas may offer relevant and profitable parallels to the modern notions of *degree vagueness* and *combinatorial vagueness* with respect to mental health and its management, offering a historical angle from which to assess the themes this volume sets out to discuss. By closely examining several key examples, this chapter will argue that Graeco-Roman physicians recognized physical and mental health as states that admit of gradation and were aware of the nuances, variations, and even relativity of the distinction between healthy and ill. When it comes to notions of physical and mental health, these nuances, as we shall see, are both quantitative and qualitative. In fact, one of the characteristics of Graeco-Roman medicine is the fundamental consideration given to a body–mind continuum as something that is subject to health and disease and can be the object of medical attention. As a consequence, it is impossible to discuss psychological or psychiatric matters in isolation, without considering the health of the individual as a whole. We shall begin, in section 2, by introducing ancient conceptions of physical health and demonstrating the relevance of degree and combinatorial vagueness in this domain. Section 3 focuses on mental health, explaining its relation to bodily health and exploring the aspects of gradation that can be traced in its representation.

2 Degrees and vagueness of physical health

2.1 Definitions of health and disease: Mixtures, balance, and imbalance

Health and illness were often (if not always)[1] described by Greek and Roman medical writers with reference to the state of various key factors composing

---

[1] The Methodist and Empiricist schools, for example, are notable exceptions to this statement.

the human body or acting upon it, in particular with regard to their 'balance' or 'imbalance'. Sources commonly refer to the compound or mixture (*krasis, mixis*) of the components or qualities of the body or of particular substances found in it.[2] When proportionately (*metriōs*) mixed and well balanced, all these were considered conducive to health; when disproportionately mixed and out of balance, they were thought to be harmful and cause illness. This representation of a mixture constantly striving for balance is reflected also by the commonly used imagery and terminology of the battle between different powers (*dunameis*) or components of the body. In such contexts, the imbalance causing illness is described in terms of one component overpowering (*kratein*) the other(s).

Thus the author of the treatise *On Regimen* (fifth-early fourth centuries BC) emphasized the balance between the food and drink taken into the body, on the one hand, and the amount of exercise performed by the body, on the other; 'for it is from the overpowering of one or the other that diseases arise, while from them being evenly balanced comes good health'. According to the author, establishing 'whether [in a given individual at a given time] food overpowers exercise, whether exercise overpowers food, or whether they are duly proportioned' will enable the doctor to recognize in advance the onset of illness.[3] The author of the treatise *On the Nature of Man* (fifth century BC) referred instead to a balance between humours, of which he held the human body to be composed:

> The body of the human being holds in itself blood, phlegm, yellow bile and black bile; these for him are the nature of the body and through them he feels pain and enjoys health. He is therefore most healthy, when these substances are duly proportioned to one another in respect of compounding, power and quantity, and when they are perfectly mixed. He suffers pain when one of these substances is in defect or excess or separated in the body and not compounded with all the other substances.[4]

The author of *On Ancient Medicine* expressed himself in very similar terms:

> There is in man bitter, salty, sweet, acid, astringent and insipid and numerous other things, which hold powers of all kinds, both in quantity and strength. These, if mixed and compounded with one another, are not apparent, nor do they hurt the human

---

[2] This was the case from the very beginning of Greek medical thought, as demonstrated by the 'Hippocratic texts', i.e. a corpus of heterogeneous texts that were transmitted under the name of Hippocrates, a collection whose doctrinal core can be dated to the fifth and early fourth centuries BC. For a history of the notion of health in Greek medicine, see Wöhrle (1990), King (2005), Bartoš (2015).

[3] Hippocrates, *On Regimen* 3.69 (Joly 200,30–202,2 = L. 6.606.5–9), translated by Jones (1953) slightly modified.

[4] Hippocrates, *On the Nature of Man* 4 (Jouanna 172,13–174,3 = L. 6.38.19–40.6), translated by Jones (1953), modified.

being; but when one of them is separated and stands alone, then it is apparent and hurts the human being.[5]

This representation remains fundamental throughout the history of ancient medical thought and takes the form of a particularly complex theory in the works of Galen of Pergamum, the illustrious second-century AD Greek physician who worked for a long time in Rome and at the side of the Roman emperor. As most fully articulated in his treatise *On Mixtures*, Galen's theory concerns the balance of the qualities in the body, where various mixtures determine its physical condition. For Galen, the 'mixture of the body' is in fact the mixture of the four qualities (hot, cold, dry, and wet) in the body and each mixture is defined by the proportion of the qualities of which it is composed. In his theory, in addition to the perfectly balanced mixture, in which the amount of each of the four qualities is equal, there are eight further mixtures, which are defined according to their dominant quality or qualities. According to Galen, there are two possibilities: either one of the four is dominant (cold, hot, dry, or wet mixture), or a pair of opposites is: for instance, the 'hot-and-dry' or the 'hot-and-wet' mixture.[6]

2.2 Degrees of health and degree vagueness

This conception of balance as the source of health (indeed, as being identical with the state of health) might appear to allow only for degrees of illness while leaving little room for degrees of health; for it implies that, given even the smallest divergence from the perfect balance (i.e. from the healthy state), an individual must be regarded as unhealthy, in other words ill. This, however, is not the case. In fact Galen does not consider the perfectly balanced mixture to be the *only* healthy mixture: this may indeed be the 'best' and 'healthiest' one, but the eight other mixtures, in which the balances are imperfect and even labelled as forms of *duskrasia* (literally 'bad mixture'), are still regarded by him as healthy conditions.[7]

We find further confirmation of these concepts of degree and gradation of health in Galen's treatise *On Matters Concerning Health*, which discusses the so-called *hugieinon*, that is, the part of medical art concerned with the maintenance

---

[5] Hippocrates, *On Ancient Medicine* 14 (Jouanna 136,10–16 = L. 1.602.9–13); see also ibid. 16 (Jouanna 139,6–8 = L. 1.606.19–20) for hot and cold having to be mixed. See also Aristotle, who claims that that health and well-being consist of a 'balanced compounding (*krasis*) of hot and cold [in the body], in relation either to each other or to the environment' (*Physics* 8.3, 246^{b}4–5).

[6] See in particular *On Mixtures* 1.2–3 (Helmreich 2–10 = K. 1.510–23).

[7] We shall see later that Galen thinks that these various mixtures also shape the mental condition of the body and that this theory of mixtures is crucial for his theory of mental health.

of health and the prevention of disease (as opposed to the *therapeutikon*, which focuses on the treatment of diseases).[8] The treatise is written as a 'handbook' for doctors on the topic of maintaining health and the first book engages directly with our topic—the definition of health. From the outset, Galen places great emphasis on the idea that health is a relative condition, characterized by varying degrees of latitude:

> Let our hypothesis be that the healthy condition is determined by activities occurring naturally; and that this is the optimum (*aristē*) and, as one might say, the fulfilment and height of health; and that that which is defective and incomplete and imperfect also has great latitude (*platos*).[9]

He later adds:

> [The different forms of health] do not differ in respect to their common form, for the forms of health are not different; they differ only in degree. For as the whiteness of snow does not differ from that of milk in so far that it is white, but only in the degree of whiteness, so in the same way the health of Achilles, for example, is the same as that of Thersites in so far that it is health, but differs in another respect, and that is in degree.[10]

Like the physiological compositional theory exposited in *On Mixtures*, here too Galen argues that alongside perfect health we find a great variety of imperfect conditions that can nevertheless be considered healthy. This notion, moreover, is apparent in several earlier Greek sources. Take for instance the passage cited earlier from *On the Nature of Man*, in which the adjective 'healthy' is qualified precisely with reference to degree. The reference there to being 'most healthy', which is also found in other sources of the classical period, implies that one can still be deemed healthy even if one is not the 'health*iest*'.[11] It suggests, therefore, the existence of a *scale* of healthy states: one can be healthy to a greater or lesser extent. The notion of degree of health is also found in a Hippocratic aphorism claiming that some have a 'more morbid' health, others a 'healthier' health.[12] Furthermore, some people were recognized as having a weaker constitution and hence as being

---

[8] For a commentary on this Galenic text, see Grimaudo (2008).

[9] Galen, *On Matters Concerning Health* 1.4.11 (Koch 7,34–8,3 = K. 6.12.7–12), translated by Green (1951), modified.

[10] Ibid. 1.5.18 (Koch 9,29–35 = K. 6.17.1–6). This has consequences for the topic of disability and health, even though this is not directly mentioned: one can be both 'disabled' and healthy and, conversely, it is true that one can have exceptional capacities and still enjoy greater or lesser health according to one's own standards.

[11] Hippocrates, *Regimen in Health* 2 (Jouanna 208,20 = L. 6.76.4–5); *On the Nature of Man* 4 (Jouanna 172,15 = L. 6.40.2–3 cf. *On the Sacred Disease* 5 (= 8 Jones) (Jouanna 13,4 = L. 6.638.15): 'healthiest head'.

[12] Hippocrates, *Aphorisms*, 6.2 (L. 6.562.10–11).

more prone to becoming sick whenever their regimen was changed—as in the case of those 'closest to sick men' who, while more vulnerable than others, are still stronger than the truely sick and are themselves not yet sick.[13]

The idea that there were different degrees of healthiness was not exclusive to medical writings. Aristotle, too, held health to be a gradual and relative state, allowing for variation and degree. He claimed, for instance, that health may change over time and went as far as to say that, since 'some diseases cause the same effects as old age', it is 'justifiable to define disease as "acquired old age" (*epiktēton gēras*) and old age as "natural disease" (*phusikos nosos*)'. Changing conditions and different regimens could result in a person being less or more healthy, regardless of his or her age.[14] Alongside these conceptual distinctions, Aristotle also offers an explicit theoretical discussion:

> health is definite although it admits of degrees . . . for it does not consist in the same proportion in everyone, nor is it even always the same one proportion in the same person, but even when it is fading it remains up to a point, and differs in degree.[15]

In addition to degree vagueness, early medical texts also attest to the complexity and the ensuing, partial nature of certain conditions, to which an exclusive label of either 'healthy' or 'ill' could not be attached. So, for example, patients who had recovered from complex fractures but remained disfigured or permanently disabled were still considered to be 'adequately healthy as far as the other things (in their body and its functions) were concerned', despite being unhealthy in the disfigured or impaired part.[16] The author of *On the Sacred Disease* recognizes that some parts of the body may be healthy at the very same time that other parts are diseased: 'seed is from all the body: healthy seed from the healthy parts, diseased seed from the diseased parts'. [17]

Galen's position is in tune with these earlier medical sources and introduces a concrete classification into his medical theory. He argues that there is an intermediate state between health and disease, for which he uses the term 'neither'— *oudeteron*.[18] An *oudeteron* body may be (1) both healthy and ill at the same

---

[13] Hippocrates, *On Ancient Medicine* 10 (Jouanna 132,12–14 = L. 1.596.3–4).

[14] Aristotle, *History of Animals* 9(7).1, 581^{b}29–2^{a}3; *Generation of Animals* 5.4, 784^{b}33.

[15] Aristotle, *Nicomachean Ethics* 10.3, 1173^{a}24, translated by Crisp (2000), slightly modified.

[16] Hippocrates, *On Joints* 56 (L. 4.244.8–9).

[17] Hippocrates, *On the Sacred Disease* 2 (= 5 Jones) (Jouanna 10,16–18 = L. 6.364.1–20).

[18] This concept of *oudeteron* originated with Herophilus' tripartite division of medicine into parts concerning health, disease, and neither health nor disease. The last one dealt with the means of treating disease (drugs and their components, surgery etc.). On Herophilus' conception and its elaboration before Galen, see von Staden (1989), 89–112; on the medieval debate concerning this question, see van der Lugt (2011), 13–46.

time; (2) neither healthy nor ill; (3) sometimes healthy and sometimes diseased, 'as, for example, happens to those who are healthy in childhood, but become diseased in their adolescence'. [19] The first kind of body is one that has 'a simultaneous share in both opposite conditions [*sc.* morbid and healthy] in either one or two parts', while the second kind 'is precisely in the middle between the healthiest and the most morbid'. Bodies of both types may remain constant from birth or fluctuate between the two during the course of life. [20] Galen's conception of an intermediate or combined state of health and disease is a telling example of the difficulty encountered by ancient physicians in determining whether an individual is sick or healthy. As a practicing physician, Galen prefers a flexible classification that could accommodate the variety he encounters in his patients. The practical manifestation of the different degrees of health, as he explains, can be found in the activities, *energeiai*, of the body and their qualitative scale:

> [healthy people] do not [all] hear equally with their ears, but . . . there is a great range of more or less. Nor do they run equally with their legs, nor grasp with their hands, nor function equally with all their organs, but one better and one worse. [21]

The healthy functioning and the quality of activities such as sense perception or locomotion vary not only from person to person, but also within each particular individual with the changes brought about by age. The level of health in each individual is measured not only against a general standard for his or her age group, but also against one's own personal standard of functional quality with respect to any given activity:

> whereas the age of adolescents is best for all vigorous activities, that of infants is inferior on account of its moisture, and that of old people on account of its dryness and frigidity. Yet in other so-called physical functions, such as growth, digestion, distribution and nutrition, infants are superior to all the other ages . . . . All, however, can be healthy at all ages. Therefore, as far as ages are concerned, you will find that in the same way the difference in constitutions is enormous; so that, for example, of two children having the same age, one will be much moister than the other and one drier, and likewise one warmer and one cooler. [22]

Nevertheless, these many 'healths'—these degrees that are found horizontally, so to speak, across humanity and vertically across the ages, stages, and different functions within each individual—are still considered to fall under a unitary concept of health. Given this broad conception of health, the question

---

[19] Galen, *Ars Medica* 1 (Boudon 279–81 = K. 1.311–12), our translation.

[20] Ibid. (Boudon 276–81 = K. 1.307–12), translated by Singer (1997), slightly modified.

[21] Galen, *On Matters concerning Health* 1.5.7–8 (Koch 8,34–9,4 = K. 6.14.16–15.4), translated by Green (1951), modified.

[22] Ibid. 1.5.50–2 (Koch 13,17–28 = K. 6.25.16–26.11), translated by Green (1951), modified.

arises: Where does the spectrum of health end and where does that of disease begin? More to the point, if imperfection and functional deterioration or impairment may still fall under the definition of health, how might a physician or patient recognize disease and label a state as being unhealthy? A key criterion for distinguishing the two is subjective: the perceptibility of the functional impairment. As Galen says:

> Sense perception is always the criterion, as it is with respect to functions of life; thus, we judge also the good constitution (*eukrasia*) and bad constitution (*duskrasia*) by means of sense perception. Similarly, we must deem each impairment of activity as disease whenever an impairment arising contrary to nature [*sc.* not from natural causes such as old age] reaches a perceptible degree.[23]

In order to overcome the vagueness of his definition of health and its operative problems, Galen introduces here a perceptible and very definite, albeit subjective, criterion: the feeling of pain. Like the functioning of bodily activities, pain is a direct and tangible manifestation of the patient's condition, as opposed, for instance, to the qualitative mixture of the body. However, whereas a functional impairment may not necessarily render the individual unhealthy and necessitate treatment, the appearance of pain or of a (subjective) feeling of suffering or damage (*lupeisthai*) does:

> since health is a sort of symmetry, and since all symmetry is accomplished and manifested in a twofold fashion, first in coming to perfection and truly being symmetry, and second in deviating slightly from this absolute perfection; so health should also be a twofold harmony, one exact, optimal, absolute and perfect; the other deviating slightly from this, but not so much so that the animal may suffer.[24]

At a practical level, therefore, health is a condition of satisfactory functioning, in which an individual is not afflicted by pain or severe impairment. If health were only the complete perfection that few (if any) can enjoy, then human life would amount to endless suffering. Allowing instead for a broad spectrum of healthy conditions while at the same time setting criteria for distinguishing the healthy from the sick is key to legitimizing the function and importance of medical doctrine and of medicine as a profession. Moreover, pain, *lupē*, reveals the role of perceptibility and subjectivity in Galen's discourse on health—the subjectivity of the suffering patient *and* of the visiting physician. Health can only be measured on the basis of real cases and what can be experienced.[25]

---

[23] Ibid. 1.5.43–44 (Koch 12,17–22 = K. 6.23.10–15), translated by Green (1951), modified.

[24] Ibid. 1.5.1–3 (Koch 8,15–20 = K. 6.13.9–16), translated by Green (1951), modified.

[25] Galen's insistence is to be understood also in the context of a polemic with those (philosophers?) who believed in one abstract, unitary, monolithic idea of 'Health' with a capital H, outside of which only illness exists, making life a state of perpetual suffering (see ibid. 1.5.23–5 [Koch 10 = K. 6.18]).

The gradualist view of Galen, to conclude, appears to have both a pragmatic component and a more philosophical one. The first reflects a fundamental pragmatism of purposes: the physician's view has to take into account, first of all, the actuality of real human beings, the patients he meets and visits. And it must therefore compose a picture for the purpose of his professional practice rather than produce an abstract model. Health is not an extreme ideal, a 'complete perfection', but rather a perceived good balance, an approximation within the range contained between the two extremes, which can be achieved and maintained through the exercise of an adequate lifestyle.

The second, philosophical component of Galen's theory of health lies in the centrality of the subject-relative concepts of 'function' and 'pain', *energeia* and *lupē*. To be healthy is, somehow unambitiously, both to find oneself above the threshold of 'pain' and to enjoy an acceptably good functioning of one's body. The assessment of these two concepts is necessarily subjective and approximate: observability and measurability of health, Galen states quite clearly, are the epistemological conditions for the very existence of the concept and make it, of necessity, relative. This, perhaps the most modern element of his entire discussion, is fundamental because it ties in deeply with Galen's psychology and his specific views on the relationship between mental health and moral life, 'happiness', and the health of the body, which appears to be the first priority of a physician. By drawing *lupē* to the fore, Galen brings subjectivity to the centre of the medical discourse, even in his deliberations on the definition of health. This makes Galen's outlook closer to concepts such as 'life quality' and 'perceived health', which ancient medicine otherwise notably does not have.

3 Degrees and vagueness of mental health

As one might expect, these discussions of physical health as varying in degree and being relative to a variety of factors also impinge upon ideas about mental health. This is the case both with reference to the activities and functions that depend on mental faculties, such as cognition, sensation, and locomotion, and in the domain of ethics. Before exploring the place of gradualism in the mental sphere, we will examine the tight connection between mental and corporeal health in ancient thought, perhaps the most significant point of dissonance in relation to modern conceptions.

3.1 Mental health and its dependence on the body

Contrary to philosophers such as the so-called Presocratics, Plato, and Aristotle, early medical writers (at least as far as we can judge from the works that have survived intact) hardly discuss the mental qua mental and the soul qua soul.[26] Indeed, the absence of a clear-cut 'mental' area of investigation appears to be a characteristic feature of early medicine; for the focus always returns to the dependence of mental capacities or activities (e.g. sense perception, cognition, and the like) on bodily conditions and to the association of proper diseases of mental import (e.g. *phrenitis*)—or of syndromes that have mental consequences (e.g. melancholic affections)—with corporal pathologies.

Despite variations in terminology and in physio-anatomic concepts, medical authors throughout antiquity remained faithful to this physiological explanation of mental health. One common explanatory model posited the complete or partial obstruction of the passages through which motor and sensory impulses were thought to be transmitted (e.g. veins, arteries, or nerves)—a phenomenon that prevented the healthy and natural execution of motion or the perception of sensory inputs.[27] Another common aetiologic explanation focused on humoural or qualitative imbalances in the organ or bodily component involved in perception and reasoning (most commonly the heart, the brain, or the blood). Such imbalances would affect the organ's ability to process and assess sensory information; they would hinder its ability to determine the appropriate reaction and to transmit the required impulses to different parts of the body (e.g. the arms, the vocal apparatus); and they would elicit a number of mental symptoms ranging from what we would call neurological dysfunctions, such as spasms or fainting, to derangement, hallucination, and delirious speech.[28]

While in the Hippocratic texts the bodily origin of mental life is mostly left implicit and rarely discussed openly, the connection between the body's condition and mental health is explored extensively in Galen's work, in particular in the treatise with the telling title *The Capacities of the Soul Depend on the Mixtures of the Body*. We have explained in section 2.1 what Galen means by 'mixtures of the body'; among the 'capacities of the soul' he lists memory, thought, locomotion, and sense perception.[29] The main aim of the treatise is

---

[26] On this, see Bartoš (2006); prior discussions are Hüffmeier (1961) and Hankinson (1991); see also Singer (1992) and Gundert (2000).

[27] See, for instance, Hippocrates, *On Wind* 13–14 (Jouanna 120–4 = L. 6.110–14); *On the Sacred Disease*, especially chs 4–7 (= 7–10) (Jouanna 12–16 = L. 6.368–74); Diocles frs 83, 95, 98, pp. 154–5, 170–3, 176–7 van der Eijk (2000); Praxagoras frs 70 and 73, pp. 80–1 Steckerl (1958).

[28] See, for instance, Hippocrates, *On the Sacred Disease* 14 (= 17 Jones) (Jouanna 26,9–27,2 = L. 6.388.3–10); Diocles, frs 72, 74–5, pp. 142–3, 146–9 van der Eijk (2000); Praxagoras frs 62, 69, 72, pp. 76, 80, 81 Steckerl (1958).

[29] Galen, *The Capacities of the Soul Depend on the Mixtures of the Body* 5 (Müller 48 = K. 4.788).

to prove that the soul's condition, its activities, and the ability to perform them not only are affected by but even dependent on the body's condition. Galen therefore stresses the important role played by the medical profession and the ability of its practitioners to preserve a healthy mental condition in patients and, when necessary, to treat mental illness. To demonstrate this, he draws on a multitude of examples and appeals to earlier authorities who are central to his arguments: Hippocrates, Plato, and Aristotle.

Galen describes *phrenitis, melancholia,* and *mania* as conditions that reveal how 'the soul is overpowered (*dunasteuesthai*]) by the ills of the body'. These conditions entail an impairment of the soul's sensory capacities and may in turn cause sensory malfunctions (e.g. seeing triple or not recognizing acquaintances) attributable to problems of the 'visual capacity' (*dunamis*) rather than to an impairment in the sensory organ (as would be the case in cataracts, for instance).[30] Galen also cites other examples of the effects of the body on the soul: an abundance of yellow and black bile in the brain, for instance, causes derangement (*paraphrosunē*) and *melancholia* respectively, both of which are associated with mnemonic and cognitive impairments; consumption of certain foodstuffs and drinks may cause stupefaction (*mōria*) or, as in the case of wine, relief from distress and low spirits;[31] the excessively cold mixture characteristic of old age is a root cause of the impaired cognitive capacity observed in the elderly,[32] and so on.

3.2 Degrees of mental health: Mental life in the Hippocratic *Regimen* 1.35–6

In light of the ancients' approach to human health and their general view of human physiology as an integrated body–mind continuum, an analysis of the mental sphere should inevitably encompass bodily, cognitive–emotional, and ethical data. In fact we find neither psychiatric nor even psychological discussions of human health in medical texts before the first centuries of our era[33]—and, even then, the discussions deviate substantially from what we now

---

[30] Ibid. (Müller 48–49 = K. 4.788–9).

[31] Ibid. 3 (Müller 39 = K. 4.776–7).

[32] Ibid. 5 (Müller 47 = K. 4.786–7).

[33] There is an important lacuna in the medical material that has survived. The works of most physicians and philosophers who wrote between the second half of the fourth century BC and the second century AD have been lost, surviving only as fragmentary citations and reports in the works of later authors. It is precisely in this period that, largely influenced by philosophical reflections, the soul and the *psuchē* became objects of medical (and not just philosophical) research and discussion.

consider to be the disciplinary domains of psychiatry and psychology. Our first example of gradualism in mental health is an extreme illustration of this. It posits a strong physiological basis of mental faculties and, given its emphasis on the 'basic constituents' of the soul (*psuchē*), it even resonates with the doctrines of naturalist philosophers on the principles or fundamental elements that constitute reality. We are, again, far removed from our understanding of psychology as a discipline dedicated to the study of human cognitive processes, emotional drives, or ethical life.[34]

The Hippocratic treatise *On Regimen* is easily the most important text in the medical corpus of the classical period when it comes to discussions of the *psuchē* and its health and/or disorder.[35] The main aim of this work is to instruct physicians and laymen how to manage one's health through the adoption of an appropriate diet. The treatise discusses in detail important aspects of human lifestyle and physiology. Although it appears to be a major digression from the text's very practical orientation, the author includes a long and fascinating account of the 'types of soul' that can be found among human beings and of the variations in their faculties and qualities. The author also assigns various features of what we would today broadly recognize as mental characteristics to discrete aspects of physiology.[36]

What emerges is a proper, fully articulated theory of mind. In fact the topic of this passage is advertised from the outset as concerning so-called 'intelligence' (i.e. *phronēsis* in an approximate and conventional translation from the Greek) and its opposite (*aphrosunē*). We shall see that this 'intelligence' entails a variety of faculties that go far beyond intellectual performance. The following discussion illustrates the existence of six possible 'psychic constitutions' or types of *psuchē*. These types depend on the varying proportions of two fundamental constituents, namely fire and water on the one hand, dryness and moisture on the other. These two can blend in different ways to produce a diverse landscape of cognitive capacities, sensorial reactivity, emotional responses, and even something resembling 'character', which deserves closer examination.

---

[34] See Harris (2013) for a rich illustration of ancient approaches to mental disorders; see especially Simon's and Hughes' chapters there for a dialogue with current medical paradigms (Simon 2013; Hughes 2013).

[35] As for most of the treatises traditionally ascribed to the so-called Hippocratic Corpus, we cannot identify the author of *Regimen* with the historical Hippocrates, although we can ascribe it to the late fifth century–early fourth century BC.

[36] On this important passage, see van der Eijk (2011) and Jouanna (2012).

The ideal balance of fire and water—a perfect case of balance between a natural quality and its opposite, since fire is 'the moistest' and water 'the driest'—makes the soul 'most intelligent and endowed with the best memory'. As the disproportion between the two elements widens, the soul loses *phronēsis* and the author identifies six possible imbalanced constitutions of the soul. (1) If the amount of water is only slightly (*oligon*) greater than the amount of fire, this results in souls that are 'intelligent too, but that fall short [of the well-blended soul previously described]; but, [with the right regime,] this type of individual can become 'more intelligent and sharper in nature'. Such souls are also characterized by dull senses, since a lack of fire slows down sensorial perceptions. (2) In the second blend, where fire is significantly overcome by water, the sensory faculties are affected in such a way that the individuals 'perceive as well as others the sensations of cold, hot and so on, but they cannot perceive sensations of sight or hearing unless they are already familiar with them'. On the whole, these humans constitute 'a slower kind' and 'are called silly'. (3) The third type, where fire is 'even further (*epi pleion*) mastered by water', comprises the so-called 'senseless' or 'thunder-struck/stupid'. Their mental impairment—their *mania*—is said to 'tend towards the slow': it is a kind of dullness, a more relaxed insanity. Their judgement and their control over their emotions are affected: they 'weep for no reason, fear things that should not be feared'; they 'are pained at what does not affect them, and their sensations are not really what a sane person should feel'. (4) The fourth combination, in which the power of water is instead insufficient, results in a kind of soul that is 'intelligent' and 'perceives quickly'; in general, this is 'a good soul' that might still improve or deteriorate, depending on the adopted regime; its fundamental nature is an intelligent one (*phronimos*). (5) The next type is that of an even quicker soul, but less constant, in which the power of water 'is further (*epi pleion*) mastered by fire': this soul 'strikes its sensations more rapidly, but is less constant than the previous type of soul, because it more rapidly passes judgement on the things presented to it, and on account of its speed rushes on to too many objects'. Souls of this sort can be made more intelligent by reducing the flesh in the body, as excessive flesh can elicit *mania* in them. (6) Finally, if water is even further (*eti pleon*) mastered by fire, the resulting *psuchē* is excessively quick and sharp: individuals are 'half-mad' (*hupomainesthai*), indeed are 'the closest to mania' and prone to dreaming or wet dreams.[37]

Drawing together his views on human mental life, the author goes on to expand the picture by accommodating a few additional qualities of the soul that do *not* depend on the mixtures of fire and water, but rather on the nature

---

[37] Hippocrates, *On Regimen* 1.35 (Joly 150–6 = L. 6.512–22), translated by Jones (1953), modified. On this, see van der Eijk (2011), 255–70.

of the passages through which the soul moves as it enters the body, the *poroi*. The *psuchē*, in fact, appears to be able to breathe in or out of the body, 'but in the following cases the blend [between fire and water] is not the cause of the characteristics: for example, irascibility, indolence, craftiness, simplicity, quarrelsomeness and benevolence. In all these cases the cause is the nature of the passages through which the soul passes.'[38] These qualities or experiences are also psychological, but the author sees them as somehow complementary to the data qualifying the six types of soul. They are set aside and declared impervious to dietary intervention: 'it is not possible to change these through regime', while the different balances of fire and water, instead, were described in such detail precisely for the practical purpose of prescribing the most appropriate diet for each one.

These fascinating passages illustrate the different ways in which the ancient author acknowledged a subtle quality in the mental sphere. First of all, he opens by recognizing that the definition of his own topic, 'intelligence'—or 'what people call' intelligence—is elusive. His cautious words expose a constitutive vagueness and a shifting nature characteristic of the sphere he is about to discuss, a sphere that in many ways overlaps with the physiology of the body and comprises disparate features. Then, as we look at the six patterns of variation, it is interesting to notice that psychological diversity is not determined by a great diversity of substances or a wide range of proportions; instead it is determined by the slight variation, the progressive shifting of balance: 'when the fire overcomes the water *slightly*'; 'when the water is *even further* mastered by fire', and so on. These gradual variations in the constituents correspond to subtle and composite variations in psychological make-up that are not clearly ranked by their desirability: there is quickness and sharpness in perception and clarity of judgement; there is emotional distress; there is veracity in the appraisal of reality; stupidity pure and simple; activities such as dreaming; vulnerability to *mania*. In particular, mania is presented here not as a full-fledged pathological state that befalls a soul by virtue of its own nature, but as a potential risk against which a diet can protect the individual, or a state adjacent to a certain type of *psuchē*. The author writes that certain souls are 'half-mad' or 'almost mad' and even creates a verbal form, *hupomainesthai*, to express this concept, which must have been important to his construct.

Thus, a view of mental life as a composite comprised of very different faculties and experiences and as varying both from one individual to the next and, most interestingly, within each individual, depending on the mental feature under

---

[38] Hippocrates *On Regimen* 1.36 (Joly 156 = L. 6.522–4), translated by Jones (1953), modified.

observation, plays a fundamental role here. These features remain anchored to a physiological, elemental organization: the proportion between the constituents (fire and water) and the bodily, material nature of the 'passages' through which the soul enters the body from the outside.

3.3 Degrees of mental health: Mental life in Galen

This view of mental faculties and mind, indissolubly linked to the physiology of the body, will be fundamental throughout the Greek medical tradition, even though that tradition did not adopt the water–fire model, which remains peculiar to the author of *Regimen*. If we look at Galen's take on this discussion, the fundamental framework remains the same: physiological and centred upon the idea of a balance to be preserved.[39] Balance accommodates variations among individuals, among age groups, and among different mental faculties and can be both perfect and wanting in various respects and yet still satisfy the requirements for 'mental health'.

Thus the management of mental health is a twofold sphere of action: as a matter of medical competence, with a physiological frame, it necessitates bodily cares; but its composite, varying, and relative nature also leaves scope for ethical self-improvement of a 'psychotherapeutical' kind. In fact Galen also wrote extensively about caring for one's character and the importance of exercising self-control and philosophical reflection in order to overcome vices such as anger and excessive grief, or the desire for pleasures and the attachment to material goods.[40]

As far as the first aspect is concerned, Galen's expansion and development of the outlook expressed in the Hippocratic text is evident in the very basis of his discussion of health of mind in relation to the body. For Galen, mental capacities (as well as ethical virtues and flaws) are determined by the individual's physiological nature—his or her bodily mixture—although they may also be affected by education and lifestyle. In the opening chapter of his treatise *The Capacities of the Soul Depend on the Mixtures of the Body*, Galen states that it is from the 'good mixture of the body', which is achieved by means of 'what we eat and drink, and also through our daily practices', that we achieve 'virtue (*aretē*) of the soul'.[41] Still, the deeper nature of each soul is

---

[39] For an introduction, see the commentaries by Singer and others to the translations of Galen's psychological works in Singer (2013). On ethical aspects, see the extensive works of Gill (2010, 2013).

[40] On anger, see von Staden (2011).

[41] Galen, *The Capacities of the Soul Depend on the Mixtures of the Body* 1 (Müller 32 = K. 768), translated by Singer (2013).

innate in the individual: for Galen, children are the perfect illustration of this principle, because their character differs from one child to another even before they are educated:

> If the substance of the soul [of children] were indistinguishable, then they would per-
> form the same actions and undergo the same affections, given the same causes. And
> therefore it is evident that children differ from each other in the substances of their
> souls to precisely the same extent that they differ in their activities and affections; and
> if in this respect, then also in their capacities.[42]

He later adds that the 'different degrees of shrewdness and foolishness depend on the mixtures in the rational soul' and that differences in the mixtures explain 'the difference in character traits, which obviously vary between spirited and lacking in spirit, intelligent and unintelligent'.[43] It is clear that Galen is thinking of children who are mentally healthy but who differ among themselves not only in character but also, as happens in *On Regimen*, in the degree of their cogni-tive abilities: his discussion, *mutatis mutandis*, responds to concerns similar to those of the Hippocratic author.

Variation also accompanies different phases of life, since over time people may become 'bad' or 'unjust' because of change in the mixtures of their bodies as well as in their education. There is, however, a threshold of severity and curabil-ity that Galen recognizes: although the mixtures of the body and the substance of the soul may be affected positively or negatively by regimen and education, in some cases mental health and ethical soundness are so badly damaged that they render some individuals 'incurably evil' (*aniatos poneroi*). These individu-als, according to Galen, are rightly sentenced to death in order to be prevented from harming the living and to deter other knaves. Most importantly, perhaps, they should be eliminated in their own best interest: 'it is better for them to die, since they are so corrupt in their soul that they cannot be educated even by the Muses, nor can they receive any improvement from Socrates or Pythagoras'.[44]

For everyone else, there are practices of self-improvement and philosophical teachings that Galen recommends. The effects of these practices are comple-mentary to those of the medical treatment, which addresses the physiologi-cal imbalance that might be causing mental disturbance. Most famously, in *The Affections and Errors of the Soul* and in the epistle *On Avoiding Distress*, Galen provides examples of such philosophical practices of caring for the self, and especially of counteracting the anger, grief, and anxiety that may follow

---

[42] Ibid. 2 (Müller 33 = K. 4.769), translated by Singer (2013).

[43] Ibid. 11 (Müller 78–9 = K. 4.821), our translation.

[44] Ibid. 11 (Müller 74 = K. 4.816), our translation.

a personal loss. These practices are in many respects comparable to what we would nowadays define as forms of cognitive therapy: they involve using reason to self-motivate the distressed individual and to train him or her to control his or her strong emotions; or practising thoughts of a sapiential kind aimed at emphasizing the unimportance of material possessions or human rewards such as fame and glory and at limiting one's dependence to what is necessary for a dignified but modest life. These classic themes of consolatory philosophy sound, to the modern ear, entirely at odds with the deterministic and body-centred view expressed in *The Capacities of the Soul Depend on the Mixtures of the Body*—two approaches that hardly appear to establish any form of dialogue between them. This contradiction remains fundamentally unresolved in Galen, and the definition of mental insanity in medical texts will remain, along these lines, divided between its underlying physiology on the one hand, its ethical treatment and normative construction on the other.[45]

In the rather heterogeneous texts we have just surveyed, we can observe Galen's underlying interest in establishing some form of order or ranking among cases of impaired mental health. Although not committing himself to a taxonomy, he adopts a grid of shifting distinctions between various degrees of severity: between cognitive shortcoming and moral depravity, notably, and between underlying anatomo-physiological disorders and mental output. On the whole, as is well known, he chooses to remain flexible and to use different explanatory and therapeutic models in different contexts.

This lack of distinct and fixed categories for mental disorders should not be taken as a lack of sophistication concerning the possibilities of taxonomy, but rather as an admission of the difficulty, in this domain, of establishing firm indicators for illness versus health. Galen's awareness of the questions and problems posed by a definition of mental disorder is evident elsewhere, for example in his remarks on Hippocrates, whom he praises for what he sees (with characteristic aggrandizement)[46] as great terminological precision in his attempt to name degrees and types of insanity:[47]

> [Hippocrates] says that on the first day Python had two symptoms accompanied by acute fever: tremor of the hands and a short *paraphrosunē* [derangement]. For he usually indicates, using different terms in different situations, the degree (*poson*) of *paraphrosunē*, saying *lērēsai* [to speak nonsense] and *paralērēsai* [to speak nonsense] and *paraphronēsai* [to be deranged] and *parenechthēnai* [to be carried away] and again

---

[45] See Nutton (2013) on this topic.

[46] See on this Thumiger (2016).

[47] This compliment grossly overplays the use of this vocabulary in Hippocrates, where the terminology is very far from the clarity Galen attributes to it; but this is not at stake here (see Thumiger 2015 on this point).

parakopsai [to be hit] and *ekstēnai* [to be out of oneself], *manēnai* [to be manic] and *ekmanēnai* [to have an attack of *mania*]. So if he says that Pythion *elērēsen*, it is clear that he *parephronēsen* in a mild way/for a short time (*metriōs*).

Although appreciative of this terminological and medical precision in identifying levels of mental pathology, on the operational level of dealing with actual patients—which seems to have concerned him most—Galen is well aware of the difficulty of distinguishing between the mentally healthy and the mentally ill in the case of people who fake a mental disease, for instance *mania*. Just as some people faked swellings and internal bleeding by applying harmful drugs to the skin or by inflicting wounds to their mouths, others attempted to fake *mania* by talking nonsense or acting foolishly. Apparently lay people expected physicians to be able to recognize such faked conditions, and Galen agrees that it is indeed possible for an experienced physician to distinguish such patients from the truly ill. In the case of physical symptoms such as spitting blood or swellings, the experienced physician can distinguish whether the perceptible phenomena are genuine or manipulated by the patient (e.g. whether the blood spat out truly originates in the stomach or lungs, or whether the swelling arises from an inner condition of the body). Presumably the consistency, shape, or colour of the blood or swelling were indicative signs that physicians with vast practical experience would recognize. In the case of symptoms of mental illness, however, there are no such perceptible phenomena to observe and Galen refers, in a somewhat cryptic remark, to the existence of an intolerably intense pain as a criterion, presumably for those who are genuinely ill.[48] As we have seen above (section 2.2), pain served Galen as a defining criterion of illness and as a means for distinguishing it from the multitude of ambiguous states of health. This physical sensation of pain seems nevertheless also to have served as a disambiguating criterion for distinguishing the mentally healthy from the mentally ill.

The examples discussed in this chapter bring to light the theoretical and practical challenges with which ancient physicians and philosophers were confronted in their attempts to define health and illness and to determine the condition of their patients, as well as the means by which they attempted to overcome these challenges. They recognized the vagueness of the concepts of health and disease in two senses: with regard to the respective degree of these states and with regard to the criteria by which each one can be defined and distinguished from the other. In recognizing the existence of a broad spectrum of healthy states and of conditions that indicated the presence of both health and illness in the

---

[48] Galen, *How to Detect Malingerers* (Deichgräber–Kudlien 113,3–18 = K. 19.1.1–2.12).

same subject (and at the same time), as discerned by criteria such as pain and maladaptive activity, physicians solved a problem posed by some philosophical approaches: the paradox of unavoidable perpetual suffering and illness in the absence of a state of perfect health. More importantly, they provided a flexible and 'user-friendly' framework for distinguishing physically and mentally ill individuals who required medical attention from those physically and mentally healthy individuals who did not.

Acknowledgement

This research was made possible by the generous funding of the Alexander von Humboldt foundation. We are grateful to Julien Devinant for his comments on an earlier version of this paper; to the editors of the volume for their useful comments; and to the organizers of the conference that originated this volume.

References

Bartoš, H. 2006. 'Varieties of the ancient greek body–soul distinction'. *Rhizai* 3 (1): 59–78.

Bartoš, H. 2015. *Philosophy and Dietetics in the Hippocratic On Regimen: A Delicate Balance of Health*. Leiden: Brill.

Crisp, R. (ed. and trans.). 2000. *Aristotle: Nicomachean Ethics*. Cambridge: Cambridge University Press.

Gill, C. 2010. *Naturalistic Psychology in Galen and Stoicism*. Oxford: Oxford University Press.

Gill, C. 2013. 'Philosophical therapy as preventive psychological medicine'. In *Mental Disorders in the Classical World*, edited by W. V. Harris, pp. 339–60. Leiden: Brill.

Green, R. M. (ed. and trans.). 1951. *A translation of Galen's hygiene. De sanitate tuenda*. Springfield, Ill.: Thomas.

Grimaudo, S. 2008. *Difendere la salute*. Naples: Bibliopolis.

Gundert, B. 2000. 'Soma and psyche in Hippocratic medicine'. In *Psyche and Soma: Physicians and Metaphysicians on the Mind–Body Problem from Antiquity to Enlightenment*, edited by J. W. Wright and P. Potter, pp. 13–36. Oxford: Oxford University Press.

Hankinson, R. J. 1991. 'Greek medical models of mind'. In *Psychology: Companions to Ancient Thought*, vol. 2, edited by S. Everson, pp. 194–217. Cambridge: Cambridge University Press.

Hüffmeier, F. 1961. 'Phronesis in den Schriften des Corpus Hippocraticum'. *Hermes* 89: 51–84.

Harris, W. V. (ed.). 2013. *Mental Disorders in the Classical World*. Leiden: Brill.

Hughes, J. C. 2013. 'If only the ancients had DSM, all would have been crystal clear: Reflections on diagnosis'. In *Mental Disorders in the Classical World*, edited by W. V. Harris, pp. 41–58. Leiden: Brill.

Jones, W. H. S. (ed. and trans.). 1953. *Hippocrates: Vol. IV: Regimen, On the Nature of Man*. London and Cambridge, Mass.: Harvard University Press (The Loeb Classical Library).

Jouanna, J. 2012. 'The theory of sensation, thought and the soul in the Hippocratic treatise Regimen: Its connections with Empedocles and Plato's Timaeus'. In *Greek Medicine from Hippocrates to Galen: Selected papers*, edited by J. Jouanna, P. J. van der Eijk, and N. Allies, pp. 195–228. Leiden: Brill.

King, H. (ed.). 2005. *Health in antiquity*. Cambridge: Cambridge University Press.

Nutton, V. 2013. 'Galenic madness'. In *Mental Disorders in the Classical World*, edited by W. V. Harris, pp. 119–28. Leiden: Brill.

Simon, B. 2013. ' "Carving nature at the joints": The dream of a perfect classification of mental illness'. In *Mental Disorders in the Classical World*, edited by W. V. Harris, pp. 27–40. Leiden: Brill.

Singer, P. N. 1992. 'Some Hippocratic mind–body problems'. In *Tratados hipocráticos (estudios acerca de su contenido, forma e influencia): Actas del VIIe Colloque international hippocratique (Madrid, 24–9 de septiembre de 1990)*, edited by F. J. A. López, pp. 131–43. Madrid: Universidad nacional de educación a distancia.

Singer, P. N. (ed. and trans.). 1997. *Galen: selected works*. Oxford: Oxford University Press.

Singer, P. N. (ed.). 2013. *Galen—Psychological Writings: Avoiding Distress, Character Traits, The Diagnosis and Treatment of the Affections and Errors Peculiar to Each Person's Soul, The Capacities of the Soul Depend on the Mixtures of the Body*. Cambridge: Cambridge University Press.

Steckerl, F. (ed. and trans.). 1958. *The Fragments of Praxagoras of Cos and his School*. Leiden: Brill.

Thumiger, C. 2015. 'Mental insanity in the Hippocratic texts: A pragmatic perspective'. *Mnemosyne* **68** (2): 210–33.

Thumiger, C. 2016. 'Mental disability? Galen on mental health'. In *Disability in Antiquity*, edited by Ch. Laes, pp. 267–81. London: Routledge.

van der Eijk, P. J. 2011. 'Modes and degrees of soul–body relationship in *On Regimen*'. In *Officina Hippocratica: Beiträge zu Ehren von Anargyros Anastassiou und Dieter Irmer*, edited by L. Perilli, A. Anastassiou, D. Irmer, and V. Lorusso, pp. 255–70. Berlin: De Gruyter.

van der Eijk. P. J. (ed. and trans.). 2000. *Diocles of Carystus*, vol. 1. Leiden: Brill.

van der Lugt, M. 2011. 'Neither ill nor healthy: The intermediate state between health and disease in medieval medicine'. *Quaderni Storici* **136**: 13–46.

von Staden, H. 2011. 'The physiology and therapy of anger: Galen on medicine, the soul, and nature'. In *Islamic Philosophy, Science, Culture, and Religion: Studies in Honor of Dimitri Gutas*, edited by F. Opwis and D. Reisman, pp. 63–87. Leiden: Brill.

Von Staden, H. 1989. *Herophilus: The Art of Medicine in Early Alexandria*. Cambridge: Cambridge University Press.

Wöhrle, G. 1990. *Studien zur Theorie der antiken Gesundheitslehre*. Stuttgart: F. Steiner.

Chapter 3

Disease as a vague and thick cluster concept

Geert Keil and Ralf Stoecker

1 Introduction

Trying to define 'mental disease' is one of the least rewarding businesses in the philosophy of medicine. The multifaceted question of what distinguishes the pathological from the non-pathological in psychiatry does not seem to admit of a conclusive answer. Obstacles pile up and it is not even clear whether the task is worth pursuing in the face of the multitude of phenomena, purposes, and conceptual intuitions waiting to be captured.

Many of the difficulties are not specific to psychiatry. A large number of competing disease theories have been developed in medical nosology and in the philosophy of medicine.[1] Defining 'mental disease' poses additional problems, however. In contrast to other areas of medicine, here the difficulty is not merely finding a property or a set of properties that all diseases share, but also addressing scepticism about whether there are such things as mental diseases, that is, states or medical conditions that are both mental and diseases (Szasz 1961; Kendell 1993).

This chapter relates the problem of demarcating the pathological from the non-pathological in psychiatry to the general problem of defining 'disease' in the philosophy of medicine. In section 2 we begin by briefly revisiting three prominent debates in medical nosology: on naturalism versus normativism; on the three dimensions of illness, sickness, and disease; and on the demarcation problem. In sections 3–5 we reformulate the demarcation problem in terms of semantic *vagueness*. As it will turn out, the vagueness of the term 'disease' takes two forms. First, 'disease' exhibits *vagueness of degree* because it draws no sharp line in a continuum. Second, it is *combinatorially vague* because there are several criteria for the term's use that might fall apart. The latter kind of vagueness helps to explain why the other two debates mentioned in section 2

---

[1] For a short but comprehensive overview, see Hofmann (2001).

appear so hopeless: Should we construe 'disease' in a naturalistic or in a normative way? Neither answer is satisfactory, since there are natural as well as normative criteria for something's being a disease. How should we balance the three dimensions of pathology, which are sometimes distinguished as 'illness', 'sickness', and 'disease' (in a narrow sense)? We do not have to, because these are non-competing criteria for the application of the cluster term 'disease' (broadly speaking).

The view of disease as a cluster concept that is not only vague but also normatively 'thick', as sketched in section 6, explains why the notorious disputes on whether or not certain intermediate states are pathological are deadlocked. It also accounts for the practical concerns behind the demarcation problem: The social and normative implications of being diagnosed are best addressed if we deliberate directly on the normative question of how to treat people in the intermediate states, without relying on some pseudo-scientific solution to the demarcation problem. Section 7 applies the thick cluster conception of disease to the recent debate on *DSM 5*'s abandonment of the 'bereavement exclusion' rule for diagnosing major depressive disorder.[2] In section 8 we discuss a legal policy issue and criticize the inclination of lawgivers and decision makers to misuse a non-clustered, binary notion of disease in order to defer the responsibility for hard decisions to medical experts. Finally, a brief outlook (section 9) widens the scope of our suggestion, compares 'disease' with other thick concepts, and draws novel conclusions for medical ethics on the basis of the more general hypothesis that a number of perplexing difficulties in applied ethics can be solved as soon as it is realized that some of its dominant concepts are thick cluster concepts.

Let us begin then by linking our subsequent considerations back to three prominent debates in medical nosology.

2 The background: Three prominent debates in medical nosology

2.1 Naturalism versus normativity

Naturalistic conceptions of disease usually hold that diseases are biological malfunctions, that is, deviations from the natural biological functions of bodily organs. According to the naturalistic view, influentially endorsed by

---

[2] The difference between 'mental disease' and 'mental disorder', however defined, will not play a role in this chapter. We are aware that this is not merely a dispute about terminology, but we do not wish to take a stand on how to distinguish the two notions. In most places we will simply use 'mental disease' as a shorthand for 'mental disease or disorder'.

Christopher Boorse (1975; 1997), determining such malfunctions or abnormalities is an objective matter best left for biology and medical science to deal with. Whether and how this approach can be transferred to psychiatry is a controversial issue. If the prospects for finding biological criteria for the majority of mental diseases are dim, then reductive naturalistic theories of disease are less promising in psychiatry than in general medicine. Boorse's own view is that the missing link between psychiatry and the rest of medicine is provided by evolutionary theory: Mental abilities have inherited adaptive functions. Mental diseases are malfunctions with respect to the normal functional organization of the human mind, which is fixed by species design (Boorse 1976).

Non-naturalist theories claim that 'disease' is basically a *normative* or *evaluative* notion in the sense that what counts as a disease varies with norms, evaluations and human interests. Hence, biological facts leave underdetermined whether a certain bodily or mental condition of an individual counts as a disease (e.g. Szasz 1961; Reznek 1987; Fulford 1989; Cooper 2005). One strand of criticism is that naturalist analyses, although defining the notion of disease in a value-free way, continue to use the term with evaluative connotations (Fulford 2001).

Non-naturalistic theories are sometimes labelled as 'constructivist'. What unites these theories is the 'denial of the naturalist thesis that disease necessarily involves bodily malfunction, [while] the positive constructivist claim varies across theories and is often elusive' (Murphy 2015, § 2). There also exist hybrid theories that combine both biological and normative elements. A case in point is Wakefield's influential 'harmful dysfunction' analysis according to which a condition is a disease or disorder 'if it is negatively valued ('harmful') and it is in fact due to a failure of some internal mechanism to perform a function for which it was biologically designed (i.e., naturally selected)' (Wakefield 2007, 149).

2.2 The relationship between sickness, illness, and disease

It has often been observed that the notion of disease oscillates between biological irregularity or dysfunction, subjective suffering and social impairment. Hence one recommendation has been to disambiguate the broad and vague notion of disease and use other terms instead. A well-known suggestion is to restrict the term 'disease' to the first dimension, biological dysfunction, while using 'illness' for the second, suffering, and 'sickness' for the third, social impairment, leaving 'ailment' as a generic term covering all three usages.[3] However,

---

[3] According to Hofmann (2002), this threefold distinction was first used in 1967 by Andrew Twaddle in his doctoral dissertation.

the use of 'ailment' as an umbrella term has not found wide acceptance, and relinquishing the notion of disease to the naturalistic camp has met with resistance. An alternative suggestion is to explicitly integrate the three dimensions into a single, complex conception of disease: the 'biopsychosocial (BPS) model', which was proposed by Engel as an alternative to the biomedical model because the latter 'leaves no room within its framework for the social, psychological, and behavioral dimensions of illness' (Engel 1977, 130). Engel held that the concept of disease is best understood as a combination of these three factors and that 'all three levels, biological, psychological, and social, must be taken into account in every health care task' (Engel 1978, 180). Engel's primary concern was psychiatry. However, the biopsychosocial conception was not his invention; the idea had been in the air since the 1950s. (The term 'biopsychosocial' was used first by the psychiatrist Roy Grinker in 1954.)

From a theoretical point of view, the BPS model has been criticized as unscientific and eclectic because merely adding further dimensions to the biomedical model does nothing to clarify the conceptual or constitutive *relations* between the three dimensions. What is lurking behind this difficulty is the age-old mind–body problem. The BPS model promised, but did not achieve, a genuine theoretical integration of the three perspectives on disease. Itemizing factors and switching between them ad hoc for various explanatory purposes or interests has pragmatic value but little scientific merit.

If we turn to *mental* diseases and disorders, the additive character of the BPS model is even more problematic and the importance of the mind–body problem particularly conspicuous. In order to find out what distinguishes *mental* diseases, you need to know what the 'mental' is and how it relates conceptually, constitutively, or causally to the physical. Biomedical orthodoxy has it that the search is in vain; there are no such things as mental as opposed to bodily diseases because the mental sphere is not distinct from the body. Mental diseases are ultimately diseases of the brain (Kendell 1993, 3).

2.3 The demarcation problem

The recent scientific and public debates on psychiatric overdiagnosis and 'diagnostic inflation' in psychiatry (Frances 2013; Paris 2015) have highlighted a notorious problem in psychiatric nosology that can be called *the demarcation problem*: the problem of where to draw the line between the pathological and the non-pathological. It is a rarely disputed fact that, for many mental disorders and diseases, there is a *continuum* between 'normal' and 'pathological' states, however defined. The example of progressive dementia may suffice to illustrate this point. Rita Hayworth, Charles Bronson, and Ronald Reagan did not suffer from dementia all their lives, yet in their later years they did. Since they did not catch Alzheimer's overnight, there must have been prodromal and intermediate stages—which raises the question of whether these stages already belonged to dementia or not.

The demarcation problem can be reframed in terms of *vagueness*. Both the concept of disease in general and the concepts of (many) particular diseases are *vague* notions in the technical sense of 'vague', as linguists and philosophers of language use the term. Vague terms draw no sharp line between their extension and their anti-extension but rather admit of borderline cases and gradual transitions. So the problem is how to categorize states in the intermediate area.

All three challenges to crisp definitions of 'disease' in general and of 'mental disease' in particular have been discussed individually in the nosological literature, but not yet synoptically. What is missing is an exploration of their co-occurrence and interplay. The problems of naturalism versus normativity, the relationship between sickness, illness, and disease, and the demarcation problem interlock in poorly understood ways and the complexity of their interrelations still seems to be underestimated. While there is little reason to expect that any theorist will ever come up with superior, non-stipulative general definitions of 'mental disease' and 'mental disorder', taking a synoptic view of the three challenges will help us better understand which aspects of the definitional problems are tractable and which are not.

The first thing to note is that the demarcation problem has two independent sources. Delimiting pathological states from non-pathological ones is problematic on at least two counts: first because mental disorders and diseases come in degrees and, second, because the line can be drawn in more than just one dimension. The first subproblem may be dubbed *the threshold problem*. Stated in terms of vagueness: 'Health' and 'disease' are vague notions because they don't set a sharp lower threshold where pathological states begin.[4] The demarcation problem's second subproblem is that there are a number of dimensions that must be considered and perhaps weighed against one another in order to demarcate disease from normality. This problem can also be framed in terms of vagueness: the notions of mental disease and disorder exhibit 'multidimensional' or 'combinatorial' vagueness. Generally, we hope to show that concepts, distinctions, and insights from the philosophy of language can contribute to a better understanding of the complexities of the demarcation problem.

---

[4] Rachel Cooper (2013, 606) describes the 'threshold problem' as 'the problem of determining the boundary of disorder in cases that shade into normality'.

3 Disease as a soritically vague concept

Philosophers of language and linguists have described vagueness as a seman-tic property of linguistic expressions. Vague terms, it is said, tolerate marginal changes, admit of borderline cases, give rise to the paradox of the heap (the sorites paradox), and thus challenge bivalence—the logical principle that every proposition is either true or false. Psychologically, semantic vagueness mani-fests itself in the speaker's uncertainty about what to say, as Grice's much quoted working definition of 'vagueness' puts it:

> To say that an expression is vague (in a broad sense of vague) is . . . to say that there are cases (actual or possible) in which one just does not know whether to apply the expression or to withhold it, and one's not knowing is not due to ignorance of the facts. (Grice 1989, 177)

It is useful to distinguish the *phenomenon* of semantic vagueness from the *problems* that the phenomenon allegedly gives rise to. The phenomenon is undeniable; countless expressions in natural languages simply *are* semanti-cally vague. As explained in the introduction to this book (Chapter 1.2), only part of the discussion in the philosophy of language is relevant to demar-cation problems in the philosophy of medicine. What is important for our inquiry, however, is the distinction between two kinds of vagueness: the kind of vagueness that we discuss in this section is called 'degree vagueness' or 'soritical vagueness'. The second kind, 'combinatorial' vagueness, will be dis-cussed in section 5.

Soritical vagueness is named after the sorites paradox. It can be traced back to the ancient philosopher Eubulides of Miletus, who used the examples of 'heap' (*sōros*) and 'bald man'. Colour terms are another classical example of soritical vagueness: on the one hand, the move 'if the colour in area #1 is red, then the neighbouring, perceptually indistinguishable area #2 is also red' seems unob-jectionable. On the other hand, a series of incremental steps will allow you to extend *ad absurdum* the predicate 'red' from clear cases through borderline cases of 'red' to clearly non-red areas. If, by this kind of 'soritical reasoning', you can 'prove' that a yellow area is red, then something went wrong, even if it is notoriously hard to tell exactly what. Likewise, 'proving' by soritical reason-ing that a fatally ill person is as fit as a fiddle is fallacious. What makes soritical conclusions paradoxical is that 'seemingly impeccable reasoning from seem-ingly impeccable premises yields a patent falsehood' (Raffman 1994, 42). Yet the question is how to escape the paradox.

The challenge of the sorites paradox is to explain where soritical reasoning goes astray. Logicians and philosophers of language have devised various *theories* of vagueness that try to eliminate the paradox and to demonstrate why soritical reasoning is only seemingly impeccable.[5] The first step seems to be flawless: a perceptually indistinguishable neighbour of a clearly red area is also red. A first stab at the fallacy is to note 'the nontransitivity of marginal difference: a series of insignificant differences 'add up' to a significant one' (Raffman 1994, 42).

As we said, soritical vagueness is, first and foremost, a linguistic phenomenon, that is, a semantic property of linguistic expressions. Being vague, just like being precise, is an attribute that pertains only to representations and not to worldly items.[6] However, the unquestionable vagueness of countless predicates in natural languages prompts the question whether this linguistic feature reflects a corresponding non-linguistic feature of the reality represented. In recent years, a growing minority of philosophers have suggested that there is an 'ontological' or 'metaphysical' kind of vagueness, either in addition to semantic vagueness or in elucidation of it. Are the terms 'heap', 'red', 'bald', 'dementia', and 'post-traumatic stress disorder' perhaps vague *because* the areas of reality that they partition exhibit continuous transitions rather than sharp cut-offs? We shall not take a stance on this question in this chapter.[7]

Not all terms with soritically vague extensions exhibit the same *amount* of vagueness. Some terms admit of more borderline cases than others. A plausible explanation for this fact is that nature is not everywhere equally continuous. 'Bone fracture' is less vague than 'dementia' because bone fracture is a threshold phenomenon: fractures suddenly occur when the amount of stress exceeds a certain value. Partial fractures also occur, but they are clearly distinguished both from complete fractures and from non-fractures. While the range of stress values is seamless, there is no corresponding continuous range of fracture phenomena. By contrast, the distribution of dementia phenomena is more even, and there is no sharp lower threshold where dementia begins. Clinicians have ordered the stages of progressive dementia along the five-stage Clinical Dementia Rating (CDR) scale; but, if asked, few psychiatrists would deny that this classification exhibits a considerable amount of arbitrariness and that the stages do not correspond to real thresholds in nature.

Soritical vagueness bedevils the classification both of dynamic processes into *stages* (as with dementia, depression, or cancer) and of static phenomena into *kinds* (unipolar depression or bipolar disorder? dementia or delirium?

---

[5] For an overview, see Keefe (2000) and Sorensen (2016).

[6] '[V]agueness and precision alike are characteristics which can only belong to a representation. They have to do with the relation between a representation and that which it represents' (Russell 1923, 85).

[7] But see the introduction to this volume (Chapter 1), sections 2.2 and 2.3. For an overview of the debate on semantic vs ontic vagueness, see Keil (2013).

attention deficit hyperactivity disorder or Asperger's?). Moreover, it also concerns the notion of disease itself, over and above the classification of particular disease entities. Let us discuss the cases in turn:

(1) *Progressive diseases* provide the clearest and least controversial cases of gradual transitions. There are no sharp cut-offs between the various stages of impairment of cognitive abilities in progressive dementia. The CDR rating dubs the five stages 'none', 'questionable', 'mild', 'moderate', and 'severe', but its proponents might as well have distinguished more stages, as the seven-stage Global Deterioration Scale for Assessment of Primary Degenerative Dementia (GDS) does. Numerals abound, adjectives are cheap, and symptoms can be described in more or less fine-grained ways.

(2) The case of differential diagnosis is more controversial. Major depressive disorder (MDD) shows high co-morbidity rates with anxiety disorder and personality disorders. How do we know that these are really distinct disorders? The Norwegian mass murderer Anders Breivik was diagnosed with paranoid schizophrenia in his first psychiatric evaluation and with narcissistic personality disorder in his second (see Chapter 10). Perhaps one of the assessment teams was simply wrong. Disagreement among equally competent assessors may often just indicate that differential diagnosis is difficult. It is more plausible, however, that in many cases adjacent diagnostic categories do not carve nature at its joints because there are no joints to be carved. But we must keep in mind that the uncertainty of a diagnosis can be attributed to the vagueness of diagnostic categories only if it is not solely due to a lack of information or to factual errors.

(3) The soritical vagueness of the concept of disease itself concerns the fuzzy boundary between the pathological and the non-pathological. Stating that a person has *a* disease can be regarded as tantamount to the disjunctive judgement that one of a large number of particular diseases ('disease entities') is present in her. Seen this way, the vagueness of the concept of disease itself has no independent source, but instead derives from the vagueness of the definitions of particular diseases. Alternatively, one may try to give a general definition of 'pathological' that bypasses the intricacies of defining particular diseases. Plausibly such a general definition will be disjunctive. One elaborate suggestion is that a state is pathological if it is either immediately lethal or life-shortening in the long run; or if it is painful, if it is a condition of infertility, if it impairs one's ability to live together with others, or if it disposes one to develop or manifest a condition that is pathological according to one or more of these criteria (see Chapter 4). However, such an elaborate disjunctive definition of 'pathological state'

does not eliminate vagueness, because the fulfilment of each of the criteria admits of degrees: Just how much pain, impairment, and so on makes a state pathological?

Later in this chapter we will consider and defend a stronger and philosophically more comprehensive disjunctive approach to the definition of disease. That approach involves normative considerations and analyses the concept of disease as displaying a special kind of combinatorial vagueness. Before explaining this second kind of vagueness, let us take a look at three common reactions to the soritical vagueness of the concept of disease.

4 Three common reactions to soritical vagueness

4.1 But there are lots of clear cases!

This is true enough, but holding that a concept is vague does not commit you to denying that clear cases abound. Baldness is a classic example of vagueness, despite the fact that there are clear-cut cases, like Yul Brynner or James Dean, for whom there is no doubt as to whether they are bald or not. Still, it is possible to construct a sorites series between the two hairdos. It is precisely characteristic of sorites series that neither the smoothness of the transition, nor even the perceptual indistinguishability between neighbouring elements bar the blatant difference between the starting point and the end point. The same holds for mental diseases: as a response to the threshold problem, insisting that there are clear cases of mental disease and non-pathological states is simply beside the point.

It is worth noting that, with respect to the non-availability of sharp thresholds, all theorists are in the same boat. Take as an illustration Allen Frances' campaign for 'saving the normal'. Frances warned that *DSM-5* would promote 'diagnostic inflation' in psychiatry: the new manual

> will dramatically increase the rates of mental disorder and cheapen the currency of psychiatric diagnosis. The DSM 5 proposals do this in two ways: (1) by reducing thresholds for existing disorders; and (2) by introducing new high prevalence disorders at the boundary with normality. (Frances 2012)

The 'boundary with normality', however, is notoriously hard to pinpoint. One may think that, if Frances defends 'the normal' so vigorously, he must be prepared to say exactly where normality ends. But he neither defines normality nor purports to do so (see Frances 2013, 3–34). In order to preserve the intuition that not all of us have mental diseases or disorders, one does not have to deny or belittle demarcation problems. The sorites paradox is so perplexing precisely because the undisputed existence of clear cases is compatible with the non-existence of sharp boundaries in the transitional region. And this is why the reminder that clear cases exist is beside the point. We turn to the second common reaction.

4.2 Introducing degrees of severity, stages, prodromal phases, and subthreshold disorders alleviates the demarcation problem

Introducing intermediate stages of diseases is useful in clinical contexts and for epidemiological statistics. It should be obvious, however, that merely *stipulating* thresholds and stages does not make natural continuities discontinuous. Stages, phases, and degrees of severity are poorly individuated. The common classifications of five stages of dementia, or of cancer, or of diabetic nephropathy (why always five?!), suggest the existence of steps or thresholds where there are none. Suffering from a progressive disease is not like descending steps on a staircase but rather like slipping down a slope. Whatever the merits of fiat boundaries are, they do not transform slopes into stairs.

In general, the interpolation of intermediate stages and borderline areas as a reaction to soritical vagueness *multiplies* demarcation problems rather than solving them. Compare the problem of the heap: originally, the question was how many grains make a heap. After having realized that there are amounts that are difficult to classify, one might be tempted to classify them as borderline cases of heaps. If we do, however, we are confronted with two questions, namely what distinguishes a borderline case from a clear case of a heap and what distinguishes a borderline heap from a clear non-heap. The same holds for the vagueness of diagnostic categories. Trying to account for borderline cases by adding 'subthreshold disorders' and 'prodromal phases' not only makes psychiatric classification more fine-grained, but also multiplies the demarcation problems: '[s]o-called subthreshold disorders require the definition of two thresholds'—one upper and one lower (Helmchen and Linden 2000, 1).

In the philosophy of language, this phenomenon is called 'higher order vagueness': borderline cases themselves have borderline cases. The phenomenon of higher order vagueness reminds us of the fact that the vagueness of a diagnostic category does not merely raise the practical problem of *where* to draw the line, but also the *conceptual* problem that, wherever the line is drawn, it will yield borderline cases and that finer classifications will yield more borderline cases.

Fine-grained classifications of stages of disease and degrees of severity may even be intellectually harmful in that they lead one to believe that diagnostic distinctions always stand for real differences. Fine-grained classifications can also suggest an amount of precision that does not actually exist. They can prompt what the linguist Manfred Pinkal calls 'intuitively untenable overprecisifications'

(Pinkal 1995, 162). Such pseudo-precision does not remove, but rather obscures, the continuous nature of the underlying phenomenon.

4.3 The vagueness of diagnostic categories is merely epistemic

'Many psychiatrists and psychologists believe that much of the vagueness in psychiatry is epistemic. Their hope is that yet to be discovered information involving biomarkers, endophenotypes, and underlying mechanisms will lead to increased diagnostic clarity' (Zachar and McNally, Chapter 9.1). While some of these hopes may materialize, they have little bearing on the vagueness issue. Grice's working definition of 'vagueness' makes it clear that the uncertainty about whether to apply a vague expression is not due to an epistemic deficit that can be remedied through additional empirical information: vagueness-induced uncertainty 'is not due to ignorance of the facts' (Grice 1989, 177). Given the vagueness of the term 'heap', a speaker may know the exact number of grains and still wonder whether or not the amount is a heap. Likewise, a clinician may know the exact medical condition of a patient and still wonder whether the condition should qualify as a disease or not. So, strictly speaking, the term 'epistemic vagueness' is a misnomer. Uncertainty that can be eliminated by collecting empirical information is *not* due to semantic vagueness. The reaction expressed by 4.3 is best seen as a claim about the underlying reality that psychiatry's diagnostic categories try to capture. The claim—or hope—is that mental diseases are perfectly individuated entities that fall into clean-cut natural kinds, even if human scientists do not (yet) know their true nature. This view is not felicitously expressed through the term 'epistemic vagueness'.

5 Disease as a combinatorially vague concept

As mentioned, not all of the vagueness of the term 'disease' and of particular names for diseases is soritical. Over and above admitting of degrees, 'disease' oscillates between various dimensions. It is a cluster concept that exhibits 'combinatorial' vagueness.[8] There is no consensus among philosophers of language as to what exactly a cluster concept is. A number of overlapping definitions have been suggested since Wittgenstein wrote about 'family resemblance' concepts. In our usage, a cluster concept is *explicitly or implicitly defined on the basis of an open or closed list of criteria, such that none of these criteria and no combination thereof are both necessary and jointly sufficient* for the phenomenon's

---

[8] The expression 'combinatorial vagueness' goes back to Alston (1967). The term 'cluster concept' was probably coined by Gasking (1960).

falling under that concept. Wittgenstein compares the conceptual cluster to a thread woven with many criss-crossing fibres, where 'the strength of the thread does not reside in the fact that some one fibre runs through its whole length, but in the overlapping of many fibres' (Wittgenstein 1953, § 67). Wittgenstein's famous example of a family resemblance concept is 'game', Alston's example of combinatorial vagueness is 'religion'.

The concept of disease as well as the terms for particular diseases have been claimed to be combinatorially vague. With respect to the latter, the idea is that the cluster concept of disease combines the dimensions of biological malfunctioning, subjective suffering, and impaired ability for social interaction. (This combination echoes the BPS model of disease.) As regards particular mental diseases and disorders, many are defined *polythetically*, that is, on the basis of a minimum number of features or symptoms drawn from a list. For a diagnosis of major depression, *DSM-5* requires five out of nine symptoms. Post-traumatic stress disorder (PTSD) can be diagnosed if six symptoms from a list of 20 are present, so that 'two people can both be diagnosed with PTSD and have no symptoms in common' (Zachar and McNally, Chapter 9.7).

The clustered nature of the concept of disease has received considerable attention in general medical nosology because it is in fact responsible for most nosological vagueness, although soritical vagueness and combinatorial vagueness often go hand in hand. The twilight zone between health and disease is inhabited, among many other things, by old-age impotence, menopause, being gap-toothed, Down syndrome, intersexuality, paedophilia, alcoholism, antisocial personality disorder, internet addiction, pregnancy, unwanted childlessness. Which of these states and conditions qualify as diseases and why? There are extensive and sometimes heated debates about each of these borderline cases. In some of them, the claim that they even border on being diseases or disorders has been indignantly rejected. We take no stand on any of these particular cases. Instead we want to point out that the divergences of opinion are nicely explained by reference to the combinatorial vagueness of the concept of disease. Consider again the three dimensions of biological malfunctioning, subjective suffering, and impaired social abilities. Seven combinations of these three strands of the cluster are logically possible: a person may be regarded as ill on any one of the three counts, on any combination of two counts, or on all three counts. Plausibly a person is less likely, or more controversially, to be considered ill the fewer of the criteria she fulfils. (For the moment, let us ignore the fact that criteria can be fulfilled to a higher or lesser degree and that they can be fulfilled entirely or partially, that is, that combinatorial and soritical vagueness overlap.) It is tempting to argue that, in order for someone to qualify as ill, at least two criteria should be met. However, advocates of the biomedical model hold that the dimension of biological malfunctioning is 'more equal than the others': How could someone be ill just by feeling so, or just by being assigned the sick role?

Both ideas have some initial plausibility, yet both are at odds with the cluster conception. First, if biological malfunctioning or organic irregularity, unlike the other criteria, were a necessary condition, then disease would *not* be a cluster concept, since biological malfunction would constitute a necessary condition. Countless ordinary language concepts include several optional and at least one necessary element. As such, these concepts do not count as clustered according to standard definitions of 'cluster concept'. If some specification of the concept of disease in terms of necessary and jointly sufficient conditions were available and accepted, then we could dispense with the cluster view.

In fact there seem to be cases where one of the strands of the cluster is sufficient and 'trumps' the absence of the other criteria: a person with undiagnosed pancreatic cancer clearly has a disease. This is why the rule of thumb that at least two criteria should be met is also at odds with the cluster conception. And indeed, biological dysfunction often is what makes the difference. Lovesickness can be terribly painful, but is not a disease, while short-sightedness (myopia) counts as a disease although the social impairment and suffering are negligible. There are other cases, however, where the suffering and the social impairment are so massive that they trump the biological criterion. There may even be cases, such as antisocial behaviour, where the condition of social impairment suffices.

None of these cases contradicts the cluster view. What matters is that no single condition or combination of conditions is both sufficient and necessary. Sometimes organic irregularity suffices, but, as long as no sufficient condition is shared by all instances of diseases (i.e. is also necessary), 'disease' remains a cluster concept with combinatorially vague boundaries. It is typical of cluster concepts that some stricter conditions work strikingly well for particular cases, so that they blind us to counterexamples. Wittgenstein anticipated this tendency to overgeneralize working definitions when he advised philosophers against an unbalanced diet—against 'nourishing one's thinking with only one kind of example' (Wittgenstein 1953, § 593). The problem with the narrower proposals that compete with the cluster view is that, while they evidently capture something important about the concept of disease, for each of them there are intuitively clear cases of diseases that do not meet the criteria, as well as cases of non-diseases that meet them.

To sum up, biological dysfunction, subjective suffering, and social impairment are part of our ordinary understanding of disease. They constitute strands of the cluster concept of disease.

6 Disease as a thick normative concept

The observation that 'disease' is vague in both ways, soritically and combinatorially, explains perfectly well why many authors disagree about the correct application of the term in various borderline cases. What still needs to be explained is why figuring out whether or not a certain condition is a disease appears to be worthwhile in the first place.

Let us begin with soritical vagueness again. Remember that in both kinds of vagueness the speaker's uncertainty as to 'whether to apply the expression or to withhold it . . . is not due to ignorance of the facts' (Grice 1989, 177). The speaker may have counted the grains and still be unsure whether they make up a heap or not. This uncertainty, however, need not worry him. He is allowed, and knows that he is allowed, to exercise discretion in classifying borderline items. It is part of the linguistic competence of ordinary speakers that they are free to go either way. In particular, they do not have to choose a particular stopping place in a sorites series (see Raffman 2014). If a colour is somewhere in the middle between blue and green, then there is no fact of the matter as to how to classify it. Usually nothing hinges on what we say in such cases, and nobody will care whether a particular arrangement of grains is called a heap, as long as the audience can identify the object that the speaker refers to and no fact is misrepresented. As Wittgenstein remarked: 'Say what you like, as long as it doesn't prevent you from seeing how things are' (Wittgenstein 1953, § 79).

With 'disease' it is different because we often care very much. But why? The difference between 'disease' and 'heap' is not that diseases are natural kinds with underlying essences, so that there is always a fact of the matter, known or unknown, as to which conditions are diseases and which are not. Nor is the difference that the medical, psychological, or social facts are so hard to know, or even inaccessible. A trained psychiatrist may have deep insight into a patient's condition and know perfectly well the relevant details without making up his mind about whether the condition is really a disease. So why not agree that you can draw the line in the borderline area wherever you like?

Evidently, the main reason for distinguishing diseases from non-pathological states lies in the social and normative consequences of being diagnosed. Despite its fuzziness, the distinction plays an eminent role in our social practice. Much hinges on whether a person is diagnosed with a disease: you might not have to go to school, you might not even be obliged to wash the dishes. Society has also attached a vast array of economic and legal consequences to the distinction: Who is offered and who is denied reimbursable treatment? Who gets disability benefits? Who is allowed to stay off work? Which defendants can argue diminished responsibility? The consequences need not be positive, however: besides being free not to work, you may also not be allowed to continue your work. You can lose your driver's license. You may be denied a life insurance policy. You can be involuntarily hospitalized. Some psychiatric diagnoses have stigmatizing effects. And so on.

Moreover, it is usually assumed that having a disease has *moral* implications, some of which *justify* the social and legal consequences. For example, our moral evaluations change considerably when a person's drug abuse gets classified as addiction or her shyness as social phobia, that is, as pathological conditions. It is not just a social fact that we treat sick people differently, rather we do so for good reasons: it is *morally just*, they *deserve* to be treated differently.

In philosophical ethics and meta-ethics, a number of authors have suggested that not only social and moral consequences follow from having a disease: there is normativity and value already 'built into' the concept of disease. 'You better visit him, he's ill', is reasonable advice because being ill entails a certain increase in a person's rights to attention and help. It also carries another evaluative claim: having a disease involves being in a state that is not normal, but defective. Something is wrong with the person, her condition is not as it should be, regardless of how these norms or standards are spelled out. Concepts that have a descriptive content combined with a prescriptive or evaluative element are called *thick normative concepts*, in short *thick concepts*.[9] Standard examples are 'cruel', 'truthful', 'fair', and 'coward'. Thick concepts are used neither to simply describe some state of affairs nor to evaluate or prescribe, rather their descriptive part is 'loaded' with evaluation. According to the view of disease as a thick concept, it is not merely a contingent social fact that being seen to be ill has certain consequences, for instance having a claim to protection. The point is rather that the consequences are somehow 'built into' the concept. Not all such consequences and reactions, however, need to be morally justified or justifiable. The stigmatization associated with certain psychiatric diagnoses surely can't be. Unlike other, simpler thick concepts, the thick concept of disease carries both morally justified and morally unjustified evaluations.

But the very idea of a concept that has evaluative connotations as part of its *meaning* is not without problems. Also, it is not easy to understand how a concept can have 'prescriptive content' or 'prescriptive force'. Surely concepts as such do not prescribe, stigmatize, evaluate, praise, blame, and the like. Concepts, unlike minded creatures, do not have the power to perform such acts. No evaluation takes place unless a thick concept is being *used* by a speaker. The point of thick concepts is perhaps that their evaluative aspects are not at the

---

[9] For an overview of the debate on thick concepts, see Roberts (2013) and Kirchin (2013).

speaker's disposal, so that he must reckon with the audience's drawing inferences about his attitudes. A related suggestion is that a thick concept's connotations are so strong that the speaker cannot 'cancel' them, as linguists say. It is virtually impossible for a speaker to address someone as a 'sadist' or as 'brutal' without conveying disapproval, regardless of how the speaker himself thinks about that person. Antisocial personality disorder as characterized in *DSM-5* is a case in point: it would be odd to describe a person as showing a 'lack of concern for feelings or problems of others; lack of guilt or remorse about the negative or harmful effects of one's actions on others; aggression; sadism; use of dominance or intimidation to control others', and so on (APA 2013, 301.7) and then add: 'this is not to say that I find his behaviour objectionable'.

In order to circumvent these worries about thick concepts as conventionally defined, we wish to leave open the question of whether the normative consequences of being diagnosed are due to the *meaning* of the term 'disease' (or of terms that denote particular diseases) rather than either just to widespread and plausible social or moral reactions to the term's descriptive content, or just to certain default assumptions about a shared background of normative attitudes, perhaps conveyed through Gricean conversational implicatures or something akin to them.

The normative consequences of being diagnosed also help to explain why we care so much about distinguishing diseases from non-pathological states. People engage in heated debates about whether a particular condition is a disease or not; the question seems to be a matter of pivotal importance. Given that, first, the prospects for solving the demarcation problem are dim and, second, a clear-cut demarcation is not indispensable either for psychiatric science or for clinical practice (more on this later), it needs to be explained why defining the notions of 'disease' and 'disorder' does not admit of the same nonchalance that speakers show with 'heap', 'bald', or 'blue'. The normative consequences of being diagnosed nicely explain this asymmetry.

At the same time, normative considerations can help us respond to the challenge from soritical vagueness, in other words to deal reasonably with the threshold problem. One lesson from soritical vagueness was that, when classifying borderline items, we are free to go either way. Now, for all their arbitrariness, thresholds may be more or less wisely chosen.[10] Decisions that are arbitrary from a conceptual or theoretical perspective need not be arbitrary

---

[10] This is very much the lesson that Wittgenstein drew from vagueness: 'We do not know the boundaries because none have been drawn. To repeat, we can draw a boundary—for a special purpose. Does it take that to make the concept usable? Not at all! (Except for that special purpose.)' (Wittgenstein 1953, § 69).

from normative, therapeutic, or broadly pragmatic perspectives.[11] If diagnostic criteria allow discretion as to where to set the threshold, then it is very reasonable to let the normative consequences of being diagnosed take up the slack. So, if we are only interested in normative consequences, then we should better ask why diseases are supposed to have these consequences and draw the line accordingly. If for example what is crucial is the fact that diseases hurt, then the line should be drawn where suffering starts.

Now the concept of disease is not only soritically vague, but also combinatorially vague. Biological, psychological, and social criteria form a cluster. And, since in borderline cases only some of these criteria apply, vagueness results. So, again, from a normative perspective we might ask where to draw the line. At first glance, the solution is the same as in cases of soritical vagueness: we might simply check which of the criteria that form the cluster is responsible for the normative consequences, and then focus on whether the person is ill in the relevant sense. If, for example, the normative consequences were merely due to the subjective feelings of pain and sorrow, we could confine ourselves to distinguishing pathological from non-pathological states on the basis of subjective experience and simply ignore the other elements that comprise the cluster concept 'disease'.

However, this suggestion turns out to be much too simple to do justice to the problem of distinguishing pathological cases from non-pathological ones. The reason is that a thorough examination of the normative consequences of having a disease will probably reveal that not only one, but all elements in the cluster can contribute to these consequences.

Consider for example two women who, for biological reasons, are unable to have children. Both suffer from this inability, so they are equally ill with respect to their subjective pain. However, since one of them is 60 years old and the other 25, it might be argued that only the second woman is sick (i.e. takes on the role of being sick), and hence that society has an obligation to help only the second woman. It is bad luck, one might say, not to be fertile at 25, but it isn't so at 60. And, since society has some responsibility to compensate its members

---

[11] 'Deciding the exact cut-off point for the threshold is often an arbitrary decision, in the sense that frequently there are no natural divisions to be mapped. Still, a choice may be more or less wise. Where possible, the threshold should be set such that the benefits of diagnosis (which may include benefits that accrue from treatment that aims to reduce the risk of future harm) will usually outweigh the disadvantages. Many of the controversies that emerged during the period of proposed changes to DSM-5 can be seen as being rooted in worries that cut-off points for some diagnoses may have been selected unwisely, such that people who could more profitably be considered normal would be considered disordered' (Cooper 2013, 610).

for undeserved bad luck, the second woman is in a stronger normative position than the first.

The example illustrates how other elements in the cluster, besides subjective feelings, can also become normatively relevant. But then we again face combinatorial vagueness and the normative implications of being pathological: a state could count as pathological in one normatively relevant respect, yet non-pathological in another normative respect. We seem to be back at square one.

Fortunately, though, the situation is not that desperate. We need not conclude, from the observation that several dimensions of disease have normative effects, that combinatorial vagueness must still somehow be overcome in order for us to crisply and unambiguously define 'disease'. We may instead conclude, if just interested in the normative implications, that it does not matter whether someone has a disease or not, as long as we know which of the criteria is fulfilled and what normative consequences are appropriate. If, say, a person's suffering is regarded as entailing certain societal obligations, those obligations hold regardless of whether the person has a disease or not, and likewise for the other criteria that constitute the cluster concept of disease.

As already mentioned, there are other reasons for wanting to define 'disease' aside from accommodating the normative and social consequences of being diagnosed. From the perspective of normative concerns, however, the observations that 'disease' is a cluster concept and that a considerable part of the vagueness between pathological and non-pathological states is combinatorial provide a more soothing explanation of our inability to clearly demarcate diseases from non-pathological states. There is simply no answer to the question of what exactly diseases are. The question marks neither an open scientific nor an open conceptual problem. It is not a good question to ask in the first place. Hence not being able to define 'disease' in terms of necessary and sufficient conditions need not worry us, given that the interests that motivated the quest were broadly practical.

In the following section we illustrate this view by considering a debate that was stimulated by the recent revision of the *DSM*: the question of whether or not bereavement-related grief should qualify as a mental disease.

7 The case of bereavement-related grief

DSM-IV advised clinicians not to diagnose MDD if the patient who met the criteria had suffered the loss of a beloved person recently, that is, within the past two months (APA 2000, 356). In *DSM-5* this so-called bereavement exclusion criterion was deleted. It is therefore now possible, although not mandatory, to diagnose MDD shortly after bereavement, as long as the criteria are met.

DSM-5 facilitates diagnosing major depression, but at the same time has added some guidelines designed to help clinicians differentiate normal loss-related grief from loss-related major depression. Still, many commentators felt uneasy with the change.

Consider a mourning widower who shows symptoms of major depression. In this case we are torn between viewing his state as pathological and viewing it as normal. Both views are plausible: on the one hand, deeply mourning a loss is something perfectly normal and human rather than defective, therefore loss-related grief could hardly be a mental disorder or disease. To suggest to a person in mourning that he is in a sort of defective state is embarrassing, because the mourner sees his grief as being inseparably bound up with his love for the deceased. And love, in turn, goes to the very heart of our human individual personality. To suggest that someone's grief is a disease is to attack his identity at its core.

The embarrassment of the mourner also has a second, social aspect. From the perspective of society, a lover's behaviour as a grieving lover is a decent way of living. To say that you lead a decent life means that you deal adequately with such situations of loss. If it is suggested, however, that the mourner is in some sort of defective or diminished state, his being a decent person is called into question. He is not taken seriously. In this sense, it is an expression of respect not to call grief a disorder or disease. The *DSM-5* authors agree with this view in their general definition of 'mental disorder', stating that an 'expectable or culturally approved response to a common stressor or loss, such as the death of a loved one, is not a mental disorder' (APA 2013, 20). It is rather the absence of grief in circumstances of bereavement that may count as pathological.

On the other hand, however, the widower is probably in need of medical support. Hence there is a good reason for classifying his deep grief, which resembles clinical depression, as a disorder or disease.[12] Deep grief involves a lot of pain and suffering that might very well be alleviated, either through medication or through other therapeutic measures.

The observation that the concept of disease is a thick cluster concept helps alleviate the tension between these views: on the face of it, they contradict each other insofar as the first one denies what the latter affirms, namely that the widower's state is pathological. But on closer inspection both refer to different elements of the thick concept of disease. They base their evaluations on different aspects of what it is to be a disease. The concern that loss-related grief might

---

[12] The *DSM* avoids the term 'mental disease' in favour of 'mental disorder', in accordance with most contemporary usage in psychiatry. In this chapter we do not take a stand on how disorders can or should be distinguished from diseases (see above, note 2).

not be a disease because it is a normal, useful, decent reaction relies on the idea that diseases are not normal but defective, while the view that grief must be a disease because it obliges us to alleviate the suffering of the mourning person is based on the subjective illness portion to the concept of disease. These different aspects are, in fact, different strands that make up the cluster concept of disease.

Our proposal has two further advantages. First, it makes it possible to respond to an argument for giving up the bereavement exception. Kenneth Kendler, a prominent member of the *DSM-5* depression task force, has pointed out that there are other stressful life events that might result in symptoms similar to those of deep forms of grief, for example being physically assaulted or raped. The manual has no exclusion rule for any of these other stressors, so why should it make an exception for bereavement?[13] One possible reaction to this argument is that it works in both directions, as Kendler himself admits: 'Either the grief exclusion criterion needs to be eliminated or extended' (Kendler 2010). Wakefield and Horwitz (2016, 185) argue that, since the cases excluded by the bereavement exclusion are 'not disorders, the similarity to analogous reactions to other stressors meant that those reactions to other stressors are not disorders either'. The *DSM* authors took the opposite line: given the similarities, there is no reason to privilege one of the stressors, hence the bereavement exclusion rule must be abandoned.[14]

In the light of our suggestion, however, there is no need either for treating grief as thoroughly exceptional or for treating it on a par with all other stressors. Instead, we can allow for variable attitudes towards different cases. After all, there are crucial and normatively relevant disanalogies between grief and PTSD, and perhaps also between different triggers for PTSD. If a woman develops depressive symptoms or PTSD after being raped, these symptoms are much more alien to her than those arising from grief. Grief over a loss is ours; it is or becomes part of us. Although not intentionally chosen, loss-related grief belongs to us like the fatigue after having climbed a mountain—and unlike being in pain during the extraction of a tooth or suffering flashbacks from a

---

[13] Kendler, Myers, and Zisook (2008); Kendler (2010).

[14] Some psychiatrists go so far as to hold 'that the presence of the DSM's depressive symptoms themselves, regardless of context or type, constitutes a disorder' (Wakefield and Horwitz 2016, 186). Maj, for instance, argues that 'a person meeting the severity, duration, and impairment criteria' for MDD should not be denied the diagnosis 'just because the depressive state occurs in the context of a significant life event', the more so since 'response to antidepressant medications is unrelated to whether or not major depression is preceded by a life event' (Maj 2008, 1374). These authors reject the bereavement exclusion rule because 'situational' major depression, as they claim, does not differ qualitatively from 'nonsituational' major depression, so that the distinction is arbitrary.

trauma. This difference is reflected in the fact that we do not regard it as deplorable that the widower is mourning after the death of his beloved wife (although, of course, we pity him for having lost his wife), while we do not hesitate to deplore that a woman has developed a stress disorder after being raped. Both the rape and the wife's death are irrevocable, but the woman would have been better off without the disorder, while the mourning widower would not be better off without his grief. Compare: if the woman could somehow switch off her traumatic flashbacks, she would probably choose to.[15] If, on the other hand, the widower could switch off the bittersweet memories that make him weep, he would probably not.

Still, we can grant that the PTSD after rape is different from the PTSD of, say, an engineer after his train hits a suicidal person. The humiliating and degrading character of rape renders some of the PTSD reactions understandable and less alien. There need be no general rules about what reactions to different kinds of traumatic experiences are 'normal' or 'appropriate', and there can be vast individual and cultural differences. As soon as we realize that disease is a thick cluster concept and hence we abstain from pressing borderline cases into the dichotomy 'pathological–not pathological', we can handle the normative demands of the different cases more sensitively and in an ethically more satisfying manner.

A second advantage of our proposal is that it relieves pressure from another strand in the debate about the bereavement exclusion. It has been argued that one has to distinguish symptoms of bereavement-related grief that, although *resembling* a depressive episode, are normal responses to a loss from cases where a person *develops* a MDD on top of, and perhaps also as an effect of, his or her non-disordered grief. Therefore the *DSM-5* authors have added a note to the MDD diagnostic criteria that advises the clinician to consider the possibility that loss-related grief develops into a genuine disorder.[16]

---

[15] In her book about living with PTSD after suffering a violent rape, Susan Brison writes: 'Not to wear glasses (or contact lenses) would be viewed as crazy. Why? Because treatment is available to bring me (almost) up to the norm . . . . Not to treat my PTSD would strike me as just as crazy' (Brison 2002, 82–3).

[16] 'Responses to a significant loss . . . may include the feelings of intense sadness, rumination about the loss, insomnia, poor appetite, and weight loss . . . which may resemble a depressive episode. Although such symptoms may be understandable or considered appropriate to the loss, the presence of a major depressive episode in addition to the normal response to a significant loss should also be carefully considered' (APA 2013, 161). Critics of the elimination of the bereavement exclusion rule object that this note comes without diagnostic criteria, that it will probably be ignored by researchers as well as by most clinicians, and that, in effect, the MDD criteria 'risk pathologizing all forms of suffering' (Wakefield and Horwitz 2016, 190 and 197).

As philosophers without special psychiatric expertise, we are not competent to assess the difficulties of making a valid differential diagnosis between bereavement-related grief that resembles a depressive episode and grief that leads to major depression. If the latter case is clearly different from the former, the case need not worry us, because MDD is indisputably a disorder. We are, however, somewhat wary of the distinction. After all, particular instances of diseases or of grief are not well-individuated entities.

What we have tried to show is that our general account of how to deal with the vagueness of the concept of disease helps alleviate the problem of whether grief should be diagnosable as disease at all. Grief is a perfectly normal, adequate reaction to a severe loss, but at the same time it may require medical treatment. Hence it matches some, but not all, of the different strands of the thick cluster concept of disease. But, as soon as we feel forced to choose between calling it a disease or not, we get either all or none of the normative consequences of disease. The thick cluster concept of disease 'inherits' the evaluations that stem from the respective strands of the cluster; therefore by applying the concept we convey the associated evaluations as a whole. This is unproblematic as long as we deal with paradigmatic cases of disease that fall squarely into the extension of the concept. But in the twilight zone, where we find grief and other problematic cases, things are different. We get the feeling that whatever we say is wrong. And the feeling is true, since either choice leads us to make a false normative statement about someone.

But there is no need to make such a choice. There is always the alternative of focusing directly on the normative issues: it is deeply embarrassing for the mourning widower if his grief is classified as defective or pathological, because he sees this grief as being inseparably bound up with his love for the deceased; and yet we still might have social obligations to assuage his suffering.

To be sure, in many medico-legal environments it is true that 'judging that a condition is not a disease commits one to preventing its medical treatment' (Reznek 1987, 171). But then the flaw is in the system that forces such a morally dubious choice. In a decent healthcare system nothing should prevent doctors from helping people who would not find a way out of their mourning without risking their stigmatization.

8 The importance of accepting that disease is a thick cluster concept

According to our view, the various normative implications of either being or not being diagnosed are connected to different strands in the cluster concept of disease. Hence, in borderline cases, we are well advised to disentangle the conceptual bundle in order to prevent our ethical judgement about a given problem from being interfered with by connotations that, although tied to other strands in the cluster, do not apply to the case at hand. The misleading consequences of applying the concept of disease to borderline cases can be avoided, it seems, if we downgrade the notion of disease, or even abstain from using it wherever possible: many of the things one wishes to say by using the terms 'disease' or 'disorder' can be said without using them.

This brings us back to the caveat that our proposal is confined to practical interests: if you are interested in normative consequences, you had better give up asking whether a certain borderline state is a disease or not. That leaves other possible interests, for example scientific ones. After all, it is not evident from the outset that the term 'disease' does not denote a natural kind. Although few researchers would claim that the 157 diagnoses listed in *DSM-5* carve nature at its joints in the same way in which inanimate stuff divides into 118 chemical elements, we still expect scientific progress to reveal phenomena and distinctions that allow for empirical validation. In some cases psychiatric research might even end up with a disease entity that one can fully explain from more fundamental biological processes.

But, on closer examination, appealing to scientific curiosity does not explain why the demarcation problem is so hotly debated, both in and out of science. We have learned from the debate on the threshold problem and on soritical vagueness that there will always remain cases in which the scientific search for a lower threshold where the pathological begins is futile, because there is no matter-of-fact answer. The scientific respectability of psychiatry should better not depend on whether non-arbitrary thresholds can be found. Science aims at understanding and explaining phenomena. Apt classifications and demarcations contribute to these aims. In the end, they constitute the terminology of scientific theories and allow reliable explanations and predictions. The development and refinement of a diagnostic manual can therefore be seen as a project within medical science, for instance in psychiatry. This project, however, should not be expected to provide a general threshold that defines where the pathological begins. In particular, it should not be expected that one can smuggle in, through the back door, a naturalistic solution to the demarcation problem. Elaborate scientific classifications of particular diseases and disorders pick out just one of the different strands in the cluster concept of disease, and hence cannot do justice to all of its normative connotations.

It is especially important to emphasize the narrowness of a scientifically restricted understanding of pathologies, because there is a strong inclination on the part of decision makers in our societies to misuse the scientific concept of disease in order to defer responsibility to medical experts and thereby avoid the embarrassing task of weighing up interests, legitimate concerns, and incommensurable goods. After all, such a strategy offers a number of advantages for decision makers:

(1) It involves non-partisan experts who usually have a higher reputation than other authorities, notably policy makers.

(2) The social and legal consequences of medical diagnoses are already institutionalized and often legally codified, for instance in labour law, criminal law, insurance law, and guardianship law.

(3) In legal and administrative contexts, the distinction between health and disease follows a binary logic, in spite of its questionable scientific legitimacy. The employee, the veteran, the defendant either have a disease that warrants the respective consequences or they don't.

But, when it comes to hard decisions, deferring to medicine, in particular to psychiatry, has major drawbacks. The following example illustrates how passing the buck turned out to be particularly problematic. In 2009 the European Court of Human Rights (ECHR) ruled that Germany violated the European Human Rights Convention by holding a perpetrator in preventive detention after he served his sentence. The person had repeatedly been convicted of violent felonies and had escaped from prison four times. After his last offence, the Marburg Regional Court convicted the person of attempted murder and further ordered his placement in preventive detention (*Sicherungsverwahrung*) under Article 66 § 1 of the German Criminal Code. As the ECHR explained:

> The court found that the applicant still suffered from a serious mental disorder which could, however, no longer be qualified as pathological and did not have to be treated medically . . . . However, he had a strong propensity to commit offences which seriously damaged his victims' physical integrity. It was to be expected that he would commit further spontaneous acts of violence and he was dangerous to the public.[17]

According to German law, however, preventive detention is only admissible if its aim is 'to rehabilitate detainees and to lay the foundations for a responsible life outside prison'.[18]

In response to the verdict from the European Court, the German legislature enacted a law that allows convicted offenders to be detained if 'they are suffering from a mental disorder and if a full assessment of their personality, life-history, and personal circumstances reveals that, as a result of their mental disorder, there exists a high probability' that they continue to pose a danger to the public.[19]

---

[17] European Court of Human Rights (2009).

[18] Ibid.

[19] Bundesministerium der Justiz n.d., § 1, 1.

This law effectively created a new and undefined category of 'mental disorder', which has no basis in diagnostic manuals and is solely designed to justify the preventive detention of persons who are considered to pose a threat to the life and physical integrity of others.[20]

In enacting the new law, as urged by the European Court, German legislature has thereby put considerable pressure on forensic psychiatrists, who are called as expert witnesses. If the high risk of reoffence is due to a 'disorder' that is unknown in professional psychiatry, the implicit expectation obviously is that the expert bases her assessment on something other than professional expertise. If the psychiatrist gives in to the pressure and, against her better judgement, diagnoses the prior offender with a mental disorder so that he can be kept in preventive detention, she violates her professional ethics. If she refuses and approves the prior offender's release, the risk of reoffence is partly her responsibility. Every newspaper reader is familiar with the shitstorm that she and the court have to face, should that risk materialize. In short, the legislature has created a lose–lose situation for the forensic psychiatrist.

No doubt the legislator himself was in serious trouble. No established methods are available for weighing up the risks to public safety against an individual's right to freedom. These are incommensurable goods. Liberal societies should surely be prepared to bear some risk of a repeat offender's committing burglary or financial fraud. Risking violent felonies that threaten other people's lives is another, more serious matter.

The dilemma is real and not to be taken lightly. It is grossly unfair, however, to dump the problem on psychiatry. Tempting as it may be for the rest of society to leave hard decisions about preventive detention to forensic psychiatrists, the temptation should be resisted. A high risk of reoffending is not a mental disorder.[21] Quite generally, society is ill-advised to misuse psychiatry to dispose of conflicts that arise elsewhere and that should be dealt by other means.

This conclusion accords well with our general aim of not holding normative decisions hostage to pseudo-scientific solutions to the demarcation problem.

---

[20] To be sure, we are dealing with cases that are not covered by the German Criminal Code's diminished responsibility rule, which holds for an offender whose capacity 'to appreciate the unlawfulness of his actions or to act in accordance with any such appreciation is substantially diminished . . . due to . . . a pathological mental disorder, a profound consciousness disorder, debility or any other serious mental abnormality' (Bundesministerium der Justiz 2015, § 21 and § 20). The new legislation is meant for offenders who are *not* diagnosed with such a responsibility-diminishing disorder but 'only' continue to pose a danger to public safety, according to the forensic psychiatrists' prognosis.

[21] For this assessment, see also the statement issued by the German Association of Psychiatry, Psychotherapy and Psychosomatics (DGPPN 2011).

The concepts of disease and disorder are not designed to draw stark distinctions between the normal and the pathological across diverse contexts. Their undeniable vagueness and their clustered nature leave room for thoughtful consideration of normative issues and help us to avoid prejudging such issues. The debate about preventive detention has revealed that there are non-medical and non-psychiatric reasons for turning a blind eye to irresolvable vagueness, for treating the fuzzy boundary between disease and normality as a sharp one, and for attaching severe social and legal consequences to the distinction. But these are bad reasons. It is certainly unwise to burden psychiatry with moral, political, or legal dilemmas that are cumbersome to deal with and are only loosely connected to the problems of psychiatric classification and diagnosis. We would do better to identify the source of the relevant problem, mostly a moral dilemma, and to bring into the open the various moral intuitions, interests, and principles that are pertinent to tackling it. In cases where there are good reasons to consider people to be, in some sense, disordered or diseased, our suggestion is that we disentangle the conceptual bundle, set aside the question of whether a given person is sick *tout court*, single out the relevant strand from the cluster, and seriously examine what normative consequences are appropriate.

9 Summary and outlook

At the outset we described the quest for a crisp definition of the notion of disease as one of the least rewarding businesses in the philosophy of medicine. At the end of our deliberations, we arrive at the conclusion that this remark was quite literally true. There will be no reward because the whole enterprise can be shown to be hopeless.

In the first parts of the chapter we drew on the philosophy of language for insights about the nature of vague concepts in order to discourage the search for a sharp general definition of 'disease'. As it turned out, the non-availability of an adequate definition in terms of necessary and jointly sufficient conditions is due, first, to the vagueness of the term 'disease', in particular to its combinatorial vagueness, and, second, to its normative character. In short, it is due to the fact that 'disease' is a thick and vague cluster concept. This conception of disease *explains* the futility of many traditional attempts to define the term.

Moreover, it provides a clue as to what should replace the hopeless search for an adequate general definition. The normative concerns that make the search seem so urgent are more adequately addressed if we figure out what is really at stake in the respective contexts. We should address the normative implications of the different strands that make up the cluster concept directly, for example whether people are suffering, are vulnerable, have physical deficiencies, or are impaired in their daily lives. These concerns can and should be dealt with regardless of whether the conditions count as pathological or not.

To be sure, the idea of treating the concept of disease as a normatively thick cluster concept has to be developed in much more detail. What is worth mentioning, however, is that the strategy as a whole is not confined to the philosophical inquiry into disease. Most likely, many concepts in medical ethics that raise demarcation problems are also thick cluster concepts. For example, the notion of a thick cluster has already proven to be extremely helpful in the debate on brain death, which originally focused on the question of whether brain-dead patients in intensive care units were still alive or already dead. The concepts of life and death are paradigmatic instances of thick cluster concepts and are presumably even thicker than the concept of disease. They are cluster concepts because they unite biological, psychological, and phenomenal features; and they are thick because each of the strands in the cluster contributes to the immense evaluative load that is conjoined with these concepts. Therefore, when wondering how to handle brain-dead patients, one should better abstain from asking whether they are still alive or already dead, since both alternatives would inevitably carry the evaluative weight of the whole, traditional concept (much like in the case of the mourning widower). What is advisable instead is to go back and examine one by one the moral principles that flow from the different strands of the cluster, specifically whether one can still harm or benefit someone, what it would mean to respect them in their dignity, and whether being a biologically functioning organism is still of value (see Stoecker 2010). One has to go beyond the concepts of life and death in order to develop an adequate ethics for brain death. Likewise, we suggest that one has to go beyond the concept of disease in order to behave adequately in light of severe grief. We are confident that this strategy—which works so well with disease and with life and death—can also help to solve other demarcation problems in applied ethics.

References

Alston, W. P. 1967. 'Vagueness'. In *Encyclopedia of Philosophy*, vol. **8**, edited by P. Edwards, pp. 218–21. New York, NY: Macmillan.

APA (American Psychiatric Association). 2000. *Diagnostic and Statistical Manual of Mental Disorders, Fourth Edition, Text Revision: DSM-IV TR*. Washington, DC: American Psychiatric Association.

APA (American Psychiatric Association). 2013. *Diagnostic and Statistical Manual of Mental Disorders, Fifth Edition: DSM-5*. Washington, DC: American Psychiatric Association.

Boorse, C. 1975. 'On the distinction between disease and illness'. *Philosophy and Public Affairs* **5**: 49–68.

Boorse, C. 1976. 'What a theory of mental health should be'. *Journal for the Theory of Social Behavior* **6**: 61–84.

Boorse, C. 1997. 'A rebuttal on health'. In *What is disease?* edited by J. M. Humber and R. F. Almeder, pp. 3–143. Totowa, NJ: Humana Press.

Brison, S. J. 2002. *Aftermath: Violence and the Remaking of a Self.* Princeton, NJ: Princeton University Press.

Bundesministerium der Justiz. 2015. German Criminal Code, translated by M. Bohlander. https://www.gesetze-im-internet.de/englisch_stgb/englisch_stgb.html (accessed 26 May 2016).

Bundesministerium der Justiz. n.d. 'Gesetz zur Therapierung und Unterbringung psychisch gestörter Gewalttäter (Therapieunterbringungsgesetz - ThUG)'. http://www.gesetze-im-internet.de/thug (accessed 27 May 2016).

Cooper, R. V. 2005. *Classifying Madness: A Philosophical Examination of the Diagnostic and Statistical Manual of Mental Disorders.* Dordrecht: Springer.

Cooper, R. V. 2013. 'Avoiding false positives: Zones of rarity, the threshold problem, and the DSM clinical significance criterion'. *Canadian Journal of Psychiatry* **58** (11): 606–11.

DGPPN (Deutsche Gesellschaft für Psychiatrie, Psychotherapie und Nervenheilkunde). 2011. Stellungnahme der Deutschen Gesellschaft für Psychiatrie, Psychotherapie und Nervenheilkunde (DGPPN) zum Gesetz zur Neuordnung des Rechts der Sicherungsverwahrung (Therapieunterbringungsgesetz/ThUG) in Kraft seit 01.01.2011. http://www.dgppn.de/fileadmin/user_upload/_medien/download/pdf/stellungnahmen/2011/stn-2011-02-10-sicherungsverwahrung.pdf (accessed 27 May 2016).

Engel, G. L. 1977. 'The need for a new medical model: A challenge for biomedicine'. *Science* **196**: 129–36.

Engel, G. L. 1978. 'The biopsychosocial model and the education of health professionals'. *Annals of the New York Academy of Sciences* **310**: 169–81.

European Court of Human Rights. 2009. 'Case of M. v Germany (Application no. 19359/04)'. http://hudoc.echr.coe.int/eng?i=001-96389 (accessed 27 May 2016).

Frances, A. 2012. 'DSM 5 and diagnostic inflation: Reply to misleading comments from the task force'. Posted 23 January 2012. https://www.psychologytoday.com/blog/dsm5-in-distress/201201/dsm-5-and-diagnostic-inflation (accessed 27 May 2016).

Frances, A. 2013. *Saving Normal: An Insider's Revolt against Out-of-Control Psychiatric Diagnosis, DSM-5, Big Pharma, and the Medicalization of Ordinary Life.* New York, NY: William Morrow.

Fulford, B. 1989. *Moral Theory and Medical Practice.* Cambridge: Cambridge University Press.

Fulford, B. 2001. '"What is (mental) disease?" An open letter to Christopher Boorse'. *Journal of Medical Ethics* **27** (2): 80–5.

Gasking, D. 1960. 'Clusters'. *Australasian Journal of Philosophy* **38** (1): 1–36.

Grice, H. P. 1989. *Studies in the ways of words.* Cambridge, MA: Harvard University Press.

Helmchen, H., and Linden, M. 2000. 'Subthreshold disorders in psychiatry: Clinical reality, methodological artifact, and the double-threshold problem'. *Comprehensive Psychiatry* **41** (2 Suppl. 1): 1–7.

Hofmann, B. 2001. 'Complexity of the concept of disease as shown through rival theoretical frameworks'. *Theoretical Medicine and Bioethics* **22** (3): 211–36.

Hofmann, B. 2002. 'On the triad disease, illness and sickness'. *The Journal of Medicine and Philosophy* **27** (6): 651–73.

Keefe, R. 2000. *Theories of Vagueness*. Cambridge: Cambridge University Press.

Keil, G. 2013. 'Introduction: Vagueness and ontology'. *Metaphysica* **14**: 149–64.

Kendell, R. E. 1993. 'The nature of psychiatric disorders'. In *Companion to Psychiatric Studies*, 5th ed., edited by R. E. Kendell and A. K. Zealley, pp. 1–7. Edinburgh: Churchill Livingston.

Kendler, K. S. 2010. 'Statement on the proposal to eliminate the grief exclusion criterion from major depression'. *DSM-5 Mood Disorder Work Group*. http://www.dsm5.org/about/Documents/Forms/AllItems.aspx (accessed 3 January 2016).

Kendler, K. S., Myers, J., and Zisook, S. 2008. 'Does bereavement related major depression differ from major depression associated with other stressful life events?'. *American Journal of Psychiatry* **165**: 1449–55.

Kirchin, S. (ed.). 2013. *Thick Concepts*. Oxford: Oxford University Press.

Maj, M. 2008. 'Depression, bereavement, and "understandable" intense sadness: Should the *DSM-IV* approach be revised?'. *American Journal of Psychiatry* **165**: 1373–5.

Murphy, D. 2015. 'Concepts of disease and health'. In *The Stanford Encyclopedia of Philosophy*, edited by E. N. Zalta. http://plato.stanford.edu/archives/spr2015/entries/health-disease (accessed 12 May 2016).

Paris, J. 2015. *Overdiagnosis in Psychiatry: How Modern Psychiatry Lost Its Way While Creating a Diagnosis for Almost All of Life's Misfortunes*. Oxford: Oxford University Press.

Pinkal, M. 1995. *Logic and Lexicon: The Semantics of the Indefinite*. Dordrecht: Kluwer.

Raffman, D. 1994. 'Vagueness without paradox'. *The Philosophical Review* **103**: 41–74.

Raffman, D. 2014. *Unruly Words. A Study of Vague Language*. Oxford: Oxford University Press.

Reznek, L. 1987. *The Nature of Disease*. New York, NY: Routledge.

Roberts, D. 2013 'Thick concepts'. *Philosophy Compass* **8** (8): 677–88.

Russell, B. 1923. 'Vagueness'. *Australasian Journal of Philosophy and Psychology* **1**: 84–92.

Sorensen, R. 2016. 'Vagueness'. In *The Stanford Encyclopedia of Philosophy*, edited by E. N. Zalta. http://plato.stanford.edu/archives/spr2016/entries/vagueness (accessed 26 May 2016).

Stoecker, R. 2010. *Der Hirntod* (2nd edn). Freiburg: Alber.

Szasz, T. S. 1961. *The Myth of Mental Illness: Foundations of a Theory of Personal Conduct*. New York, NY: Hoeber–Harper.

Wakefield, J. C. 2007. 'The concept of mental disorder: Diagnostic implications of the harmful dysfunction analysis'. *World Psychiatry* **6** (3): 149–56.

Wakefield, J. C., and Horwitz, A. V. 2016. 'Psychiatry's continuing expansion of depressive disorder'. In *Sadness or Depression? International Perspectives on the Depression Epidemic and Its Meaning*, edited by J. C. Wakefield and S. Demazeux, pp. 173–203. Dordrecht: Springer.

Wittgenstein, L. 1953. *Philosophical Investigations*, translated by G. E. M. Anscombe. Oxford: Basil Blackwell.

Chapter 4

Disease entities and the borderline between health and disease: Where is the place of gradations?

Peter Hucklenbroich

1 Background and introduction

Everyone knows that there are very different degrees of illness and disease. There is a broad continuum extending, for example, from a mild case of the common cold to a malignant cancer in the stage of metastatic dissemination. Even the same disease may exhibit very different degrees of severity in different cases; for instance an allergy can range from a mere disposition of itchiness to severe asthma attacks and even lethal anaphylaxis. From this basic truth, many people draw the conclusion that the *transition from health to disease* is a matter of degree, or even that the borderline between health and disease is vague and imprecise. As a consequence, they take the general concepts of health and disease to be graduated. But this conclusion is wrong, at least as far as the concepts of contemporary scientific medicine are concerned. This is not to say that medicine is unaware of grades, levels, and stages of disease. On the contrary, medical theory takes them systematically into account and has developed a host of specific conceptual methods for dealing with them. However, the difference between being healthy and being in any sense diseased continues to be a sharp, categorical distinction that corresponds to a clear-cut borderline, or at least to a borderline with some known and definite exceptions and special cases.

   This apparent paradox is resolved by taking into account the fact that the central theoretical concept of medicine is not the general concept of a plain disease or a plain illness, but rather the concept of specific *disease entities*. This concept is a theoretical one, in the same sense in which concepts like *elementary particle, isotope, genome,* or *evolution* are theoretical concepts of science. It is part of the ontology of contemporary medicine and it allows for categorical distinctions, in contrast to mere gradations. In what follows I will give a more detailed account of this concept.

Recent philosophical discussions about the concept of disease, particularly of mental disease, refer to the question of whether the borderline between health and illness/disease may be blurred and fuzzy and whether the proper conceptual tool for dealing with disease should be gradualism.[1] This discussion was stimulated, additionally, by the ongoing debate over the revision of the *Diagnostic and Statistical Manual of Mental Disorders* (*DSM*; see APA 2013). Gradualism is proposed as a solution to controversies about the existence of some—allegedly—newly defined kinds of mental disorder, for example 'subthreshold disorders' and 'prodromal stages' of diseases or disorders. The psychiatrist Allen Frances, for one, worries that 'diagnostic inflation' will ensue and lead to a pathologization of normal mental states (Frances 2013). But the concepts of thresholds, subthresholds, unapparent courses, and prodromes are common, widespread, and indispensable tools in medical concept formation. Nobody, at least in somatic medicine, argues that, because of the existence of such types of pathological conditions, clinical nosology has to be abandoned and replaced by gradualism; nor has anyone suggested that these concepts foster 'diagnostic inflation'. Why, then, should medicine change its conceptual foundation and theoretical strategy in the case of psychiatry?

In what follows I shall give, first, a condensed and partial reconstruction of the concept of disease entity, because this theoretical medical concept has hitherto been widely neglected in philosophical accounts that deal with the notions of disease and illness. Then I will show how the phenomenon of different degrees of severity is dealt with in this theoretical framework. Finally I will argue that the conceptual and methodological place of gradations in medicine is not at the demarcation point between health and disease in general, but rather in the internal differentiation of disease entities and their pathological parameters. In the final section I will also illustrate my position by discussing some paradigmatic features of psychiatric nosology.

2 The structure of general nosology and the concept of disease entity: A sketch in ten principles

The theoretical concept of disease entity (or disease unit) is a result of three ideas that emerged in medicine over the past four centuries:

- first, the idea of the existence of distinct *types of disease* (*species morborum*) that might be seen as analogous to the types of plants and animals in botany and zoology and that form a taxonomy, namely a nosology. The notion of a

---

[1] See Chapter 2. Recently S. Andrew Schroeder (2013) has proposed a 'comparativistic' approach to the demarcation between health and disease that is akin to gradualism.

clinically defined disease entity or 'clinical disease entity' (CDE) is linked to the work of Thomas Sydenham and François Boissier de Sauvages de Lacroix in the seventeenth and eighteenth centuries respectively;

◆ second, the discovery and empirical proof of the existence of *external and internal causes* of disease that are specific to each type of disease. This discovery is linked mainly to the origin and development of bacteriology during the nineteenth century (Louis Pasteur, Robert Koch) and is reflected in the origin of the discipline of *aetiology*. It stimulated a broad methodological discussion about the concepts of 'cause' and 'condition' in the first decades of the twentieth century (see Engelhardt and Schipperges 1980, 102–9);

◆ third, the conception that diseases have a *natural history* or *natural course*, which extends from their causes to their manifestations and outcomes, consists of a pathologically altered physiological (i.e. pathophysiological) process, and involves morphological alterations and lesions of cells and tissues (Claude Bernard, Rudolf Virchow). This pathologically altered process and development of life is called *pathogenesis* or, insofar as it includes causal origins, *aetiopathogenesis*.

These three ideas merged and eventually formed the concept of an aetiopathogenetically definable and explainable disease entity—in short, an 'explainable disease entity' (EDE). Over the course of the twentieth century, this theoretical concept spread throughout medicine and ultimately constituted the foundation of theoretical and clinical nosologies in almost all medical disciplines. The only specialty that still awaits a nosology of EDEs is psychiatry. This historical background should be kept in mind when disputing the concept of disease in psychiatry.

In spite of the widespread application of EDE in medicine, its full and precise meaning is seldom explicitly outlined and analysed. Therefore I am going to describe and briefly reconstruct its main features, together with the conceptual structure of general pathology and nosology (GPN)—in other words the medical theory of disease. First, there are some principles that govern the overall structure of GPN.

2.1 All the pathological phenomena we experience are cases of disease entities or, better put, cases of partial manifestations (symptoms, signs, findings) of disease entities

'Disease entity' is a category used for the theoretical interpretation and explanation of individual cases of being ill. The system of disease entities must satisfy a *principle of completeness*: every single abnormal or pathological phenomenon and every case of being ill is (i.e. must be conceived as) an *instance* or *case* of one disease entity (or multiple concomitant disease entities).[2] Or, to put it the other way round, in clinical experience there are no 'isolated' pathological conditions or symptoms that are not an instance or a part of a disease entity or are not themselves a proper disease entity. Symptoms, findings, or dysfunctions that appear to be isolated need to be scrutinized diagnostically or through further research in order for us to detect or discover their pathogenesis, and hence their underlying disease entity.

EXAMPLE: A case of chest pain may be conceived of as an instance of the disease entity coronary heart disease (CHD), or of angina pectoris as a symptom of CHD. Alternatively, it may be a symptom of variant angina (Prinzmetal), of cardioneurosis, or of a different disease of the heart, lung, pleura, thoracic muscles, or some other organ; but it cannot be an 'isolated' chest pain without cause and pathogenesis and without an underlying disease that is an instance (token) of a disease entity (type).

2.2 A disease entity is the *pattern* or *type* for the entire natural course of the respective individual diseases

Individual cases of a disease entity may differ in several respects. Particularly, they may differ in the symptoms and signs they exhibit, in the time and duration of these signs and symptoms and of the disease itself, and in the severity of their manifestations. The disease entity itself is not definable by one single 'typical', 'ideal', or 'normal' course, but rather by a *pattern* of courses. Logically speaking, a disease entity is a set of possible *alternative* courses; as a predicate in sentences of the form 'x has disease entity D', it renders them equivalent to a complex *disjunction* of the form '(x has course D_1) or (x has course D_2) or . . . or (x has course D_n)'. The descriptions of disease entities in textbooks are explicit formulations of these alternative possible courses, as they include information about signs and symptoms, frequencies, stages, degrees of severity or seriousness, and types of variation ('variants'). Indeed, the logical structure of the description and definition of a disease entity must be even more complex than a mere disjunction of atomic clauses, because it must embrace for example conditional clauses like 'if condition C is given, x may have course D_x'. Furthermore, it must allow for the existence of different primary causes, or even different *sets* of primary causes, which nevertheless share a common pathogenesis and hence belong to the same disease entity; such a case is usually called a multifactorial or a polyaetiologic disease (or both). But here I cannot dwell further on the logical peculiarities of defining disease entities.[3]

---

[2] For convenience, the case of co-existing disease entities or multimorbidity will be omitted in this analysis. But in clinical reality it is the normal case: the majority of patients suffer from more than one disease.

[3] For a more detailed account of definitions, see Hucklenbroich (2014a), section 3.3.

2.3 Disease entities are not dispositions

There is a general disposition of the organism to fall ill that is called 'pathibility' and is triggered by specific causes of disease. These specific causes trigger a specific reaction of the organism, which develops into a specific course of disease that, in turn, is an instance of that specific disease entity. This general disposition of pathibility, a universal feature of human organisms, must be distinguished from *particular dispositional properties* of specific disease entities and from *specific dispositional disease entities* that are *defined* by a pathological disposition, for example an allergy.[4]

2.4 A disease entity covers not only signs and symptoms over time, but also the underlying causal structure: aetiopathogenesis

This principle expresses the insight that any disease entity that is clinically discovered and defined—any CDE—is in need of a scientific *explanation* that reveals the corresponding EDE—its underlying mechanism of causal pathogenesis. Therefore disease entities are able to form the basis for a causal (aetiopathogenetic) explanation of symptoms and other manifestations or findings. As long as the aetiopathogenetic definition of any disease entity is not completely known, the epistemological status of this (alleged) entity must be conceived as 'preliminarily proposed' and requiring proof of its existence as a proper disease entity. Further research may discover that, in reality, there are different disease entities that underlie the same clinical picture.

2.5 Disease entities are defined by specifying necessary and sufficient conditions

In medical terminology, these are *obligatory* and *pathognomonic* conditions or properties. Such properties may be clinical signs, lab findings, underlying alterations of tissues and cells, altered functions of organs, or specific pathomechanisms. The process of discovering, identifying, and explaining disease entities and their natural history is a gradual and piecemeal process of empirical research. It leads from clinical observation and pattern matching (i.e. from CDEs), through causal analysis and identification of causes and *pathomechanisms*, to etiopathogenetical explanation (i.e. to EDEs).

EXAMPLE: Myocardial infarction (MI) is defined by necrosis (i.e. death) of at least one heart muscle cell caused by oxygen shortage. This definition gives the necessary and sufficient condition for the disease entity MI; any other feature of

---

[4] For a more detailed account of dispositions, see ibid., section 3.5.

MI, be it pain, fear, arrhythmia, the patient's death, or anything else, is a facultative manifestation of MI, in other words it is not obligatory. Also, the particular
cause or mechanism by which the oxygen shortage is brought about does not
matter. As for the presence or absence of MI, it does not matter whether only
one single cell or the whole heart muscle is affected by necrosis. But of course
this difference, between silent infarction and imminent cardiac death, is of vital
importance for the patient and for clinical treatment.

2.6 The defining properties of disease entities form the basis for distinguishing between different disease entities and for establishing a correct diagnosis in differential diagnostics

In order to ascertain and *prove* that a disease entity is really at hand and can
be diagnosed (and treated) in a given individual case, it has to be ascertained,
in the last instance, that its defining properties are present.

EXAMPLE: If a case of MI is suspected, it is necessary to ascertain the effects
that are verifying evidence of heart muscle necrosis, e.g. pathognomonic
ECG and lab findings.

A special case is comprised by a particular set of disease entities for which
the precise aetiopathogenesis is not yet known and that are defined, accordingly, by a set of weighted features that must be summed up in order for us to
see whether they exceed a definite numerical threshold. This method of defining disease entities by 'scores' or 'indices' can be found in almost all medical
specialties for at least some of their nosological entities, but particularly in psychiatry. Some philosophers object to this method or even take it as evidence
of vagueness. But this objection is a misperception: scores of this type are not
defined *ad libitum* or by an open-ended list of features, which would turn them
into 'cluster concepts', but are (and are bound to be) constructed and continually tested through empirical, statistical methods designed to ascertain their
validity, objectivity, and selectivity. Hence their adequateness, unequivocal-
ity, and conceptual distinctness are ascertained through empirical rather than
conceptual methods. This manner of detecting and discriminating between
disease entities is a proper part of evidence-based medicine (EBM).

Additionally, in the case of many disease entities, one has to distinguish
between *defining* criteria and *diagnostic* criteria. The latter might be given by an
open-ended list of features that may or may not be present, if only their presence is conclusive for the presence of the disease entity itself. This conclusive-
ness must have been established by empirical studies that refer in the last resort
to the *defining* criteria as the *gold standard* of diagnostics.

2.7 Disease entities may exist in relationships with one another, particularly in relationships of predisposition and consequence (consecution, complication)

Because such pairs of disease entities are different by definition, they cannot be conceived of as one variant form or variant course of one single disease entity. The question of whether a given type of course *can and should* be defined as forming a proper disease entity or a mere variant of an already existing disease entity is a question of concept formation in nosology. Concept formation must be carried out in a consistent, univocal manner, which not only satisfies principles of systematic completeness and of conceptual distinctness and disjunctivity but also respects the medical meaning and importance of the corresponding object or entity.

EXAMPLE: CHD is a predisposition for MI. But MI is not a mere variant course of CHD, because (1) there are several different predispositions for MI, (2) MI may occur without a predispositional disease entity, and (3) the eminently vital importance of the event of MI justifies its definition as a separate disease entity.

2.8 The different courses that are variants of one aetiopathologically defined disease entity may be distinguished by their *degree of severity* (or seriousness)

There may even be courses without any symptoms or signs—so-called clinically silent or *inapparent* courses. Whether the disease entity is at hand or not is not decided by the degree of severity of its course but by the existence (and diagnostic proof) of its defining properties. Thus, as long as the defining properties are given, someone can be diseased (ill) in the medical sense and can 'suffer' from a well-defined disease entity, even though he or she does not experience any subjective complaints or symptoms. The existence of different degrees of severity, and even inapparent courses, of defined disease entities implies that it would be misleading to conceive of, and reconstruct, the diagnosis in a gradualist manner, if this implies that *being in any way diseased* is only a matter of degree or percentage. Instead the diagnosis may be supplemented with information about the *degree of severity of this instance of the disease entity* (mild, moderate, severe, inapparent). Of course, any adequate *therapeutic* treatment must also take this information into account. Gradualism takes place only *inside* disease entities, not between them and a state of healthiness: in the context of theoretical medicine, health should be defined as the absence of any instance of a disease entity.

2.9 Disease entities have temporal characteristics

But, in different kinds of disease entities, these characteristics may differ widely in shape, length, and degree of variability. Additionally, one must distinguish between the temporal characteristics of the entire entity and those of its clinical signs. But here, too, gradualism is found only inside disease entities. One important temporal characteristic involves the existence of prodromes and prodromal states (or stages) for many disease entities. This case is given if, at least in some instances of the entity, physiological alterations that are clinically inapparent, or even clinical signs and symptoms that are diagnostically unspecific, occur before specific, typical manifestations emerge and can be diagnosed.

EXAMPLE: In the case of the common cold and some other infectious diseases, the patient usually experiences lassitude and abnormal fatigue some days before the typical symptoms and exanthemata arise. In some other cases, the prodromes themselves are typical (and can be diagnosed), but are called 'prodromes' because they occur before the main, more severe manifestations appear. But in all these cases prodromes are a proper part of the disease entity and are pathological.

2.10 The defining property of a disease entity is always a pathological condition

Therefore the reconstruction of the concepts 'pathological' and 'pathologicity' is key to understanding the nature of disease entities. The natural course of an instance (case, token) of a disease entity (type) is the whole set of causally connected states and events of the affected organism, from the primary cause to the final outcome, *as far as they are pathological* or *pathologically* altered (in the sense explicated in what follows).

3 Reconstruction of the concept of pathologicity: Seven steps

I. The concept of pathologicity can be characterized by a *system of criteria*. These criteria stem from a pre-scientific, lifeworld intuition about disease, illness, and abnormality but are refined and rendered more precise in a stepwise process of theoretical clarification. They are thereby adjusted to the theoretical, medico-scientific description of the human organism.

II. The first and primary step or level of the criteria of pathologicity (or, for short, of the disease criteria) may be said to consist of five intuitive criteria (CR1). A condition of the human organism is pathological if it is

(1) immediately lethal or life-shortening in the long run;

(2) a condition of pain, suffering, or other specific complaints (to be enumerated);

(3) a condition of infertility (incapability of biological reproduction);

(4) a condition that destroys or impairs one's ability to live together in human symbiotic communities, or

(5) a specific disposition of an individual organism to develop or manifest a condition that is pathological according to one or more of these criteria.

Of course, these basic intuitive criteria need a more precise and somewhat technical formulation if we are to avoid circularities and misinterpretations. Some refinements and restrictions on their usage are given below.[5]

III. The criteria defined as CR1 refer to life conditions that are, at least partially, attributed to the organism and are not exclusively attributable to its environment. The criteria are restricted to life conditions that are *biologically autonomous* and independent of the volition and insight of the affected person (that is to say, the condition will occur and/or remain even if the person affected does not want it to and/or know about it). Interrelations and interactions between organism and environment, involuntary desires and imaginations, illusions, misperceptions, hallucinations, and delusions are generally attributed to the affected organism.

IV. CR1 are independent of one another. Each criterion is a sufficient condition of pathologicity. They can, however, apply simultaneously to the same case.

V. There are some more preconditions of applicability that, from the perspective of common sense and medical understanding, may be more or less self-evident, but that need to be stated explicitly in order to avoid misinterpretations. Some of them are conditions of applicability (CA):

(1) CR1 apply exclusively to the *untreated* state and *natural* course of the life condition that is being evaluated as healthy or pathological.

(2) In evaluating a life condition C, the entire range of possible alternative natural states and courses is taken into account. The content of the range of possible alternatives is determined by empirical (medical) knowledge. If this range is empty, that is, if C is *inevitable* (like mortality and natural death), C cannot be judged pathological. The same holds true if the only possible alternatives are *artificial* ones, or if the range of possible alternatives contains only conditions that are not (in a medical sense) better than C according to CR1.

(3) In particular, sexual dimorphism and the existence of phases and stages of ontogenetic development, including gravidity and intrauterine life, are natural and inevitable stages. Neither they themselves nor their peculiar features are therefore pathological.

---

[5] For more detail on the criteria and their application in medical pathology, see Hucklenbroich (2007; 2010; 2012; 2013—in German; 2014a; 2014b—in English).

(4) CR1 do not apply to a person's actions, provided that his or her cognitive, emotional, and volitional abilities are pathologically unchanged.

VI. All life conditions that satisfy CR1 are *pathological in the primary sense*. On the basis of these conditions, further pathological life conditions can be defined in a derivative, *secondary* sense. This is done according to a second criterion (CR2). CR2 picks up a life condition that, although not pathological in the primary sense, is *pathological in the secondary sense* if:

(1) it is a causal consequence of pathological life conditions (i.e. conditions that are already known to be pathological in the primary sense or pathological in the secondary sense), and

(2) its absence is not pathological.

VII. There are some very 'special' cases of pathologicity that need to be mentioned but cannot be discussed here in greater detail: the *facultative* pathologicity, the *ambivalence* of health and disease, the *neutrality* of health and disease (i.e. a condition that is not pathological no matter whether it is present or absent), and perhaps *paradoxical* pathologicity (e.g. 'the disease of not being able to be diseased', as in the title of Müller-Eckhard 1955).[6]

4 Genetic distributions, variance, and threshold values

Many of an organism's phenotypical traits show a distribution and a variance of their value or expression that are caused by the variance of genetic factors or dispositions. Now, *genetic variance and variability* is a precondition of biological life and development: it is an inevitable condition, even if it leads to inequality by working to the advantage or disadvantage of an individual. It has to be accepted that differences within this range, if genetically contingent, are inevitable and thus *not pathological*.

Therefore one individual may, due to genetic variation, bear the expression or value of a property that, in another individual, is caused by disease (and is pathological in the secondary sense), for example concerning body height or mass. In such cases the condition of the first individual is never pathological; the condition of the second individual is pathological because its *expected value* is changed by disease.

Nevertheless, there are genetic conditions that lead to phenotypical conditions that are definitely pathological in the primary sense. Insofar as they are

---

[6] Examples of all these special cases are given in Hucklenbroich (2014a), section 4.3.

sufficient causes or dispositions for pathological (phenotypical) conditions, these genetic conditions are themselves pathological in the primary sense.

The second criterion in CR1 refers to pain, suffering, and any number of specific complaints. There are two kinds of complaints: the first kind is always pathological, the second kind is pathological if the degree of the sensation, the quantity of the stimulus, or the intensity of the organism's response exceeds a definite threshold value. This threshold value, although in many cases felt intuitively, must be determined empirically for every form of complaint of this second kind.

The first kind of complaint, without a threshold, encompasses, besides the sensation of *pain*, sensations such as nausea, dizziness, pruritus (itching), dyspnea, tinnitus, tussive irritation, and many more. These sensations all involve *suffering*, be it mild or severe; by contrast, their absence goes unnoticed. Their threshold value is zero.

The threshold value of the second kind of complaint is not zero. Sensations of fear, grief, lust, and pleasure undergo permanent undulations that are triggered by internal, physiological rhythms and oscillations, as well as by reactions to external events. But there are threshold values that mark the changeover to pathological forms: angst and panic, depression, frigidity, and anhedonia. To determine the objective threshold value for this changeover, detailed knowledge and a thorough analysis of the morphological foundations, physiological regulations, and other aetiologically relevant circumstances of the subjective sensation are needed. Even individual, biographical experiences and culturally influenced personal learning histories may be taken into account. If it is possible to demonstrate the existence of a temporal regulation or homeostasis that is directly correlated to the sensation and that can be disturbed, we will have found an objective criterion for the existence and value of the threshold.

EXAMPLE: In the sensations of warm/hot and cool/cold, there is a changeover from the excitation of the receptors of heat and cold to that of the receptors of pain, if a definite degree of (objective) temperature is exceeded. This degree of temperature marks the objective threshold value of pathologicity for these parameters.

There are domains of medical knowledge in which the objective foundations of many threshold values are not known or not yet fully understood. This is particularly the case in psychopathology. Nevertheless, the existence of threshold values is strongly supported by clinical experience. Therefore clinicians usually rely on scores and indices as surrogates for this knowledge (see further, section 6). Many definitions of psychiatric disorders in the International Statistical Classification of Diseases and Related Health Problems (ICD)-10 and in *DSM-IV* and *DMS-5* are of this kind. Identifying the real thresholds *and the real disease entities* will likely require years and decades of ongoing aetiopathological research.

5 Non-diseases requiring medical treatment

There are many states and life conditions that are in need of treatment from physicians but are not diseases (disease entities) or pathological conditions. In medical practice this is a known and accepted fact. But in policy and in ethical discussions about healthcare this fact seems to be underestimated, if recognized at all. Thus the treatment of such conditions is frequently disguised (for example, as prevention) and not openly discussed as treatment for a non-disease. Sometimes this practice is mistakenly granted legitimacy as a result of inaccurate notions of disease. To be sure, treatment or prevention is not treatment or prevention of a disease in the case of the following conditions:

- discomfort of ageing, that is, decreasing abilities and increasing vulnerability caused by the very process of ageing;
- inevitable pain, as in childbirth, teething, and menstruation;
- gravidity, when there is no medical indication for contraception or abortion;
- bodily attributes that are not pathological, but that elicit negative reactions from other people or society in general;
- conditions that represent extreme values in a statistical distribution but are not caused by pathogenic factors, for example low values of intelligence or talent;
- mental and emotional problems attributable to difficult life circumstances (see section 7).

In many of these cases medical assistance and advice are considered appropriate, if requested and available. But, because these are not pathological conditions, the justification for medical treatment must rely on the *analogy* or *equivalence* between these conditions and genuine pathological conditions, and on some principle of *justice* regarding access to help and assistance. In this area a clarification in social legislation and health policy is long overdue.

6 Conceptual methods of dealing with gradation in medicine: A few examples

As mentioned in sections 1 and 2, medical theory is well aware that diseases manifest different degrees of severity, and it has developed numerous conceptual tools for dealing with them. There is, however, no unique technique of describing and representing gradation. Rather there are very different methods, which are adjusted to the particular type of disease or problem. I shall offer here only a few examples, in order to illustrate the existence and diversity of these conceptual techniques.

I. *Modal attributes*. The simplest form of dealing with degrees of severity is to apply adjectives like *inapparent, mild, moderate, severe*, and the like. In many clinical situations this method is sufficient.

II. *Subclassification*. Some disease entities or pathological conditions are subclassified according to their severity. This subdivision may or may not correspond to the temporal pattern of development. For example, the pathophysiological state of congestive heart failure (CHF) is classified, according to the functional criteria of the New York Heart Association (NYHA), into four subclasses (I–IV), which range from inapparent forms (I) to forms that manifest severe complaints even at rest (IV).

III. *Objectively measurable functional parameters*. This method includes, for example, the measurement of blood pressure (in millimeters mercury or torr) for determining the degree of hypertension, or the measurement of a joint's flexibility (in angular degree) for determining pathological restrictions and their severity.

IV. *Indices and scores*. Many methods are used for evaluating and assessing artificially the 'degree of health' in typical clinical situations such as childbirth or reanimation. Closer inspection reveals that this 'degree of health' always means the severity or degree of either health *problems* or disease states. For example, the APGAR score is a simple method for evaluating a newborn child by using five simple criteria on a scale from 0 to 2 and then summing up the five values. The five criteria are **a**ppearance, **p**ulse, **g**rimace, **a**ctivity, **r**espiration, forming the acronym APGAR. It is worth noting, by the way, that what is measured is the degree of *reduction* of these functions. Another example is the Karnofsky score, a method for assessing cancer patients' quality of life, particularly their ability to survive chemotherapy. The Karnofsky score runs from 100 to 0, where 100 represents 'perfect' health and 0 is death. What is measured here is the degree of *health reduction* or *diseasedness*, not the degree of health. Scores of this kind are used for recognizing medical problems and assessing their prognosis and are empirically established and tested through statistical methods.

These examples show that gradations in medical theory are specific to types of diseases, to pathological conditions, or to clinical problems and are not related to an intermediate range between health and disease/illness. As far as disease entities are concerned, medical gradations do not affect or disrupt the sharp distinction between the presence and the absence of a disease entity. But it may well be that philosophical methods of treating gradations and vagueness can provide useful tools for the further conceptual development of our notions concerning the degree of severity of disease entities and of pathological conditions generally.

7 The case of psychopathology

Most fields and subdisciplines of medicine have a fully developed nosology of disease entities—not only CDEs but also a lot of EDEs. Even where the full system of EDEs is not known, we do know the principal pathogenetic pathways leading from causes and primary alterations of morphology, structure, and function to clinical manifestations and symptoms. The situation is different in psychopathology: there is a deep and broad gap between our knowledge of the structure and physiological function of the body and brain on the one hand, and the clinical phenomenology of psychiatric 'disorders' on the other. Hence we cannot define EDEs. This is a *prima facie* limitation of concept formation in psychiatry. ICD-10, *DSM-IV*, and *DSM-5* use the notion of *disorder* explicitly as a provisional solution, to be improved and replaced later on by a final nosological concept like *disease* or *disease entity*. Disorders are defined by clinical symptomatology instead of causal aetiopathogenesis. Thus they resemble very early stages in the conceptual development of CDEs, not to mention EDEs. The term *diseases* is currently being completely avoided because we do not know which disorders will develop into proper disease entities, which will have to be conceptually rearranged, and which will vanish altogether. This cautious approach must be respected. Nevertheless, we might consider what the principal possibilities of categorizing disorders nosologically are. In my view, there are essentially three possibilities:

(1) Further research on the aetiology and pathogenesis of known psychiatric disorders may clarify and explain their causes, conditions, and courses to the point where proper disease entities become definable. This will probably happen, at least for some of the known disorders, for example psychotic (schizophrenia), bipolar, depressive, anxiety, and obsessive–compulsive disorders. This nosological classification will likely improve the current differentiations and distinctions and will allow us to identify predispositions, inapparent and subclinical courses, and prodromes as certain stages and phases of authentic nosological entities.

(2) A number of disorders might turn out to form a group of 'suboptimal adaptations' to the social environment. Disorders of this kind may, in some cases, remain apparently normal and completely without pathological behaviour. These are inapparent courses, but they are pathological because of the restrictions they impose on behaviour and experience. Other cases may

bear the risk of decompensation if the person is put under mental and emotional pressure—'decompensation' meaning the occurrence of obviously abnormal, deviant behaviour. Because of this risk, such cases of adaptation are generally suboptimal, although in everyday situations they present no abnormal or deviant symptoms. They may turn out to form a group of *dispositional* disease entities: they show asymptomatic and symptomatic phases depending on the degree of seriousness and on the occurrence of 'stressors' as triggers. Some examples are conversion, eating, and personality disorders.[7] If this interpretation is correct, these are proper CDEs waiting for an aetiopathogenetic explanation and definition.

(3) A third group of disorders may be categorized as 'non-pathological problems and conflicts of individual and social life'. Disorders in this group do not originate from pathological or pathogenic causes. But they may accompany the stresses and strains of daily life and may require professional help and support. If this support requires the competence of a psychiatrist or psychotherapist, we should speak of mental 'non-disease' in need of treatment and support. Consider for example the problems of mental development (in school and education), of sociocultural integration (clashing cultural traditions), or of civil partnership (marital and family conflicts). Disorders of this kind might be dubbed 'non-diseases' if they require professional help and should be distinguished on the one hand from proper diseases (group 1 and 2), and, on the other, from major problems and conflicts in or between whole societies such as unemployment, pauperism, industrial conflict, racism, or war.

If we accept this distinction between three types or groups of disorders, two different tasks for future research can be defined. First, we need more and deeper investigations into the multifactorial aetiology of mental disorders, which should turn them into proper psychiatric disease entities. But, second, we also need a hard and fast definition of 'mental non-disease in need of professional help'. We should develop a proper classification of problems and conflicts that are not diseases (disease entities) yet might or should nevertheless be treated by psychiatrists and psychotherapists if the clients demand it. The result of this work should be an 'international classification of non-diseases': an 'ICN' analogous to the ICD classification. Ultimately this should lead to corresponding national legislation concerning the rights and duties that flow from the 'diagnosis' of a non-disease. But I suspect that the path to such legislation will be long and thorny.

---

[7] Some very impressive case studies are contributed by Doering (2013).

8 Conclusion: Six theses concerning the debate about gradualism in health

(1) In medical theory and pathology, the conceptual distinction between healthy or normal and diseased or pathological is conceived of as a qualitative, sharp, and objective demarcation and not as a matter of degree. *Within the realm of pathological conditions (including symptoms and incompletely described states) and of completely described disease entities* there are gradations, namely degrees of severity of symptoms, manifestations, and courses, which include inapparent yet pathological courses (see Hucklenbroich 2016). These gradations are consistent with the diagnostic classification of a case as being an instance of a definite disease entity, provided that the defining property of this entity is present. But in practical medicine the exact aetiological diagnosis must frequently be left open because aetiologically oriented diagnostics are judged inappropriate or unacceptable to the patient, particularly in mild cases. Nevertheless, this abandonment of aetiological diagnosis for practical reasons is not to be confused with conceptual vagueness or fuzziness. In addition, some borderline cases of diagnosis result from insufficient knowledge about aetiopathogenesis, especially in psychopathology. In these cases medical theory is in need not of conceptual gradualism, but of empirical research in order to identify the causes and thresholds of disease.

(2) The concepts 'ill/diseased/pathological' and 'normal/healthy' in medical pathology are not 'family resemblance concepts' or 'cluster concepts'. The central theoretical concepts are concepts for disease entities. These concepts must be introduced and justified by exact, aetiopathological definitions (i.e. by recourse to EDEs) or at least by necessary and sufficient clinical findings (i.e. by recourse to CDEs), and not by family resemblance or an open-ended list of features. The defining conditions refer to criteria of pathologicity. These criteria are not totally unequivocal if assessed intuitively; but, in the context of general and special pathology and aetiopathogenetic nosology, they become unequivocal. Because the *general* distinction between normal and pathological refers, in the final analysis, to disease entities, it is unequivocal as well. This may, however, not be the case in ordinary language and at pre-scientific or premature stages in the development of medical specialties.

(3) Individual diseases are instances of disease entities. They comprise states and processes of a living organism that meet the criteria of pathologicity and form an *individual* unit or entity by virtue of a causal, aetiopathogenetic connection. They have a temporal dimension extending from primary causes to outcome. A *generic* disease entity is the set or pattern of possible

alternative natural courses of its instances. Are disease entities natural kinds? This question must be returned to the questioner: to date, no one has suggested a definition of 'natural kind' that can satisfy the minimal preconditions of a scientifically applicable concept. I am tempted to suspect that 'natural kind' is itself not a natural kind, or—to put it non-paradoxically—'natural kind' may be simply a designation for well-established scientific concepts. If so, disease entities are obviously very well established scientific concepts in medicine, and they are as 'natural' as the table of chemical elements and the classification of biological species.

(4) Disease entities are entities without a fixed, unitary granularity. That is to say, disease entities can be defined at different levels of detail. One disease entity at a high level may comprise a number of disease entities at a lower level. For example, the disease entity 'common cold' comprises a lot of disease entities defined aetiologically by the kind of virus that causes this special kind of common cold (there are many kinds of viruses that do that). Nevertheless, all kinds of disease entities at all levels of granularity are defined by objective, scientifically established properties.

(5) Legal and forensic judgements refer not only to the pathologicity, but also to the degree of severity or impairment of a condition. There are three types of situations that pose challenges to law and jurisprudence:

(1) If the exact causal situation of a case of disease is unknown (perhaps due to lack of scientific knowledge or of information about the patient), then it may be difficult to judge the severity of that case.

(2) If the condition to be judged is not genuinely pathological but rather analogous or equivalent to a disease (e.g. ageing), then hitherto existing legal formulations neither cover the needs and rights of patients nor derive them from legal principles.

(3) The same is true for 'non-diseases' that require professional support or treatment from medical specialists—and hence probably also for a relevant subgroup of psychiatric disorders.

(6) The proper place for gradations in medical pathology is not in an alleged intermediate realm at the borderline between either health and disease or normality and disorder, but rather in the internal variance and differentiation of specific pathological conditions and disease entities, particularly concerning their degree of severity.

References

APA (American Psychiatric Association). 2013. *Diagnostic and Statistical Manual of Mental Disorders, Fifth Edition: DSM-5*. Washington, DC: American Psychiatric Association.

Doering, S. 2013. 'Anpassung und psychische Krankheit'. In *Wissenschaftstheoretische Aspekte des Krankheitsbegriffs*, edited by P. Hucklenbroich and A. Buyx, pp. 211–21. Münster: mentis.

Engelhardt, D. v., and Schipperges, H. 1980. *Die inneren Verbindungen zwischen Philosophie und Medizin im 20. Jahrhundert*. Darmstadt: WBG.

Frances, A. 2013. *Saving Normal*. New York, NY: William Morrow.

Hucklenbroich, P. 2007. 'Krankheit: Begriffsklärung und Grundlagen einer Krankheitstheorie'. *Erwägen Wissen Ethik* **18** (1): 77–90.

Hucklenbroich, P. 2010. 'Der Krankheitsbegriff: Seine Grenzen und Ambivalenzen in der medizinethischen Diskussion'. In *Endliches Leben*, edited by M. Höfner, S. Schaede, and G. Thomas, pp. 133–60. Tübingen: Mohr Siebeck.

Hucklenbroich, P. 2012. 'Der Krankheitsbegriff der Medizin in der Perspektive einer rekonstruktiven Wissenschaftstheorie'. In *Das Gesunde, das Kranke und die Medizinethik. Moralische Implikationen des Krankheitsbegriffs*, edited by M. Rothhaar and A. Frewer, pp. 33–63. Stuttgart: Steiner.

Hucklenbroich, P. 2013. 'Die wissenschaftstheoretische Struktur der medizinischen Krankheitslehre'. In *Wissenschaftstheoretische Aspekte des Krankheitsbegriffs*, edited by P. Hucklenbroich and A. Buyx, pp. 13–83. Münster: mentis.

Hucklenbroich, P. 2014a. ' "Disease entity" as the key theoretical concept of medicine'. *Journal of Medicine and Philosophy* **39** (6): 609–33.

Hucklenbroich, P. 2014b. 'Medical criteria of pathologicity and their role in scientific psychiatry: Comments on the articles of Henrik Walter and Marco Stier'. *Frontiers in Psychology* 5. http://dx.doi.org/10.3389/fpsyg.2014.00128 (accessed 25 May, 2016).

Hucklenbroich, P. 2016. 'Medical theory and its notions of definition and explanation'. In *Handbook of the Philosophy of Medicine*, edited by T. Schramme and S. Edwards, pp. 1–9, Heidelberg: Springer.

Müller-Eckhard, H. 1955. *Die Krankheit nicht krank sein zu können*. Stuttgart: Klett.

Schroeder, S. A. 2013. 'Rethinking Health: Healthy or Healthier than?'. *The British Journal for the Philosophy of Science* **64**: 131–59.

Chapter 5

Indeterminacy in medical classification: On continuity, uncertainty, and vagueness

Rico Hauswald and Lara Keuck

1 Introduction

This chapter aims to clarify the vocabulary of and relations among ontological, epistemological, and semantic aspects of indeterminacy in medical classification systems. Although classifications of diseases and of mental disorders are often characterized as having blurred boundaries, there is no consensus on what exactly this means. We want to provide some terminological clarifications that are as unambiguous as possible, as useful for as many different positions as possible, and helpful towards solving misunderstandings and entanglements in the debate on the validity of classifications of mental disorders. In brief, we claim that, ontologically, disease entities are continuous or discrete. Epistemologically, the assessment of the validity of medical classifications can be more or less secured or controversial. Semantically, disease categories are defined precisely or vaguely.

Although we will have to make some commitments in order to qualify our vocabulary, our main aim is to open up a conceptual field that allows different actors to locate their position within this field by using the terms we suggest.

In fact we do not share the same views on all issues raised in this chapter. But we do share the assumption that, as a first step, it is necessary to clarify what we are actually debating about before discussing which account may be more or less coherent or persuasive. In this sense, when we introduce notions such as 'realization gaps' or 'interest-relativity', we do so because we take the underlying positions to be particularly suitable for addressing continuity as an ontological problem of indeterminacy and interest variety as an epistemic one—and not because we find the positions necessarily persuasive in every possible respect. However, we have found it helpful to lay out the problem of medical indeterminacy in the way proposed in this chapter in order to avoid discussions that reduce the problem of classifying diseases to a 'nothing but' problem of kinds *or* interests *or* words.

Take the example of major depressive disorder (MDD). The newest edition of the *Diagnostic and Statistical Manual of Mental Disorders, DSM-5* (APA 2013), has introduced new thresholds for conditions to qualify as MDD. In particular, the relevant time span in which a person must have shown symptoms of MDD (as listed within the *DSM*) has been shortened from six to two weeks. This revision has prompted much debate, especially with regard to the potential of pathologizing depression-like symptoms of grief after the death of a loved one (see also Chapter 3). The debate includes the *ontological* question of whether or not there is a qualitative difference between symptoms that remain for two weeks and symptoms that persist for a longer time. In other words, are the different instances that shall be classified together really of one kind? This ontological inquiry is translated into the *semantic* question of whether or not the class of cases that exhibit symptoms of depression for two weeks should be labelled 'major depressive disorder'. In brief, is this category described using the appropriate terms? The ontological and semantic considerations can be put in relation to the *epistemic* problem of whether or not the phenomenon that is researched, diagnosed, and labelled in practice is sufficiently characterized to exclude the unintentional misapplication of the classification. Do the relevant actors know enough about MDD—and is there a viable consensus on this issue—to shorten the necessary time span of the diagnosing symptoms from six to two weeks?

In what follows we shall elucidate the philosophical details of the ontological, epistemic, and semantic aspects of medical classification systems (sections 2–4). Subsequently we shall analyse the relations between these aspects and draw some conclusions about how our terminological clarifications might help in elucidating and clarifying the concept of validity of medical classification systems.

2 Continuity: On ontological aspects of indeterminacy

In this section we develop the idea that ontological aspects of the indeterminacy of medical classifications can be accounted for by reference to the notions of continuity and discreteness. By disease entities or medical kinds being continuous we mean that there is a gradual transition between a disease entity and 'normal' physiological states, or between two different disease entities. Examples are disorders that come in milder and more severe forms, and everything in-between. By contrast, in cases where there is no continuity between disease entities or kinds, but rather something like a 'qualitative jump', we shall say that there is something between them that has been called *realization gaps* (Pinkal 1995, 106). Think of the infectious diseases measles and rubella. One might identify many overlapping similarities between the different forms of these diseases, but they do not (as far as we know) merge into one another. Hence we shall explain the case of continuity in medical nosology through the presence of realization gaps and the case of discreteness through their absence. This account also provides a framework for modelling the historical changeability and 'looping effects' of psychiatric classifications.

Before we elaborate on this idea in more detail, let us begin with some general reflections on the ontology of disease entities. Sure enough, the ontological nature of diseases is one of the most fundamental questions in the philosophy of medicine. And so in the following passages we can offer only some sketchy remarks about our position.

Ontology in general refers to questions about the nature of the world, that is to say the world as it is *in reality* and not necessarily as it is conceived by humans. In brief, medical ontology is about the nature of human diseases. To what sorts of entities (if any) do medical classificatory concepts correspond? What is captured by medical classifications? There is a spectrum of theoretical options for answering these questions; and it ranges from the view that diseases should be understood as natural kinds with essences (essentialism), to the view that there are no 'natural' divisions that medical concepts correspond to (eliminativism).

In what follows we adopt a causal cluster kind theory, that is, a moderately realistic view of disease entities (for a general discussion of such a theory, see for example Boyd 1991 and 2010). This view represents disease entities not as mere semantic artefacts or illusions but as particular clusters of certain characteristic properties that occur in reality as a result of causal processes. On the other hand, a causal cluster conception is not committed to the view that disease entities are real—in any interesting sense of the word—if and only if they are characterized by essences. There are two principal reasons for adopting a causal cluster kind conception. On the one hand, recent debates in medical ontology have suggested that the two extreme positions of essentialism or eliminativism are rather dubious. Many contemporary authors find moderate views more attractive, because essentialism turns out to be too demanding—at best only very few kinds, either inside or outside the domain of medicine, would still qualify as 'natural'—while eliminativism neglects the fact that there are significant differences between medical classifications and arbitrary distinctions with no scientific basis. (See for example Cooper 2005 and Reznek 1987, who defend versions of cluster theories of (mental) diseases.) The second reason for adopting a causal cluster kind theory of disease entities is that it can serve as a framework in which more extreme positions such as essentialism or eliminativism can be integrated—in the sense that natural medical kinds with essences, if they exist, can be considered a special case of medical cluster kinds. Adopting a causal cluster kind theory allows us to be quite liberal and flexible towards the ontology of disease entities. The central, paradigmatic case in causal cluster kind theory is that disease categories correspond to particular disease cluster kinds. But we can also allow for the possibility that some disease categories correspond to essentialistically defined kinds, as well as for the possibility that other disease categories correspond to nothing 'natural' at all. Haslam (2002) argued that the classificatory concepts used in psychiatry correspond to a plurality of different ontological categories (he distinguished 'non-kinds', 'practical kinds', 'fuzzy kinds', 'discrete kinds', and 'natural kinds'). In a sense we agree with this sort of ontological pluralism, but we also think that causal cluster kind theory provides a general framework in which the different forms of disease entities can be integrated (see Hauswald 2014, esp. ch. 3.3).

Importantly, causal property clusters should not be confused with cluster *concepts*. While ontologically a causal property cluster is a kind, in other words a non-linguistic entity, a cluster concept is a certain type of concept, in other words a linguistic entity. Usually cluster concepts are distinguished from analytically defined concepts in the traditional sense (like 'bachelor'), in that the latter are defined by a set of criteria, *all* of which need to be fulfilled in order for the concept to apply (in the case of 'bachelor': 'is male', 'is unmarried', 'is adult'). A cluster concept, on the other hand, is defined by a set of criteria only *some* of which need to be met in order for the concept to apply. The polythetically defined categories of the *DSM* provide illustrations. For example, in order to diagnose schizophreniform disorder according to *DSM-5* (295.40 (F20.81)), two or more of the following criteria must be met: the presence of delusions, of hallucinations, of disorganized speech, of grossly disorganized or catatonic behaviour, or of negative symptoms. Accordingly, the concept 'schizophreniform disorder' applies in the case of a person with, say, delusions and hallucinations (and none of the other symptoms), but also in the case of a person with disorganized speech and catatonic behaviour (and none of the other symptoms). Now, one might wonder whether there is one single causal property cluster in reality to which these different persons belong and which the *DSM* category somehow attempts to capture. We will immediately be a bit more explicit about what this would mean. Meanwhile let us note that, in general, there is no necessary connection between particular cluster concepts and particular causal cluster kinds. To illustrate this point, let us define a cluster concept C by the three criteria 'is blue', 'is round', and 'weighs less than one kilogram'. Let us further assume that C applies if at least two of these criteria are met. Then C applies, for example, to my blue pencil, to a blue ball, and to a small round stone. Obviously these objects are not of one kind, in the sense that they do not belong to one causal property cluster. This shows that there is no apriori reason to assume that there must be a causal property cluster corresponding to the cluster concept 'schizophreniform disorder', although it is certainly *possible* that there is one. However, at this juncture we do not want to debate this question; the main point we want to stress here is that there is a fundamental difference between this hypothetical causal property cluster (which would be a non-linguistic entity) and a cluster *concept* such as a *DSM* category (which is a linguistic entity; and in sections 4 and 5 we will return to their relationship).

Let us now turn to the notion of real or natural kinds and their analysis in terms of causal property clusters. The basic idea behind the conception of natural kinds as causal property clusters goes back at least to nineteenth-century philosophers of the empiricist tradition (for an examination of this tradition, see Hacking 1991). For example, according to the nineteenth-century philosopher William Whewell, what makes a kind natural is the presence of 'an inexhaustible body of resemblances amongst individuals . . . made by nature, not by mere definition' (Whewell 1971, 290). John Stuart Mill writes:

> a hundred generations have not exhausted the common properties of animals or of plants, of sulphur or of phosphorus; nor do we suppose them to be exhaustible, but proceed to new observations and experiments, in the full confidence of discovering new properties which were by no means implied in those we previously knew. (Mill 1973 [1843], 122)

These quotations express two core intuitions associated with the concept of natural kinds: the idea that individuals belonging to a natural kind share a great many common properties; and the idea that this similarity is a result of causal processes, not of 'mere definition'. The causal cluster conception of natural kinds captures these intuitions. Here is the basic model. Imagine a multidimensional property space (MPS) in which all existing individuals are located. In this MPS individuals are not distributed homogeneously or randomly. Instead their distribution is structured. In some areas there are many individuals; other areas are empty. We shall call the latter 'realization gaps', the former 'realization accumulations'. Roughly speaking, the realization accumulations can be identified with natural or real kinds. As an example, consider biological species. Individuals belonging to a particular species differ in many different ways. No cat perfectly resembles any other cat; thus no two cats occupy the very same location in the MPS. But at the same time all cats share a great many properties among themselves. This means that there is a relatively small region in the MPS where all cats are located, even though no two cats might occupy perfectly identical locations. Other species occupy other regions in the MPS. In-between these regions there are realization gaps, which means that there are no individuals occupying these in-between regions. There is no gradual transition between cats and dogs; no intermediate individuals exist. If there were something like 'the most dog-like cat', this specimen would still be much more like a paradigmatic cat than it would be like 'the most cat-like dog'—that is, it would share many more properties with the former than with the latter.

Three things need further emphasis. Note, first, that the causal cluster conception can account for the possibility of historically evolving kinds. The evolution of a kind can be modelled as the gradual movement of the corresponding realization accumulation in the MPS. An obvious example of evolving kinds is that of biological species (and so, when we just said that there is no gradual transition between two species, we were obviously thinking of them synchronically, as they are at a given time, and not diachronically or how they came to be; and we also excluded potential biological limitations to the species concept, such as lateral gene transfer). Arguably, psychiatric disorders may also evolve historically. On the basis of this assumption, Ian Hacking has argued in many of his writings that psychiatric disorders are prone to what he calls 'looping effects', which turn them into 'interactive kinds' (see for example Hacking 1995; 1998; 1999). Looping effects in this sense occur when self-aware subjects realize that they are instances of particular kinds or fall into certain classificatory categories, then react in one way or another. In turn, these reactions may in the long run affect the evolution of the kind itself. What may follow from this is an interesting interplay between the ontological level and the epistemological level (for more on the latter, see the following section); for how psychiatric disorders are conceived of in science and society can have a significant influence on how they are shaped and how they evolve over time. However, while Hacking conceives of interactive kinds as opposites of natural kinds, on the basis of a causal property cluster model it is possible to conceive of interactive kinds, conversely, as a special *subtype* of natural kinds. If we model the historical evolution of a kind as the gradual movement of the corresponding realization accumulation in the MPS, interactive kinds can be modelled as those kinds in which this movement is caused by special reactions of the self-aware people who are instances of these kinds (for the details, see Hauswald 2014, esp. ch. 3.4, and Hauswald 2016). In any case, we should note that looping effects and the historical changeability of disorders constitute one important source of indeterminacy in medical ontology.

A second point to emphasize is that, for the causal cluster conception, the naturalness of a kind is a gradable matter. Kinds can be more or less natural (where 'natural' means that there is a basis for some classificatory distinction that is not just a matter of mere human convention). The naturalness of a kind depends on two things: the number of properties that are shared by the individuals belonging to the realization accumulation in question, and the discreteness of that accumulation, that is, how clearly it is separated from other accumulations (how clear the realization gap is between them). In psychiatry, many conditions are not as clear-cut as they might be in other fields. Many psychiatric conditions are not separated from one another by full-fledged realization gaps, but rather by something Kendell and Jablensky (2003) call 'zones of rarity'— zones in the logical space with occasional realizations of atypical combinations of properties. When kinds are not separated by clear realization gaps, it can be more difficult to decide whether a given case is a case of mental disorder x or y. Nevertheless, on our liberal causal cluster conception many psychiatric conditions may still qualify as natural or real kinds, even if they might be less natural than the kinds studied by physics, chemistry, or even somatic medicine. Furthermore, note that, due to the gradability of psychiatric kinds, continuity and discreteness in psychiatry turn out to be the poles of a spectrum rather than mutually exclusive alternatives.

Finally, the causal cluster conception is not committed to the view that capturing realization accumulations is the only criterion when it comes to constructing useful scientific classifications or classification systems. It may well be that there are many realization accumulations, most of which are scientifically rather uninteresting (Cooper 2013 makes this point in referring to Dupré's 1993 idea of a promiscuous realism). The choice of those realization accumulations that are pertinent to a given domain of research can legitimately be influenced by pragmatic criteria as well. For example, when constructing disease classification systems, medical scientists not only attempt to identify medical realization accumulations and gaps but also make value judgements. They want to identify those realization accumulations that accompany some negative evaluations (at least this is what adherents to harmful dysfunction analysis would say; see Wakefield 1992). Furthermore, it is possible that weighting properties will influence classificatory decisions, such that the categorization of a given individual will be influenced not only by its belonging to a particular realization accumulation but also by its exhibiting some properties considered to be especially relevant. In this sense, Richard Boyd writes: 'It is an a posteriori theoretical question which of these properties and which of the homeostatic mechanisms count, *and to what extent they count*, in determining membership in the kind' (Boyd 1991, 141–2, emphasis added). This weighting of properties is often a function of particular epistemic and pragmatic interests. It enables us to reconstruct the classificatory treatment of 'freak entities' (Hawley and Bird 2011, 214), that is, of individuals who do not exhibit some properties typical of a given kind, but who are nevertheless determinately treated as belonging to that kind. The idea of weighting properties can explain this: although the 'freak entity' fails to exhibit some typical properties, it might exhibit a property that is considered of particular importance. Two examples of such properties are descent in classifying species and aetiology in medicine: in aetiology-based classification systems, if two individuals share many symptoms, they will nevertheless be classified as having two distinct diseases if the symptoms are caused by different aetiological factors. Here the property cluster model of natural kinds comes close to the micro-essentialist conception, that is, a conception according to which certain micro-structural properties—such as the atomic structure of chemical elements or the genetic structure of biological species—determine membership in a kind. With a micro-essentialist conception in mind, Putnam writes:

> there is (we presume) in the world something—say, a virus—which normally causes such-and-such symptoms. Perhaps other diseases occasionally (rarely) produce these same symptoms in a few patients. When a patient has these symptoms we say he has 'multiple sclerosis'—but, of course, we are prepared to say that we were mistaken if the etiology turns out to have been abnormal. And we are prepared to classify illnesses as cases of multiple sclerosis, even if the symptoms are rather deviant, as long as it turns out that the underlying condition was the virus that causes multiple sclerosis, and that the deviancy in the symptoms was, say, random variation. (Putnam 1975, 311)

The relevance of selecting and weighting properties in the use of medical classifications shows that the question whether a given category refers to a natural kind is not equivalent to the question whether that category provides a suitable class for the purposes of the medical classification.

3 Uncertainty: On epistemological aspects of indeterminacy

Choosing and weighting shared properties as 'medically relevant' is at the core of the epistemic enterprise of classifying diseases and mental disorders, in other words of classifying them according to what we know and what we want to know about diseases. We would like to introduce this epistemic perspective as complementing the ontological account on causal cluster kinds, arguing that realization gaps may occur in nature, but to identify, assess, weigh, evaluate, and agree on them is a human activity, namely one that belongs to science. In scientific enterprises, controversy can arise between different individuals or groups of individuals. However, epistemological aspects of indeterminacy also affect a single individual when this individual is not certain as to how to evaluate given evidence or how to classify a given condition. This uncertainty does not reflect mere ignorance about the current state of knowledge. Indeed, a single individual may want to apply a classification in different contexts, for example to characterize a clinical population for a clinical trial or to compile longitudinal epidemiological studies. There are often some hard cases that cannot be easily assigned to one category (affected) or another (unaffected). Small differences in research design (or clinical guidelines) can lead to classifications of these cases under 'affected' in one evaluation setting and 'not affected' in the other. Research protocols matter, and the acknowledgement of this fact can provide insight into more general considerations about epistemological aspects of indeterminacy in medical classification: the identification of causal cluster kinds is limited by our access to knowledge about the world, which is in turn mediated by our (technically aided) perceptive and cognitive capabilities. In this sense, revisions in the classification of diseases are fostered by new diagnostic possibilities that, ideally, allow one to capture more precisely (e.g. via imaging techniques that provide higher resolution) the property of interest (e.g. a histopathological alteration) or to identify a property (e.g. a genetic mutation) as a shared and relevant property in the first place. As we show in this section, these epistemic activities are prone to uncertainty and therefore elicit controversy about what suffices as relevant knowledge in guiding classifications. In this reading, one important reason for the fuzziness of medical classification is epistemic uncertainty and the lack of uncontroversial knowledge about diseases. In the existing debate on the current limitations and future possibilities of psychiatric classification, this issue has been addressed in various ways.

For instance, psychiatrist Ken Kendler (2012) describes the ideal process of reclassifying diseases and mental disorders as a journey towards ever greater epistemic accuracy and scientific adequacy (see Schaffner's 2012 comment on Kendler). We call this an optimistic view of classification: while existing classifications are typically acknowledged as not following this ideal (or not following it enough), the current problems of classification seem to be solvable *in principle* (see Chapter 4; also Murphy 2006 for philosophical defences of optimistic views on classification). Proponents of an optimistic view come up with a series of suggestions on how to improve the current process of revising classification manuals—suggestions that include a more science-oriented approach and less influence from economically oriented stakeholders, especially from insurance companies and the pharmaceutical industry (see also Cooper 2005).

Other philosophers and psychiatrists are more sceptical. For instance, in at least some cases that are classified as mental disorders, Derek Bolton (2008) doubts that there is *any possible* way to distinguish objectively (which here means conceptually as well as scientifically) between social deviance, normal responses to the challenges of living, and mental illness. We shall call this a pessimistic view of classification: it signifies that the indeterminacy of classification that results from a lack of secured and uncontroversial knowledge is in principle insurmountable. Bolton questions the adequacy of the general concept of 'mental disorders' and suggests replacing it with the alternative term 'mental health problems' and confining the notion of 'disorder' to more specific uses, for instance in forensic psychiatry.

Both accounts, the optimistic and the pessimistic view of classification, take borderline cases (not to be confused with borderline disorder) as their test cases. Borderline cases in psychiatry, such as 'mild neurocognitive disorder', include mild or prodromal states between what is conceived of as normal living and what is conceived of as psychopathological. We will say more about the semantics of borderline cases in the following section. What is of interest with respect to the epistemic enterprise of classification is the fact that borderline cases are inquiry-resistant cases that often provoke controversy. With Roy Sorensen (2016), we can distinguish between absolute and relative borderline cases. Proponents of the optimistic view on classification focus on *relative* borderline cases: the question to be answered is clear, but we do not have the means at hand to answer it (yet). That is to say, in principle it is possible to tell whether a given condition is pathological, and 'the unknowability of a borderline statement is only relative to a given means of settling the issue' (ibid., 2). Think of Kendler's call for a closer alignment of psychiatric classification with scientific progress.

Proponents of the pessimistic view on classification may agree that some specific cases could be solved through the development and application of new diagnostic means. But the focus of the pessimistic view is on *absolute* borderline cases: no possible method of inquiry could settle the question of whether the individual has the disorder. As Sorensen argues with respect to obesity, '[w]hen we reach this stage, we start to suspect that our uncertainty is due to the concept of obesity rather than to our limited means of testing for obesity' (ibid.). We have seen Bolton apply this strategy to the concept of 'mental disorder'.

An interesting case is the recently introduced Research Domain Criteria (RDoC) of the National Institute of Mental Health. The RDoC are presented as an alternative classificatory tool for research, but they are also thought to be useful in revising clinical classifications of mental disorders (Insel 2013; see Tabb 2015 for a philosophical analysis of this view and its limitations). In a way, optimistic and pessimistic views on classification come together here: a pessimistic view on existing classificatory tools such as the *DSM* (which is deemed to act as an 'epistemological blinder' for research; see Hyman 2010) is used to propagate an optimistic view on an alternative classificatory tool: the RDoC, which make use of another concept, namely 'research domains' instead of categorical disorders. The RDoC are thought to be in principle able to solve some of the borderline problems that provoke so much controversy in psychiatry today.

One crucial question with respect to our not knowing whether a certain condition is pathological or not seems to be this: What kind of knowing or not knowing is present? Are we faced with a relative or an absolute borderline case? Should we take an optimistic or a pessimistic view on the given problem of classification? That is to say, should we try to improve our scientific means, or do we rather need to question the whole concept that we are trying to capture? Notably, these questions can be asked with respect to both the manifestation of a condition in an individual ('Is this (already) a case of the mental disorder x?') and the concept of the condition as a pathological one ('Is x a mental disorder (at all)?'). Moreover, they can also be asked with respect to differential diagnosis, both in the concrete individual ('Is this a case of the mental disorder x or of the mental disorder y?') and in the abstract, conceptual sense ('Is x a mental disorder that differs from the mental disorder y?').

Medical classification systems are pragmatic tools that are evaluated according to the usefulness of the classification. This may involve sorting and managing patients according to the prognosis of their condition (curable/ chronic) and/or choosing (or developing) the best therapeutic option for the case in question. The therapeutic focus is, arguably, mirrored in the chase for medically relevant causal cluster kinds: causal relations are ideally manipulable (see, e.g. Woodward 2013). If we know that a property p causes y, we can use this knowledge not only to classify all y-likes as being 'of the kind that is caused by p-likes', we can also try to intervene, and hence prevent p from causing y. However, this simply pushes the question mark to the next series of issues: When is an intervention successful? How do we evaluate medical outcomes? Is, for instance, the number of years survived more important than the quality of life, or is it less important? How can 'quality of life' be operationalized, measured, and compared? What is the relationship between subjective bettering and a measurable positive outcome? In practice, these questions have been negotiated in many different forms: evaluation issues impact on and are themselves shaped by the politics of public health, the ethics and economies of clinical trial design, and the methodology of evidence-based medicine, to name but a few factors.[1]

We call these questions issues of controversy, because they require some amount of agreement on what should count as privileged knowledge. The settlement of issues of controversy is interest-relative. Let us now take a closer look at what interest-relativity means and what it implies for medical classification systems.

---

[1] For an in-depth study of these interlacements in the history of cancer trials, see Keating and Cambrosio (2012).

In the literature, interest-relativity is discussed with respect to gradable adjectives such as 'small, smaller, smallest' (e.g. Fara 2000; 2008): the appropriate application of 'small' depends upon the comparison of the subject under discussion with another case ('C is small, because she is smaller than D') or with a class of comparison ('C is small, because she is smaller than the average children of her age') and upon the question of *why* we are interested in knowing whether C is small. To answer the question of how small is something small enough to be called 'small', Delia Graff Fara argues that 'significance is determined, at least in part, by interests' (Fara 2008, 327). The basic idea is that, if we want to decide whether someone is so small that she should be prescribed growth hormones, then 'small' is evaluated against a different norm of smallness from the one we invoke when we say that someone is too small to be eligible for a pilot's licence. Fara (2000) introduces interest-relativity as a source of vagueness in language: 'the semantics of vague expressions renders the truth conditions of utterances containing them sensitive to our interests, with the result that vagueness in language has a traceable source in the vagueness of our interests' (ibid., 49). In other words, Fara argues that, if evaluative terms such as certain gradable adjectives and, arguably, medical terms like 'disease' or 'mental disorder' are used for different purposes, this impacts on the possible precision of those terms. Moreover, she stresses that it is our desires and purposes (i.e. interests) themselves that are subjected to vagueness: 'Purposes and desires can be vague because their achievement or satisfaction conditions may have vague boundaries' (ibid., 47). This resonates with the questions raised above concerning the satisfaction conditions of successful medical interventions and better quality of life. We mention interest-relativity in order to conceptualize how the interests of medical classification users and the norms they apply shape the meaning of the classifications and, vice versa, how the norms that are applied in order to shape the meaning of classifications need to be suitable (enough) for the interests of the classification users if they are to ensure the applicability of the given classification system.

For instance, the conceptualization of individual conditions as being instances of a specific medical kind may focus on the (therapeutically) relevant (causal) similarities between individual cases. The most broadly applied standardized classification systems, the ICD and the *DSM*, were, however, originally not introduced for therapeutic guidance but for statistical purposes (this is still apparent in the fully expanded names: International Statistical Classification of Diseases and Related Health Problems and *Diagnostic and Statistical Manual of Mental Disorders*). Indeed, one could argue that the very reason for their broad application is their informational use, that is, the codification of diagnoses for the purpose of gathering data for epidemiological, administrative, and reimbursement purposes (see Bowker and Star 1999). Broadly applied, classification systems are faced with different needs, depending on their use: for research purposes, the reliability and precision of classifications are crucial; in medical education, classification systems act as reference atlases of disease prototypes; in clinical practice, they ideally help to guide diagnostic and therapeutic decision-making; in administration, they are key variables in hospital management and insurance company policies. The different functions of medical classification systems are not necessarily in conflict. Yet the differing demands of classification users often lead to trade-offs: easy applicability of a manual is key to its large-scale use but usually comes at the cost of a more sophisticated subgrouping that, although usually more expensive and time-consuming, is more informative for research purposes (see Keuck 2011a). In practice, the demands of the various classification users and the implications of those demands for issues of controversy are more or less negotiated during revision processes. But they are also negotiated when existing classifications are actually applied and supplemented via more context-specific tools, such as local diagnostic guidelines or research criteria. The evaluation of medical classifications is therefore relative to interests: a classification is not per se good or bad; it is good or bad *for* a given task (see Keuck 2011b).

This brings us back to the epistemic endeavour of weighting, selecting, and classifying. Grouping individual conditions into classes necessitates the selection of classifiable characteristics. From an epistemological point of view, the selected characteristics need to be, first, *exclusive enough* to allow one to separate a disease from conditions that do not belong in the medical domain and to distinguish between diseases or disorders that differ from each other in a relevant aspect. This epistemic requirement is apparent in many different methodological strategies, ranging from the practices of differential diagnosis to statistical techniques for testing sensitivity and specificity.

Second, the selected characteristics need to be *inclusive enough* to allow for groups to be built. This draws on a point made in the previous section: no two individuals are exactly the same and, likewise, no two occurrences of a disease are the same—as they are manifested within individual bodies and minds. In this regard, 'disease' can be understood as an abstraction: irrelevant individual differences are abstracted away, cases are put in relation to each other, and abstract concepts ('disease x') are formed. The epistemic practices of abstracting common characteristics of (a specific) 'disease' should, however, not be reduced to mental operations of concept formation. Rather, mental operations are intertwined with and depend on practical operations that, literally, dissect the disease from the organism (for a related, more detailed account of abstraction in biology, see Winther 2009). The obtained abstract concept helps us to order the real world, to identify and compare alterations in different individuals (for a related account of diseases as historical abstractions, see Fleck 1979 [1935]). How to judge whether these alterations are pathological or fall within a normal range of life forms, and what kind of norms are implied by such judgements, are hotly contested issues in the philosophy of medicine and psychiatry:[2] they are, again, issues of controversy that are deemed responsible for the indeterminacy of medical classification in the epistemic context and that, in practice, are set- tled vis-à-vis more or less heterogeneous interests.

Different strategies are implemented to deal with the heterogeneity and com- plexity of individual cases and to render the classification system workable. These strategies are, first, to identify relevant properties of a disease; second, to disregard other properties that the cases under consideration do not necessar- ily share; and, third, to frame the selected properties in terms that adequately describe the phenomena with regard to the aim of classification. For example, in *DSM-IV* (APA 1994), cognitive decline was *identified* as the cardinal symp- tom of 'dementia of Alzheimer's type' (for a closer analysis of this example, see Keuck 2011b). At the same time, the previously included symptom 'personality change' was *disregarded* in *DSM-IV* not because this symptom was absent in demented patients, but because it was not found to be one of the more sensitive variables that discriminate between dementia of Alzheimer's type and control subjects (Salmon et al. 1998). Finally—and this becomes even more evident in the revised classification of 'major neurocognitive disorder due to Alzheimer's disease' in *DSM-5* (APA 2013)—the question of what is specific to this and no other disease was *framed* in terms that could be operationalized and reliably measured through neuropsychological testing in order to gain a higher inter- rater reliability (i.e. probability that two or more independent psychiatrists would come to the same diagnostic conclusion when applying the diagnostic manual to a given case)—'with lesser exclusive reliance on individual judgment' (APA 2010, 8).

The work of weighting, selecting, and ignoring is necessary in order to con- ceptualize an individual phenomenon as a case of a somehow defined abstract disease. This is of epistemic merit, because it allows one to use knowledge gained from other comparative cases. More specifically, the practices of abstracting (e.g. identifying, disregarding, and framing characteristics of a disease) enable researchers to treat diseases as scientific phenomena. While (an individual) phenomenon might be understood literally as the thing it shows itself to be,

---

[2] For an overview and comparison of the theoretical framework of most accounts, including Boorse's (1977) statistical dysfunction, Canguilhem's (1991 [1966]) biological normativity, and Nordenfelt's (1995) action theory, see Hofmann (2001).

the term 'scientific phenomenon' has been used in philosophy of science to describe what a given scientific approach tries to explain, that is, the mostly non-observable explanandum. In the words of Bogen and Woodward (1988, 306), 'well-developed scientific theories do predict and explain facts about phenomena. Phenomena are detected through the use of data, but in most cases are not observable in any interesting sense of that term.' By this reading, scientific phenomena can be understood as the epistemological counterpart to natural kinds. To quote Ian Hacking: 'we investigate nature by the use of apparatus in controlled environments, and are able to create phenomena that never or at best seldom occur in a pure state before people have physically excluded all "irrelevant" factors' (Hacking 1988, 507). Natural kinds exist in the world. Scientific phenomena are examined as part of a research enterprise.[3]

Recent studies in the philosophy of science have applied these ideas to psychological and psychiatric objects of inquiry and have analysed how key concepts of cognitive neuroscience such as 'memory' are stabilized (or fail to be stabilized) as scientific phenomena across multiple experimental settings (e.g. Sullivan 2009; Feest 2011). For, in order for researchers to stabilize a phenomenon, uniformly applicable standards must be at place. But a single standard may not serve all interests, not even solely within a specific research context. This issue is not only of theoretical interest but also of practical importance, because large-scale, distributive research endeavours such as the Alzheimer Disease Neuroimaging Initiative (ADNI) or the Cognitive Neuroscience Treatment Research to Improve Cognition in Schizophrenia (CNTRICS) initiative aim to acquire knowledge about diseases that are, at best, elusive phenomena (Huber 2015; Sullivan 2014). Characterizing diseases, 'research domains', or symptoms as scientific phenomena sheds some light on a specific epistemological aspect of indeterminacy, namely the instability of disease classifications that is due to the diversity of interests of classification users (and not to the unstable, continuous nature of diseases). Two points require further elaboration.

First, while the stabilization of scientific phenomena is important for gaining reliable experimental results, stabilization may conflict with the ontological continuity of disease kinds. For instance, when researching infectious diseases, experimental stabilization of viral or bacterial strains is necessary in order to enable the replication of the given experiment; in nature, however, high mutation rates of infectious agents are a characteristic of infectious diseases, thereby giving rise to biologically evolving disease kinds. Similarly, historically evolving

---

[3] Indeed, such abstractions abound within the highly divergent field of medical science. For an in-depth analysis of different explanatory values and their corresponding epistemologies in the medical sciences, see Lemoine (2011).

mental disorders might make it difficult to obtain comparable data. Or, vice versa, presenting psychiatric research as not depending on the time and context in which it was conducted might cloud important facts about the changeability of psychiatric kinds. Scientific strategies to acquire secured knowledge about a phenomenon can therefore themselves lead to epistemic uncertainty regarding the relationship between the stabilized phenomenon that is explained and the instable, individually manifested diseases that shall be diagnosed, classified, or treated.

Second, what we know about diseases and why we want to know something about them (e.g. to reduce the suffering of an individual or to stop the disease from spreading) are interrelated. The better disease phenomena are framed to fit our needs and expectations, the more stabilized they appear. Think about oncological classification: the category of hormone-dependent cancer focuses on a particular property shared by different cases, namely the diagnostically detectable and treatable overexpression of hormone-binding receptors on the cancer cell surface.

The answer to the 'why do we want to know' question as well as the choice of standards both involve, at least in part, issues of negotiation, resource availability, and power. In some contexts, far more effort may be put into ensuring a high degree of reliability and specificity of the classification, while in other contexts the classification is kept workable by using it only for postdiagnostic purposes, regardless of how the actual diagnosis was achieved. The degree of stability of disease phenomena and of their representation in medical classification systems is, at least in part, a consequence of homogenizing the interests and thereby reducing issues of controversy between those who revise and use the classifications. The less diverse the interests, the more specific and stable the classification will appear. If the standards are set for when small is small enough to be called 'small' across the board, the use of the word 'small' will appear to be less interest-relative and therefore less controversial. Knowledge about 'smallness' will be more reliable and seem more secured, but might be less relevant for some contexts. The same seems to be true if you replace 'small' with 'disordered'.

The epistemic practices of comparing cases and abstracting from individual phenomena to scientific phenomena and to disease categories help us to order the (pathological) world. This ordering confronts us with epistemic uncertainty concerning (absolute or relative) borderline cases—or even, drawing on Fara's understanding of vagueness, with boundarylessness—in the various senses described above: 'Is this already a case of mental disorder x?', 'Is x a mental disorder that differs from mental disorder y?', 'Is "mental disorder" at all the right concept to capture condition x?'. This brings us to the semantics of borderline cases.

4 **Vagueness: On semantic aspects of indeterminacy**

Vagueness and precision are properties of semantic entities such as concepts, predicates, or classificatory categories. Natural kinds can never be vague—not because they are natural, but because they are kinds. They are not the sort of thing that can be either vague or precise. The same holds for scientific phenomena. While kinds can be continuous or discrete and scientific phenomena can be stable or unstable, only semantic entities can be vague or precise. This ontological clarification was given as early as 1923 by Bertrand Russell:

> Apart from representation, whether cognitive or mechanical, there can be no such thing as vagueness or precision; things are what they are, and there is an end of it. Nothing is more or less what it is, or to a certain extent possessed of the properties which it possesses. Vagueness in a cognitive occurrence is a characteristic of its relation to that which is known, not a characteristic of the occurrence in itself. (Russell 1923, 85)

Nevertheless, there are important relations between semantic entities, scientific phenomena, and kinds—and thus relations between the vague–precise distinction, the stable–unstable distinction, and the continuous–discrete distinction. In order to examine these relations, we should first clarify the notions of vagueness and precision.

In the previous section we have already introduced the distinction between relative and absolute borderline cases. According to the most common definition, a term is vague if and only if it has absolute borderline cases (Sorensen 2013). An absolute borderline case is an object to which the concept neither definitely applies nor definitely does not apply. For example, the common concept 'ill' seems to be vague because there are many conditions someone can have in which it is unclear whether or not that person is ill (think of mild headaches or mild nausea). Importantly, this uncertainty is not just due to our lack of knowledge (but see the above section for epistemological problems to ascertain this condition). A genuine—that is, absolute—borderline case is such that the uncertainty remains even after the determination of all knowable facts. Vagueness occurs simply because a concept is not defined for certain situations.

There are two main types of vagueness we shall focus on in the following: degree vagueness and combinatory vagueness (Alston 1967, 219). Degree-vague concepts fail to draw a sharp line in a single dimension. By contrast, combinatory vague concepts are cluster concepts consisting of a complex of independent dimensions; and these dimensions are such that in some of their combinations it is indeterminate whether or not the concept applies. For example, the concept 'is tall (for a man)' is degree-vague because it fails to draw a sharp line in a single underlying dimension—the dimension height. Alston's example of a combinatory vague concept is 'religion'. According to Alston (1967, 219), religions are characterized by a number of striking features such as the belief in gods, the demarcation of certain objects as sacred, the presence of ritual acts, the presence of a moral code, characteristic feelings, a world view and the individual's more or less total organization of his life around it, and a social organization bound together by the preceding characteristics. The term 'religion' is vague because it is not clear how many of these characteristics, and which ones, must at least be present in order for the concept to apply. For example, it is clear that the presence of rituals alone is not sufficient. However, the presence of *all* the characteristics is not necessary either, since there are specific cases that do not exhibit all of them (for example, in Buddhism, there is no belief in gods). Where to draw the line between religions and non-religions is not completely clear.

In medical classification both types of vagueness occur. An obvious example of degree vagueness can be found in the typology of different degrees of severity of mental retardation according to *DSM-IV* (APA 2000, 42). The levels are as follows: mild mental retardation (IQ level 50–5 to approximately 70), moderate mental retardation (IQ level 35–40 to 50–5), severe mental retardation (IQ level 20–5 to 35–40), and profound mental retardation (IQ level below 20 or 25). The individual stages are vaguely defined; they overlap. An individual with an IQ of, say, 54 falls definitely neither into the category 'moderate retardation' nor into the category 'mild retardation'. Note, however, that the overlap zones themselves are precisely delimited (at the IQ levels 20, 25, 35, 40, 50, and 55, respectively). As a consequence, the levels do not exhibit higher order vagueness, that is, they do not admit of borderline cases of borderline cases. Either a person falls into the clear-cut overlap zone or she does not. Only the stage 'mild mental retardation', with an upper limit at 'approximately 70', exhibits higher order vagueness, because this border zone is not clearly demarcated.

Let us now turn to combinatory vagueness in psychiatric classification. Many definitions of disorders in the *DSM* have a polythetic—that is, cluster-like—structure. For example, according to *DSM-5*, MDD can be diagnosed if five out of nine symptoms are present. The polythetic structure alone does not make these categories vague, since there are precise and vague cluster concepts. Despite its being polythetically defined, MDD is a precise category in the sense that it has a precise threshold, lying at five symptoms' being present. Sure enough, one might still argue that each of the symptoms is not defined precisely and exhibits vagueness of degree, which, again, would turn the category MDD into a vague category. But in that case the category would exhibit vagueness of degree, not combinatory vagueness. By contrast, other *DSM* definitions do exhibit combinatory vagueness. For example, the levels of severity associated with many disorders are sometimes vaguely defined. In order to diagnose the 'mild' form of attention deficit/hyperactivity disorder, 'few, if any, symptoms in excess of those required to make the diagnosis' need to be present (APA 2013, 60). This is a vague formulation, since the term 'few' does not specify an exact number of symptoms to be met, in other words a precise threshold.

5 Continuity, uncertainty, and vagueness are theoretically independent

To illustrate the differences between ontological and semantic levels of analysis, we shall first look at the relationship between classificatory concepts and the entities that are generally classified by these concepts. Any classificatory concept has an extension, in other words there is a class that comprises all the objects to which that concept applies. In the case of vague concepts, this is a class with fuzzy boundaries. Kinds, on the other hand, also have extensional correlates, namely classes comprising all the instances of these kinds. We shall say that a classificatory category corresponds to a particular kind if the concept is intended to apply to all and only the instances of that kind. If the classificatory concept perfectly fits the kind, then the concept's extension and the class of instances of the kind are coextensive. Consider a disease entity E. There is a class C_E comprising all the individual occurrences of E. Now suppose that there is a system of medical classification that is intended to capture disease entities such as E. Suppose, further, that there is a category Cat_E in that classificatory system that is intended to capture E. If the classificatory system is similar to the *DSM*, then lists of criteria, which involve the presence of symptoms and so on, define the individual categories. In the optimal case, the extension of Cat_E will comprise exactly the individual occurrences of E (which means that Cat_E and C_E are coextensive). In the suboptimal case, some instances of E will be excluded from Cat_E or some non-instances will be included.[4]

After these preliminary explanations about the relationship between classificatory categories and disease entities, we are now in a position to turn to special questions concerning indeterminacy. As to the continuous–discrete and the vague–precise distinctions, one might suppose that continuity corresponds

---

[4] This case is analogous to, but not identical with the problem of false negatives and false positives in clinical practice. A false negative (false positive) is an individual who actually does (does not) meet the definition of a classificatory category Cat_E, but who is not classified (is classified) as falling into Cat_E by the doctor. In a similar vein, a non-fitting category is a category Cat_E that is defined (by the developers of the classification system) in such a way that some instances of E are excluded from Cat_E or some non-instances are included in it.

to vagueness and discreteness corresponds to precision in the sense that the disease entities with discrete boundaries are best matched by precisely defined categories, while those that gradually merge into one another are best matched by vaguely defined categories. However, as we have seen in section 3, disease classifications serve a variety of pragmatic needs, and the nexus just cited may not always hold. If we observe existing medical classifications, it becomes obvious that all four combinations resulting from the continuous–discrete and the vague–precise distinctions are indeed realized. The continuous–vague and the discrete–precise combinations are trivial; but the discrete–vague and the continuous–precise combinations are realized as well. For an example of the latter, consider the definition of hypertension. Arguably, blood pressure is a gradable feature. There are no realization gaps and no qualitative jumps at any point on the scale. Yet common definitions draw a sharp boundary, usually lying at 140 mm Hg systolic pressure, that distinguishes normal from pathological blood pressure. Similarly, many *DSM* categories are precisely defined categories that try to capture disease entities that arguably have somewhat unsharp boundaries. There may be various reasons to draw such a sharp line even in absence of realization gaps and qualitative jumps. One such reason is practicality. A precisely defined category may be more easily usable than a vaguely defined one, which is more time-consuming and requires the user to be more careful. Another advantage is that precisely defined categories facilitate communication because they reduce the risk that different users mean different things when using one and the same word. On the other hand, cutting a continuous reality into sharply defined pieces can also have the disadvantage of being misleading and inappropriate. Indeed, some authors state that '[d]ividing people into "hypertensives" and "normotensives" is commonplace but problematic' (Law 2012, S30). Law and Wald (2002, 1570) even recommend that '[t]erms like hypertension, hypercholesterolaemia, and osteoporosis that focus medical attention on the tails of the distributions of physiological variables are best avoided'.

In practice, the translation from ontological features of disease entities into the semantics of classification is mediated by the epistemic enterprises of identifying relevant properties of disease phenomena and disregarding other properties. We have seen that relevance is considered to be an interest-relative concept: properties of disease phenomena are not only assessed differently in different contexts but also weighted differently, depending on the uses to which they are put. We may think that vagueness maps onto controversial classification and precision onto uncontroversial classification, but this is not necessarily so. The suitability of classifications varies in practice and, moreover, their validity is assessed on the basis of pragmatic standards. Think of the current research programme on so-called bio-ontologies. Bio-ontologies such as the gene ontology are algorithm-based classifications that were developed to facilitate and homogenize communication among genetic scientists (see Leonelli 2010). Such an informatics-based classification might also improve the organization of biomedical knowledge and the classification of diseases and mental disorders (Ceusters and Smith 2010). Bio-ontologies strive for ontological discreteness (although they may allow for dimensional approaches if they are representable in a formal structure) and for semantic precision, because they can be better modelled in binary algorithms that facilitate the informatics-based design of classifications (see Jansen 2008). In the case of these 'ontologies', the selection of the relevant properties of disease phenomena is oriented towards (scientific) properties that fit well their informational use (e.g. genetic alteration existent–non-existent). From a clinical point of view, however, the properties that can be translated into neat algorithms need not necessarily be clinically significant ones. Especially in psychiatry, vague concepts such as subjective well-being may be of great clinical importance but are very difficult to reduce to hierarchical, often binary bio-ontologies from genes to organisms. If a concept is precise but no longer captures what it should represent, it might cause just as much (or more) controversy, and reflect just as much (or more) epistemic uncertainty, as a vague term that is able to accommodate the inquiry-resistant character of some cases.

6 **Conclusion**

In this chapter we have argued that the continuous–discrete, the controversial–uncontroversial, and the vague–precise distinctions apply to different sorts of entities. The first is an ontological distinction and applies to disease entities (or kinds in general), the second is an epistemological distinction and applies to knowledge about diseases, and the third is a semantic distinction and applies to classificatory categories (or concepts in general). We have tried to show that these distinctions are logically independent in the sense that there is no necessary correlation between, say, continuous disease entities, controversial knowledge, and vague medical categories. In fact there are reasons to define precise categories, and reasons to define vague categories, not necessarily depending on whether or not the corresponding disease entities are characterized by realization gaps.

Our analysis leads us to conclude that there is room for a plethora of classifications with different uses (including perhaps biomedical ontologies for the computer-aided organization of medical literature). Due to the fact that, in practice, we have no unmediated view of the actual ontological nature of our targets of interest, we cannot evaluate the validity of the classifications in question independently of our interests. Since it is often difficult to decide whether we are faced with absolute or relative borderline cases, we should be aware of the caveats, but also of the productive nature of indeterminacies in medical classification systems insofar as they enable scientific and conceptual research.

References

Alston, W. 1967. 'Vagueness'. In *The Encyclopedia of Philosophy*, edited by P. Edwards, pp. 218–21. New York, NY: Macmillan.

APA (**American Psychiatric Association**). 1994. *Diagnostic and statistical manual of mental disorders. DSM-IV, Fourth Edition.* Washington, DC: American Psychiatric Association.

APA (**American Psychiatric Association**). 2000. *Diagnostic and Statistical Manual of Mental Disorders, Fourth Edition, Text Revision: DSM-IV TR.* Washington, DC: American Psychiatric Association.

APA (**American Psychiatric Association**). 2010. *DSM-5 Development: DSM-5 Neurocognitive Criteria.* January 2010. http://www.dsm5.org/ProposedRevisions/Pages/Delirium,Dementia,Amnestic,OtherCognitive.aspx (accessed: 15 Oct 2010; no longer available online).

APA (**American Psychiatric Association**). 2013. *Diagnostic and Statistical Manual of Mental Disorders, Fifth Edition: DSM-5.* Washington, DC: American Psychiatric Association.

Bogen, J., and **Woodward, J.** 1988. 'Saving the phenomena'. *The Philosophical Review* **97**: 303–52.

Boorse, C. 1977. 'Health as a theoretical concept'. *Philosophy of Science* **44**: 542–73.

Bolton, D. 2008. *What Is Mental Disorder? An Essay in Philosophy, Science, and Values.* Oxford: Oxford University Press.

Bowker, G. C., and **Star, S. L.** 1999. *Sorting Things Out: Classification and Its Consequences.* Cambridge, MA: MIT Press.

Boyd, R. 1991. 'Realism, anti-foundationalism and the enthusiasm for natural kinds'. *Philosophical Studies* **61**: 127–48.

Boyd, R. 2010. 'Realism, natural kinds, and philosophical methods'. In *The Semantics and Metaphysics of Natural Kinds*, edited by H. Beebee and N. Sabbarton-Leary, pp. 212–34. New York, NY: Routledge.

Canguilhem, G. 1991 [1966]. *The Normal and the Pathological*, translated by C. R. Fawcett. New York, NY: Zone Books.

Ceusters, W., and **Smith, B.** 2010. 'Foundations for a realist ontology of mental disease'. *Journal of Biomedical Semantics* **1** (1). doi: 10.1186/2041-1480-1-10

Cooper, R. 2005. *Classifying Madness: A Philosophical Examination of the Diagnostic and Statistical Manual of Mental Disorders.* Dordrecht: Springer.

Cooper, R. 2013. 'Avoiding false positives: Zones of rarity, the threshold problem, and the DSM clinical significance criterion'. *Canadian Journal of Psychiatry* **58**: 606–11.

Dupré, J. 1993. *The Disorder of Things.* Cambridge, MA: Harvard University Press.

Fara, D. G. 2000. 'Shifting sands: An interest-relative theory of vagueness'. *Philosophical Topics* **28**: 45–81 (originally published under the name Delia Graff).

Fara, D. G. 2008. 'Profiling interest-relativity'. *Analysis* **68**: 326–35.

Feest, U. 2011. 'What exactly is stabilized when phenomena are stabilized?'. *Synthese* **182**: 57–71.

Fleck, L. 1979 [1935]. *Genesis and Development of a Scientific Fact*. Chicago, IL: University of Chicago Press.

Hacking, I. 1988. 'On the stability of the laboratory sciences'. *The Journal of Philosophy* **85**: 507–14.

Hacking, I. 1991. 'A tradition of natural kind'. *Philosophical Studies* **61**: 109–26.

Hacking, I. 1995. 'The looping effect of human kinds'. In *Causal Cognition: A Multidisciplinary Debate*, edited by D. Sperber, D. Premack, and A. Premack, pp. 351–83. Oxford/New York, NY: Clarendon/Oxford University Press.

Hacking, I. 1998. *Mad Travelers. Reflections on the Reality of Transient Mental Illnesses*. Charlottesville, VA: University Press of Virginia.

Hacking, I. 1999. *The Social Construction of What?* Cambridge, MA: Harvard University Press.

Haslam, N. 2002. 'Kinds of kinds: A conceptual taxonomy of psychiatric categories'. *Philosophy, Psychiatry, & Psychology* **9**: 203–17.

Hauswald, R. 2014. *Soziale Pluralitäten: Zur Ontologie, Wissenschaftstheorie und Semantik des Klassifizierens und Gruppierens von Menschen in Gesellschaft und Humanwissenschaft*. Münster: mentis.

Hauswald, R. 2016. 'The ontology of interactive kinds'. *Journal of Social Ontology* **2**: 203–22.

Hawley, K., and Bird, A. 2011. 'What are natural kinds?'. *Philosophical Perspectives* **25**: 205–21.

Hofmann, B. 2001. 'Complexity of the concept of disease as shown through rival theoretical frameworks'. *Theoretical Medicine* **22**: 211–36.

Huber, L. 2015. 'Measuring by which standard? How plurality challenges the ideal of epistemic singularity'. In *Standardization in Measurement*, edited by O. Schlaudt and L. Huber, pp. 207–15. London: Pickering & Chatto.

Hyman, S. E. 2010. 'The diagnosis of mental disorders: The problem of reification'. *Annual Review of Clinical Psychology* **6**: 155–79.

Insel, T. 2013. 'Transforming diagnosis'. http://www.nimh.nih.gov/about/director/2013/transforming-diagnosis.shtml (accessed 26 August 2014).

Jansen, L. 2008. 'Classifications'. In *Applied Ontology*, edited by K. Munn and B. Smith, pp. 159–172. Heusenstamm: Ontos.

Keating, P., and Cambrosio, A. 2012. *Cancer on Trial: Oncology as a New Style of Practice*. Chicago, IL: Chicago University Press.

Kendell, R., and Jablensky, A. 2003. 'Distinguishing between the validity and utility of psychiatric diagnoses'. *The American Journal of Psychiatry* **160**: 4–12.

Kendler, K. S. 2012. 'Epistemic iteration as a historical model for psychiatric nosology: Promises and limitations'. In *Philosophical Issues in Psychiatry II: Nosology*, edited by K. S. Kendler and J. Parnas, pp. 305–22. Oxford: Oxford University Press.

Keuck, L. K. 2011a. 'How to make sense of broadly applied medical classification systems: Introducing epistemic hubs'. *History and Philosophy of the Life Sciences* **33**: 583–602. [Originally published under the name Lara K. Kutschenko.]

Keuck, L. K. 2011b. 'In quest for "good" medical classification systems'. *Medicine Studies* **3**: 53–70. [Originally published under the name Lara K. Kutschenko.]

Law, M. 2012. 'A change in paradigm: Lowering blood pressure in everyone over a certain age'. *Annals of Medicine* **44** (Suppl. 1): S30–S35.

Law, M., and Wald, N. J. 2002. 'Risk factor thresholds: their existence under scrutiny'. *BMJ* **324**: 1570–6.

Lemoine, M. 2011. *La désunité de la médecine: Essai sur les valeurs explicatives de la science médicale*. Paris: Hermann.

Leonelli, S. 2010. 'Documenting the emergence of bio-ontologies: Or, why researching bioinformatics requires HPSSB'. *History and Philosophy of the Life Sciences* **32**: 105–26.

Mill, J. S. 1973 [1843]. *A System of Logic, Ratiocinative and Inductive. Being a Connected View of the Principles of Evidence and the Methods of Scientific Investigation*. Toronto: University of Toronto Press.

Murphy, D. 2006. *Psychiatry in the Scientific Image*. Cambridge: MIT Press.

Nordenfelt, L. 1995. *On the Nature of Health: An Action-Theoretic Approach*. Dordrecht: Reidel Publishing.

Pinkal, M. 1995. *Logic and Lexicon: The Semantics of the Indefinite*. Dordrecht: Springer.

Putnam, H. 1975. 'Dreaming and "depth grammar"'. In id., *Mind, Language, and Reality: Philosophical Papers II*, pp. 304–24. Cambridge: Cambridge University Press.

Reznek, L. 1987. *The Nature of Disease*. New York, NY: Routledge.

Russell, B. 1923. 'Vagueness'. *Australasian Journal of Philosophy and Psychology* **1**: 84–91.

Salmon, D. P. et al. 1998. 'Alzheimer's disease: Data analysis for the DSM-IV task force'. In *DSM-IV Sourcebook*, edited by T. A. Widiger et al., pp. 91–107. Washington, DC: American Psychiatric Publishing.

Schaffner, K. F. 2012. 'Coherentist approaches to scientific progress in psychiatry: Comments on Kendler'. In *Philosophical Issues in Psychiatry II: Nosology*, edited by K. S. Kendler and J. Parnas, pp. 323–30. Oxford: Oxford University Press.

Sorensen, R. 2016. 'Vagueness'. In *The Stanford Encyclopedia of Philosophy*, edited by E. N. Zalta. http://plato.stanford.edu/archives/spr2016/entries/vagueness (accessed 16 June 2016).

Sullivan, J. A. 2009. 'The multiplicity of experimental protocols: A challenge to reductionist and non-reductionist models of the unity of neuroscience'. *Synthese* **167**: 511–39.

Sullivan, J. A. 2014. 'Stabilizing mental disorders: Prospects and problems'. In *Classifying Psychopathology: Mental Kinds and Natural Kinds*, edited by H. Kincaid and J. A. Sullivan, pp. 360–96. Cambridge, MA: MIT Press.

Tabb, K. 2015. 'Psychiatric progress and the assumption of diagnostic discrimination'. *Philosophy of Science* **82**: 1047–58.

Wakefield, J. C. 1992. 'The concept of mental disorder: On the boundary between biological facts and social values'. *American Psychologist* **47**: 373–88.

Whewell, W. 1971. *On the Philosophy of Discovery*. New York, NY: Franklin.

Winther, R. G. 2009. 'Character analysis in cladistics: Abstraction, reification, and the search for objectivity'. *Acta Biotheoretica* **57**: 129–62.

Woodward, J. 2013. 'Causation and manipulability'. In *The Stanford Encyclopedia of Philosophy*, edited by E. N. Zalta. http://plato.stanford.edu/archives/win2013/entries/causation-mani (accessed 26 August 2014).

Part III

Vagueness in psychiatric classification and diagnosis

Chapter 6

Psychiatric diagnosis, tacit knowledge, and criteria

Tim Thornton

1 Introduction

For the last 50 years, both of the major psychiatric diagnostic systems—the *Diagnostic and Statistical Manual of Mental Disorders* (*DSM*; see e.g. APA 2013) and the International Statistical Classification of Diseases and Related Health Problems (ICD)—have aimed at reliability at the potential cost of validity. They have done this by codifying diagnosis in the form of criteria, being influenced by operationalism from the philosophy of physics and downplaying aetiological theory. It is an empirical question whether *DSM-III, -IV*, and now *-5* and the parallel ICD classifications have achieved this aim overall.

There have been criticisms, however, that the explicit criteria underdetermine the diagnoses made by skilled clinicians. That is, the criteria themselves have a vagueness or indeterminacy for which experienced psychiatrists have to compensate in diagnostic judgements, in response to particular patients who express particular signs and symptoms. The overall top-down or gestalt judgement is more precise than the component criteria on which it is supposed to be based.

The aim of this chapter is to address not whether this is so but rather how it could be so. In doing this, I will make two suggestions. First, diagnosis may involve an important tacit element. As a recognitional judgement, it may share characteristics of an uncodifiable form of know-how. Second, the postulation of criteriological intermediaries between the skilled clinician and his or her patients' or clients' actual conditions may distort the recognitional process. Judgement of the underlying mental states of patients and clients may be more secure than the operationalized criteria.

The first section outlines the reasons for the emphasis, since the second half of the twentieth century, on operationalism in both the main psychiatric taxonomies. The second section sets out three similar clinically based criticisms of the resulting criteriological model of diagnosis.

The final two sections set out to shed light on why these criticisms apply, first by suggesting that diagnostic judgements are an instance of a broader class of tacit knowledge and then by suggesting that the criteriological view distorts the way in which clinical signs and symptoms bespeak, to a skilled clinical, underlying pathologies directly.

2 Background: The rise of criteriological diagnosis

Over the last half century, there has been a concerted effort to improve the reliability of psychiatric diagnosis by pruning the two main diagnostic systems of possibly overhasty aetiological theory and by stressing instead more directly observational features of presenting subjects. Two main factors explain this. (For a fuller account, see Fulford, Thornton, and Graham 2006.)

First, on its foundation in 1945, the World Health Organisation (WHO) set about establishing an international classification of diseases. The chapters of the classification dealing with physical illnesses were well received, but the psychiatric section was not widely adopted. The British psychiatrist Erwin Stengel was asked to propose a basis for a more acceptable classification. Stengel chaired a session at an American Psychological Association conference of 1959 at which the philosopher Carl Hempel spoke. As a result of Hempel's paper (and an intervention by the psychiatrist Sir Aubrey Lewis), Stengel proposed that attempts at a classification based on theories of the causes of mental disorder should be given up (on the grounds that such theories were premature) and suggested that the classification should instead rely on what could be directly observed, that is, on symptoms.

In fact Hempel's paper provided only *partial* support for the moral that was actually drawn for psychiatry. He argued:

> Broadly speaking, the vocabulary of science has two basic functions: first, to permit an adequate description of the things and events that are the objects of scientific investigation; second, to permit the establishment of general laws or theories by means of which particular events may be explained and predicted and thus scientifically understood; for to understand a phenomenon scientifically is to show that it occurs in accordance with general laws or theoretical principles. (Hempel 1994, 317)

These two requirements—that terms employed in classifications should have clear, public criteria of application and should lend themselves to the formulation of general laws—correspond to the aims of *reliability* and *validity* respectively. Clear public criteria promote both test–retest and inter-rater reliability, while general laws are a step, at least, towards construct validity. But it was the former that was adopted by psychiatry as the key aim at the time. With respect to it, Hempel claimed:

Science aims at knowledge that is *objective* in the sense of being intersubjectively certifiable, independently of individual opinion or preference, on the basis of data obtainable by suitable experiments or observations. This requires that the terms used in formulating scientific statements have clearly specified meanings and be understood in the same sense by all those who use them. (Ibid., 318)

He commends the use of operational definitions (following Bridgman 1927), although he emphasizes that in psychiatry the kind of measurement operations in terms of which concepts would be defined would have to be construed loosely. This view has been influential up to the present WHO psychiatric taxonomy in ICD-10.

The second reason for the emphasis on reliability, and hence operationalism, in recent psychiatric taxonomy was a parallel influence, within American psychiatry, on drafting *DSM-III*. While *DSM-I* and *DSM-II* had drawn heavily on psychoanalytic theoretical terms, the committee charged with drawing up *DSM-III* drew on the work of a group of psychiatrists from Washington University in St Louis. Responding in part to research that had revealed significant differences in diagnostic practices between various psychiatrists, the 'St Louis group', led by John Feighner, published operationalized criteria for psychiatric diagnosis. The *DSM-III* task force replaced references to Freudian aetiological theory with more observational criteria.

This stress on operationalism has had an effect on the way in which criteriological diagnosis is codified in *DSM* manuals and in ICD classifications. Syndromes are described and characterized in terms of disjunctions and conjunctions of symptoms. The symptoms themselves are described in ways influenced by operationalism and with as little aetiological theory as possible. (That they are neither strictly operationally defined nor strictly aetiologically theory-free is not relevant here.) Thus one can think of such a manual as providing guidance for, or a justification of, the diagnosis of a specific syndrome. Presented with an individual, the diagnosis of a specific syndrome is justified because he or she has a sufficient number of the relevant symptoms, which can be, as closely as possible, 'read off' from their presentation. The underlying syndrome is connected to more accessible, epistemologically basic signs and symptoms.

3 An objection to criteriological approaches

Although the rationale for a criteriological—or bottom-up—approach to diagnosis seems clear, it has not escaped criticism. The charge outlined in this section is that combining individual signs and symptoms—understood initially in isolation from context and only assembled in the conjunctions that add up to diagnosis—makes the signs and symptoms imprecise.

In a paper called 'Phenomenological and Criteriological Diagnosis: Different or Complementary?' Alfred Kraus, professor of psychiatry at Heidelberg, argues that diagnostic systems such as the *DSM* and the ICD miss out an important element of psychiatric diagnosis (Kraus 1994). Because they assume that diagnoses are built up from a number of individual and conceptually independent symptoms, they cannot capture top-down and holistic elements of diagnosis.

One key criticism that Kraus makes of what he calls this criteriological approach to diagnosis is that, rather than providing a reliable foundation, the connection between individual symptoms and conditions lacks *specificity*.

> [S]ymptomatological/criteriological diagnosis not only makes the reality of the patient accessible in a very reduced way but also portrays the pathological phenomena in a very imprecise and broad manner . . . The reduction of phenomena to symptoms and criteria has as its consequence a loss of specificity. (Ibid., 153–4)

Taking delusions as an example of a symptom, Kraus argues that that there is no reliable connection between delusions in general and schizophrenia, which undermines a criteriological model of the diagnosis of schizophrenia. 'Delusion' is a vague term picking out a variety of psychological states. The reliable connection is between particular kinds of delusional structure and schizophrenia. But the identification of delusions with a specific schizophrenic colouring presupposes, Kraus argues, a top-down holistic model rather than a bottom-up description. The assumption, on the criteriological approach, that symptoms can be recognized and described independently of the psychopathological diagnostic categories of which they are a part introduces vagueness to their descriptions and hence undermines the specificity of their connection to diagnostic judgements.

Kraus also argues that in the bottom-up model symptoms can only be added together through conjunction. But no mere conjunction of individual symptoms—a 'Chinese restaurant menu' approach—can capture the psychological integrity up to which the individual parts add. For that, again, one needs a top-down holistic approach. This is not to say, however, that particular elements cannot be identified in a holistic diagnosis. It is just that the individual elements have a different logic.

One way (although not Kraus' own) of marking the relevant distinction involved here is to contrast parts that are independent pieces and parts that are essential aspects. The pieces of a jigsaw add up to a whole, but each piece can exist independently of the others. By contrast, a musical note has both a tone and a pitch, but neither aspect can exist independently of the other. Thus, according to a holistic approach, psychological symptoms are not independent building blocks towards diagnostic judgements but are interdependent aspects of a psychological unity.

Kraus combines these two comments on the limits of a criteriological model of diagnosis with a further philosophical explanation of the difference in approach. This is why he contrasts the criteriological with a phenomenological rather than merely a holistic model. This model concentrates not on psychiatric diseases but on the mode of being of whole persons, the 'whole of the being in the world of schizophrenics or manics' (ibid., 152). Thus the phenomenologically based diagnosis of schizophrenia turns on an overall assessment of the patient—a 'praecox feeling'—as having a very different form of 'being-in-the-world'. Whether or not that more general view is correct, Kraus' criticism suggests that the operational structure of psychiatric manuals introduces vagueness into the description of symptoms and hence undermines the specificity of the link between symptom, when properly understood, and diagnostic judgement.

Mario Maj makes a similar criticism. Again taking the example of schizophrenia, he claims:

> One could argue that we have come to a critical point in which it is difficult to discern whether the operational approach is disclosing the intrinsic weakness of the concept of schizophrenia (showing that the schizophrenic syndrome does not have a character and can be defined only by exclusion) or whether the case of schizophrenia is bringing to light the intrinsic limitations of the operational approach (showing that this approach is unable to convey the clinical flavour of such a complex syndrome). In other terms, there may be, beyond the individual phenomena, a 'psychological whole' . . . in schizophrenia, that the operational approach fails to grasp, or such a psychological whole may simply be an illusion, that the operational approach unveils. (Maj 1998, 459–60)

In fact Maj argues that this shows the weakness of the operational approach. He claims that the *DSM* criteria fail to account for aspects of a proper grasp of schizophrenia—for example, the intuitive ranking of symptoms (which have equal footing in the *DSM* account). He suggests that there is, nevertheless, no particular danger in the use of *DSM* criteria by skilled, expert clinicians, for whom they serve merely as a reminder of a more complex prior understanding. But there is a problem with the use of these criteria to encode diagnosis for those without such an underlying understanding:

> If the few words composing the DSM-IV definition will probably evoke, in the mind of expert clinicians, the complex picture that they have learnt to recognise along the years, the same cannot be expected for students and residents. (Ibid., 460)

Maj's criticism that *DSM* criteria do not capture a proper, expert understanding of the diagnosis of schizophrenia raises the question of how or why that could be the case. If the criticism is right, is it that the wrong criteria have been used—either the wrong symptoms or the wrong rules of combination? Or is there something more fundamentally wrong with the criteriological approach as applied to psychiatry?

Josef Parnas suggests the latter. In a paper describing preoperational approaches to taxonomy and diagnosis as a 'disappearing heritage', he comments on an underlying difference in attitude towards signs and symptoms of schizophrenia:

> When the pre-DSM-III psychopathologists emphasized this or that feature as being very characteristic of schizophrenia, they did not use the concept of a symptom/sign as it is being used today in the operational approach. This latter approach envisages the symptoms and signs as being (ideally) third person data, namely as reified (thing-like), mutually independent (atomic) entities, devoid of meaning and therefore appropriate for context-independent definitions and unproblematic assessments. It is as if the symptom/sign and its causal substrate were assumed to exhibit the same descriptive nature: both are spatio-temporally delimited objects, i.e., things. In this paradigm, the symptoms and signs have no intrinsic sense or meaning. They are almost entirely referring, i.e., pointing to the underlying abnormalities of anatomo-physiological substrate. This scheme of 'symptoms = causal referents' is automatically activated in the mind of a physician confronting a medical somatic illness. Yet the psychiatrist, who confronts his 'psychiatric object', finds himself in a situation without analogue in the somatic medicine. The psychiatrist does not confront a leg, an abdomen, not a thing, but a person, i.e., broadly speaking, another embodied consciousness. What the patient manifests is not isolated symptoms/signs with referring functions but rather certain wholes of mutually implicative, interpenetrating experiences, feelings, beliefs, expressions, and actions, all permeated by biographical detail. (Parnas 2011, 1126)

The claim here is that the criteriological approach has the wrong model of psychiatric symptoms and signs in two respects. Just as smoke can indicate fire or tree rings the age of a tree, the criteriological approach takes signs and symptoms to be free-standing items that merely causally indicate underlying states. Furthermore, these relations are independent of one another: they are atomic. By contrast, Parnas suggests, psychiatric signs and symptoms are both essentially meaning-laden (rather than brutely causal) and mutually interdependent wholes. It is the latter claim—the one about interdependence—that plays the more important role in his criticism.

One argument for the interdependence of symptoms and signs is that it is only in particular contexts that symptoms are reliable. Thus, for example, mumbling speech is comparatively widespread (Parnas estimates it applies to 5 percent of the population), but in—and only in—the context of other features such as 'mannerist allure, inappropriate affect, and vagueness of thought, it acquires a psychopathological significance' (ibid., 1126). So the effectiveness of the sign is context-dependent. In some contexts the sign is indicative and in others not. Excluded from context, as it is in the criteriological approach, the sign is vague. Parnas goes further by suggesting a more than merely additive view. Grasp of psychiatric symptoms is likened to seeing the figure of the duck-rabbit first as a rabbit and then suddenly as a duck: it is seeing the signs and symptoms under an overall aspect or gestalt.

> A Gestalt is a salient unity or organization of phenomenal aspects. This unity emerges from the relations between component features (part–whole relations) but cannot be reduced to their simple aggregate (whole is more than the sum of its parts) . . . A Gestalt instantiates a certain generality of type (e.g., this patient is typical of a category X), but this typicality is always modified, because it is necessarily embodied in a particular, concrete individual, thus deforming the ideal clarity of type (universal and particular). (Ibid., 1126)

So the model of diagnosis is one in which the skilled clinician grasps the right diagnosis as an integrated whole, in which different aspects can be seen as abstractions from that whole rather than as its basic building blocks. Such a view would accommodate Kraus' rejection of a 'Chinese restaurant menu' approach and Maj's suggestion that criteriological elements serve as reminders for already skilled clinicians. They do—on this view—in the sense that, after the fact, such articulations of the overall picture are possible, as a musical note may be divided into its pitch, tone, and duration while it cannot be built up from them as independent building blocks. But that does not imply that the expert judgement of the whole could be built up from the individual criteria understood in isolation.

There is a further possibility hinted at in the criticism of Kraus, Maj, and Parnas. On a criteriological view, symptoms are not merely independent of each other (as Kraus points out); they are conceptually independent of the underlying psychopathological state they indicate. But, in the case of Kraus and Parnas at least, there is a suggestion that the connection between symptoms (when correctly understood) and psychopathological state is more direct: the state is expressed directly in the signs and symptoms, at least for those with the skill to see it.

4 Diagnosis and tacit knowledge

The criticisms of the criteriological approach set out in the preceding section prompt two further questions. The bottom-up codification of diagnosis through simpler, more basic signs and symptoms suggests an explanation of how complex diagnostic judgement is possible. It is possible because it is based on simpler, more epistemically accessible building blocks. The first question concerns the nature of an overall 'gestalt' judgement if that explanation is rejected. On what is top-down judgement based, and what is its relationship to the criteriological approach? In this section I will suggest an analogy with context-dependent tacit knowledge, in order to try to make the rejection of the above explanation seem a less puzzling possibility (for a more detailed discussion, see Thornton 2013). But my analogy will also help highlight how the move from context-dependent recognition to explicit criteria introduces vagueness into the description of psychiatric symptoms.

Second, if diagnostic judgement is not based on more observational features of a clinical encounter, how can it yield knowledge of underlying mental states? In the final section I will suggest an analogy with the more general problem of 'other minds' and outline what may initially seem a counter-intuitive view outlined by the philosopher John McDowell, which inverts the epistemic priority of judgements about behavioural signs and symptoms and judgements about underlying mental states. Again, this will suggest that reliance on basic criteria comes at the cost of introducing vagueness into the description of psychiatric symptoms, which undermines the potential directness of psychiatric diagnosis, as described by Kraus, Maj, and Parnas.

I suggested at the start that the development of the theoretically minimal criteriological approach to diagnosis in psychiatry was partly influenced by operationalism in the philosophy of science in the first part of the twentieth century. The aim was to minimize uncodified elements in psychiatric diagnosis so as to maximize reliability. But there was, in the second half of the century, a contrasting view about the nature of scientific knowledge: the arguments for the importance of tacit knowledge advanced by Michael Polanyi, the chemist turned philosopher. (Polanyi himself talks of tacit *knowing* rather than knowledge. I will, nevertheless, use 'knowledge' while talking about his views but will return to emphasize the practical dimension to what is tacit.) Top-down or gestalt judgement in psychiatry can be thought of as an instance of tacit knowledge. I will use Polanyi to introduce this notion but will deviate from his account shortly.

Polanyi gives the following example: 'We know a person's face, and can recognize it among a thousand, indeed among a million. Yet we usually cannot tell how we recognize a face we know. So most of this knowledge cannot be put into words' (Polanyi 1967, 4). This is an instance of what he takes to be a general phenomenon. Indeed, he begins his book *The Tacit Dimension* with the following bold claim: 'I shall reconsider human knowledge by starting from the fact that *we can know more than we can tell* (ibid.). The broad suggestion is that knowledge can be tacit when it is, on some understanding, 'untellable'. 'Tellable' knowledge is a subset of all knowledge and excludes tacit knowledge. But the slogan is gnomic. Does it carry, for example, a sotto voce qualification 'at any one particular time'? Or does it mean: ever?

The very idea of tacit knowledge presents a challenge: it has to be tacit and it has to be knowledge. But it is not easy to meet both conditions. Emphasizing the tacit status threatens the idea that there is something known. Articulating a knowable content—that which is known by the possessor of tacit knowledge—risks making it explicit. There is a second strand through Polanyi's work that helps address this problem. At the start of his book *Personal Knowledge*, he says: 'I regard knowing as an active comprehension of things known, an action that requires skill' (Polanyi 1962, vii). These two features suggest a way to understand tacit knowledge: it is not, or perhaps cannot be made, explicit; and it is connected to action, the practical knowledge of a skilled agent. The latter connection suggests a way in which tacit knowledge can have a content: as practical knowledge of how to do something. Taking tacit knowledge to be practical suggests one way in which it is untellable. It cannot be made explicit except in context-dependent practical demonstrations. It is not that it is mysteriously ineffable but that it cannot be put into words alone or reduced to words.

Psychiatric diagnostic judgement can be thought of as an example of such a skill: the ability to recognize, in a particular context, the manifestation of psychiatric illness. Polanyi also compares recognition to a practical skill, likening it to bicycle riding:

> I may ride a bicycle and say nothing, or pick out my macintosh among twenty others and say nothing. Though I cannot say clearly how I ride a bicycle nor how I recognise my macintosh (for I don't know it clearly), yet this will not prevent me from saying that I know how to ride a bicycle and how to recognise my macintosh. For I know that I know how to do such things, though I know the particulars of what I know only in an instrumental manner and am focally quite ignorant of them. (Ibid., 88)

In both cases, the 'knowledge-how' depends on something that is not explicit: the details of the act of bike riding or raincoat recognition. While one can recognize one's own macintosh, one is, according to Polanyi, ignorant, in some sense, of how. Thus how one recognizes it is tacit. Polanyi suggests here that explicit recognition of something as an instance of a type is based on the implicit recognition of subsidiary properties of which one is focally ignorant. He explains the distinction between focal and subsidiary awareness through the example of focusing attention on what a pointing finger points to. When one is looking from the finger to the object, the object is the focus of attention, while the finger, though seen, is not attended to. It is not invisible, however, and could itself become the object of focal attention.

Polanyi seems to assume that the question of how one recognizes something always has an informative answer; and then, to cover cases where it is not obvious what this is, he suggests that it can be tacit. But, first, while the question sometimes may have an informative answer, there is no reason to think that it always has (consider recognizing that a wall is red). Secondly, even in cases where one recognizes a particular as an instance of a general kind in virtue of some further properties *and cannot give an independent account of those properties*, it is not clear that one need be focally ignorant of them. It may be, instead, that the awareness one has of the 'subsidiary' properties is simply manifested in the act of recognition. I might say, I recognize that this is a—or perhaps my—macintosh because of how it looks *here* with the interplay of sleeve, shoulder, and colour, even if I could not recognize a separated sleeve, shoulder, or paint colour sample as being of the same type. While it seems plausible that one might not be able to say in context-independent terms just what it is about the sleeve that distinguishes a (or my) macintosh from any other kind of raincoat (one may, for example, lack the vocabulary of fashion or tailoring), this need not imply that one is focally ignorant of, or not attending to, just those features that make a difference. Recognition may depend on context-dependent or demonstrative elements, such as recognizing shapes or colours for which one has no prior name. But, if anything, this suggests that one has to be focally aware, not focally ignorant, of them.

Thus Polanyi's own account of the tacit nature of recognition faces objections. But such criticism suggests the possibility of a more minimal account of tacit knowledge. Recognition is tacit because it is a skill—for example, developed through repetition and critical practice and demonstrated in applications—and because it can thus be articulated only in context-dependent terms such as 'like this!'. It cannot be explicated in words alone, independently of additional practical demonstrations in context.

If the skilled diagnostic judgement described in the previous section by Kraus, Maj, and Parnas is thought of as tacit knowledge of the kind just explicated, then it can be contrasted with criteriological diagnosis in the following way. The criteria set out in the ICD and in the *DSM* are an attempt to make psychiatric diagnosis *explicit*, to put it into words alone. They endeavour to set out context-independent descriptions of psychiatric syndromes.

Such an attempt is akin to trying to model an ability to recognize colours and shades on the general knowledge of names for colours that ordinary people have. For most people, the ability to recognize, think about, and recall (at least for some period) particular shades of colour goes beyond what they can make explicit linguistically. The ability can instead be manifested by pointing to particular instances of colour themselves. By contrast with the fine discriminations that can be made in the presence of actual colours and shades, colour *vocabulary* is generally vague.

Similarly, by contrast with the context-dependent discriminations of skilled clinicians that are made in the presence of their patients and clients, the criteria set out in diagnostic manuals are vague. Because they are fully linguistic, the criteria in the *DSM* and in the ICD are portable. There is an advantage to the communication of a linguistic codification of diagnosis that floats free of particular interpersonal relations. But it is bought at the cost of precision. By contrast, the features that play a role in the top-down diagnoses of skilled clinicians are identified in the presence of a particular patient's or client's psychological whole. Such recognition cannot be captured in words alone.

The analogy suggested in this section has been between clinical judgement made possible by the presence of a patient or client and recognition of a macintosh, either as an instance of a kind or as a particular one, or recognition of a colour or shade in its presence. The analogy suggests that the patient herself is passive and plays no active role. Since clinical judgement depends a great deal on what patients say and do, the general picture of tacit knowledge needs augmenting with a specific account of the recognition of mental states. That is the subject of the next section.

5 **Criteria and other minds**

In the previous section I suggested that tacit knowledge can be used to shed light on the idea that an overall top-down or gestalt diagnostic judgement could be more specific than a diagnosis based on general but vague criteria. A skilled clinician has a recognitional skill that can be exemplified only in context-dependent judgements, in the presence of patients or clients. That is to approach the problem from an epistemological perspective: what it is to have knowledge in this way. In this section I will complement the approach by taking an ontological view. What could the relation be between the underlying mental states and conditions that amount to mental illness or disease syndromes and the more apparently epistemically accessible criteria set out in the *DSM* and in the ICD? Addressing this question will also address the active role of patients and clients raised just now.

To sketch an answer, I will consider a debate from the philosophy of mind about whether our knowledge of other minds in general is based on behavioural *criteria*. Although the argument against this view that I will outline does not directly carry over to the case of psychiatric diagnosis, it does suggest why criteriological diagnosis is vague by comparison to top-down or gestalt judgement.

The concept of a criterion was introduced into the philosophy of mind as a solution to the problem of other minds by followers of the philosopher Ludwig Wittgenstein. The influential Wittgenstein exegete P. M. S. Hacker, writing in the *Oxford Companion to Philosophy*, defines a criterion thus:

> A standard by which to judge something; a feature of a thing by which it can be judged to be thus and so. In the writings of the later Wittgenstein it is used as a quasi-technical term. Typically, something counts as a criterion for another thing if it is necessarily good evidence for it. Unlike inductive evidence, criterial support is determined by convention and is partly constitutive of the meaning of the expression for whose

application it is a criterion. Unlike entailment, criterial support is characteristically defeasible. Wittgenstein argued that behavioural expressions of the 'inner', e.g. groaning or crying out in pain, are neither inductive evidence for the mental (Cartesianism), nor do they entail the instantiation of the relevant mental term (behaviourism), but are defeasible criteria for its application. (Hacker 1995, 171)

Key features of this definition are that the criteria of, for example, an 'inner' state like pain are fixed by convention and are partly constitutive of what we mean by the word 'pain'. Thus groaning and crying out are not mere symptoms but rather part of what we understand by 'pain', connected by definition, not by induction. At the same time, however, the criteria of pain are *defeasible*.

The reason for this qualification is the following intuition. While, in general, pain behaviour is the expression of underlying pain, on occasion behaviour that resembles pain behaviour in every detail is not the expression of pain. It may be the result of acting or pretence. (And, equally, genuine underlying pain may sometimes be stoically kept from expression.) As a result, the criterial support that apparent pain behaviour gives for a judgement that someone is in pain is taken to be defeasible. It can, on occasion, be overturned.

The idea that criteria give only defeasible support for a claim is combined with a further assumption, which the philosopher John McDowell, in his criticism of this very notion, describes thus: 'if a condition is ever a criterion for a claim, then any condition of that type constitutes a criterion for that claim, or one suitably related to it' (McDowell 1982, 462–3). In other words, criteria are types. While on most occasions, when instances of some general type of criterion are satisfied, the underlying fact for which those instances are criteria also obtains, on some occasions the type of criterion is satisfied (by some particular circumstances) but the fact does not obtain. In such cases, the criterion is satisfied but is nevertheless also defeated.

This suggests that there is an essential underdeterminination in the support that criteria, so understood, provide for judgements about mental states. In any particular case, on this picture, some expression, some sign or symptom of pain for example, may or may not actually *mean* that the person expressing it is actually in pain. Hence the behavioural expression is vague. Its meaning is imprecise.

This worry provides the basis for McDowell's criticism of the use of criteria, understood in this way, to explain how knowledge of other minds is possible. On the assumption that it is possible, at least sometimes, to know someone else's mental state, McDowell asks how such knowledge is supposed to be based 'on an experiential intake that falls short of the fact known . . . in the sense [of] . . . being compatible with there being no such fact' (ibid., 459).

The worry is this. If one knows something, then it cannot be the case that—'for all one knows'—things may be otherwise. That possibility is ruled out precisely because one *knows* what is the case. But if criteria fall short of implying the fact that they are supposed to enable one to know, then they cannot themselves rule out the possibility that the fact does not obtain. So, if our everyday concept of knowledge *does* rule this out, then such knowledge cannot be based on perception that the criteria for some mental state are satisfied. A possible alternative view in which the perceived criteria are supposed merely to be sufficient to satisfy linguistic *conventions* for the *ascription* of knowledge would not address this objection either.

> If experiencing the satisfaction of 'criteria' does legitimise ('criterially') a claim to know that things are thus and so, it cannot also be legitimate to admit that the position is one in which, for all one knows, things may be otherwise. But the difficulty is to see how the fact that 'criteria' are defeasible can be prevented from compelling that admission; in which case we can conclude, by contraposition, that experiencing the satisfaction of 'criteria' cannot legitimize a claim of knowledge. How can appeal to 'convention' somehow drive a wedge between accepting that everything that one has is compatible with things not being so, on the one hand, and admitting that one does not know that things are so, on the other? (Ibid., 458)

Imagine that there are two observers who both see that the behavioural criteria, so construed, for two other people's being in pain are satisfied but that only one of them really is in pain: the other is pretending. If the observers' experiences are the only grounds for their knowing the mental state of their respective subject, and if their perceptions are the same in both cases (seeing that the criteria for pain are met), then how can one observer know his or her subject's mental state and the other observer not? Surely, neither has *knowledge*, even if one has, by chance, a true belief. It seems merely a matter of luck that one observer's experience is of undefeated criteria while the other's is of defeated criteria, that in one case the observed subject really is in pain and in the other merely pretending. The luckier observer has done nothing extra to earn the right to knowledge. Construing criteria as defeasible in order to try to accommodate the fact that we are fallible at knowing other people's minds cannot work, because it rules out that we ever have knowledge.

There is, however, an alternative view of criteria and of knowledge of other minds that is based on them. Rather than assuming that, in the case of pretence, the criteria for mental states are satisfied but are also defeated—given that it is a case of pretence—one can instead construe pretence as a case of the criteria only *appearing* to be satisfied. This is a rejection of the idea that criteria are *defeasible types* of situation. Instead, McDowell presses the view that, when criteria are satisfied, one's experience *does not fall short of the facts*. So there cannot be cases where the criteria are satisfied without the fact for which they give criterial support also holding.

McDowell supports this interpretative possibility by considering a passage in which Wittgenstein discusses criteria in a non-mental context:

> The fluctuation in grammar between criteria and symptoms makes it look as if there were nothing at all but symptoms. We say, for example: 'Experience teaches that there is rain when the barometer falls, but it also teaches that there is rain when we have certain sensations of wet and cold, or such-and-such visual impressions.' In defence of this one says that these sense-impressions can deceive us. But here one fails to reflect that the fact that the false appearance is precisely one of rain is founded on a definition. (Wittgenstein 1953, §354)

Wittgenstein rejects the temptation to say that both the fall of a barometer and the sensations of wet and cold (or the visual impressions) are mere *symptoms* of rain. Instead, and by contrast with the barometer fall, the connection between the sensations (or the visual impressions) and rain is definitional or criterial. They are used in an explanation of what 'rain' means. This thought can, however, be interpreted in two ways:

> Commentators often take this to imply that when our senses deceive us, criteria for rain are satisfied, although no rain is falling. But what the passage says is surely just this: for things, say, to look a certain way to us is, as a matter of 'definition' (or 'convention' . . .), for it to look to us as though it is raining; it would be a mistake to suppose that the 'sense-impressions' yield the judgement that it is raining merely symptomatically—that arriving at the judgement is mediated by an empirical theory. That is quite compatible with this thought . . . when our 'sense-impressions' deceive us, the fact is not that criteria for rain are satisfied but that they *appear* to be satisfied. (McDowell 1982, 466)

Someone who steps outside his house when the lawn sprinklers are switched on may think that by having experiences of wet and cold he has experienced the criteria for rain, albeit on this occasion defeated. After all, when being taught about rain, he may have been taught it through practical definitions involving experiences that felt similar. But the experiences used in the practical definition were not just any experiences of wet and cold; they were wet and cold experiences of falling rain. Similarly, in the case of criteria for mental states, pretence can make it *seem* that the criteria for pain, for example, are satisfied when in fact they are not.

Taking the criteria to be merely *any* experience of wet and cold (for rain) or *any* experience of high-pitched cries (for pain) makes them too vague to sustain knowledge. Correcting this requires rethinking the generality and the descriptive nature of criteria. If the criteria for pain are given in general and behavioural terms, they are too vague to underpin knowledge. Such 'criteria' do not only *mean* pain. So one might think of them as particular, though still behavioural. If so, only particular instances of behavioural criteria (particular instances of crying out and rubbing knees, etc.) are valid guides to underlying pain. Such a suggestion maintains the behavioural character of criteria for mental states but denies their generality. But this threatens the idea that one can learn how to recognize pain. The alternative is to maintain (something of) their generality but deny the restriction to merely behavioural signs and symptoms. On such an account, the criteria for pain do not have in common anything that could be given in mind-free behavioural terms. Rather they share the essentially mind-involving generality of being *expressions of pain*.

McDowell offers a philosophical diagnosis of why such a view of criteria seems to go unnoticed that goes back to the influence of Cartesian dualism. If one starts from that basic picture, then that picture invites a contrast between behavioural states of other people, to which one can have direct perceptual access, and mental states, which are, in some sense, hidden behind them. According to Descartes, they even exist in different kinds of space (*res cogitans* and *res extensa*). Cartesian dualism suggests an alienated picture of human behaviour in which all that anyone else can ever see is bodily movement, which is only contingently associated with minds. Because perception of, and judgements about, such 'behaviour' are taken to be unproblematic while access to other people's *mental* states is taken to be problematic, a route is needed from one to the other. Thus it seems plausible to think that judgements about mental states have to be grounded in independent judgements about behaviour. The alienated picture of human behaviour survives in approaches to the philosophy of mind that have long since rejected Descartes' conception of the mind as *res cogitans* (or thinking stuff) existing in a different dimension from matter (*res extensa*).

This picture of the relation of mind and body is neither obligatory nor natural, however. One can instead think of mind and body as more closely linked. What one says and does *expresses* what one thinks and feels. While one person's mental states do not themselves fall within the direct experience of another, that person's expression of her mental state does. Such expression is *not* one that is consistent with the *absence* of the inner state. So McDowell replaces an account in which all that is visible to an observer is another person's intrinsically brute or meaningless behaviour, which stands in need of further interpretation and hypothesis, with one in which that behaviour is charged with expression.

This claim addresses the worry, raised at the end of the previous section, that an analogy with the tacit recognitional judgement of a macintosh or of a shade of colour suggests that patients and clients are passive in the face of a clinical gaze. If the analogy held closely, then one person's mental state would have to fall directly within the experience of another, just as a colour can. The nuanced view is that this is not so. Patients and clients have to reveal their mental states through speech and action. But, to continue to describe the nuanced view, what they say and do makes their mental lives available to others in a way that requires no inference. This account adds to the more general picture of tacit knowledge given in the previous section the further idea that recognitional judgement of others' mental states requires that the other people actively express them.

By denying that our 'access' to the minds of others must proceed through a neutrally described behavioural intermediary (their behaviour), McDowell can offer a much less technically charged account of criteria, which he summarizes thus:

> I think we should understand criteria to be, in the first instance, ways of telling how things are, of the sort specified by 'On the basis of what he says and does' or 'By how things look'; and we should take it that knowledge that a criterion for a claim is actually satisfied—if we allow ourselves to speak in those terms as well—would be an exercise of the very capacity we speak of when we say that one can tell, on the basis of such-and-such criteria, whether things are as the claim would represent them as being. (McDowell 1982, 470–1)

Knowledge of other minds depends on what people say and do. It does not require a kind of direct mind reading. The judgement is based on, emerges from, what they say and do. But the conceptualization of what they say and do need not be couched in mind-independent neutral terms. As Dowell comments:

> This flouts an idea we are prone to find natural, that a basis for a judgement must be something on which we have firmer cognitive purchase than we do on the judgement itself; but although the idea can seem natural, it is an illusion to suppose it is compulsory. (Ibid., 471)

It may be easier to see patterns and generalities in behaviour construed as essentially expressive of minds than in neutrally described bodily movement. So, even though judgements about others' minds may be based on their behaviour, the description of the behaviour may be less secure than the description of what it expresses.

I have set out two contrasting accounts of criteria from the philosophical discussion of the problem of other minds in order to shed light on the more specific issue of mental illness diagnosis. There are, however, two related important differences between the two cases, and they need mention.

First, the application of the idea of criteria to the more general problem of other minds and to the case of psychiatric diagnosis differs in one clear respect. It is merely a theoretical idea in the former case, but it is set out in practical detail in recent editions of the *DSM* and versions of the ICD in the latter case. Second, and related to this, is an important difference in the dialectical context of criticism of behavioural criteria in the two cases. The argument above assumes that it is possible to have knowledge of other minds. Since the standard model of criteria (as defeasible behavioural types) makes knowledge impossible, it cannot be the basis of our knowledge of other minds.

But one might object that psychiatry does not aspire to *knowledge* when it comes to diagnosis, but to some weaker state, such as a belief with a particular degree of probability. And, hence, an argument that shows that knowledge cannot be based on criteria, so understood, need not undermine that project. Such an objection carries risk, however. Since psychiatry is a practical discipline, diagnoses form the basis for action (concerning treatment and management). Thus clinicians need more than merely having beliefs with a particular (suitably high) probability of being true; they need to know that they have beliefs with such probabilities.

Nevertheless, even if psychiatric diagnosis need not aspire to knowledge itself but merely to some known probability of being correct, it could be based on criteria understood as behavioural types (i.e. the target of the criticism in this section). Provided that there are other methods of arriving at diagnoses, such as the considered judgement of skilled clinicians or longitudinal studies, it would be possible to make an assessment of the sensitivity and specificity—in probabilistic terms—of types of behavioural criteria. The dialectical context differs for defenders of defeasible criteria for knowledge of other minds, because they assume that there is no more fundamental way of having such knowledge, and hence no independent test of the construct validity of the criteria.

Despite these differences, McDowell's discussion of the two accounts of criteria and of the role, in the account he defends, of the idea that behaviour can directly express mental states explains the relative vagueness of criteriological diagnosis by comparison to the specificity of gestalt judgement. Both the *DSM* and the ICD stress operationalized descriptions as opposed to more essentially psychiatric descriptions couched in aetiological terms. They do this in an attempt to provide secure foundations for diagnosis. But that very strategy makes the criteria mere approximations of the underlying psychopathological states they aim to capture. As Kraus, Maj, and Parnas suggest, precision requires thinking of psychiatric symptoms as abstractions from a diagnostic whole rather than built up from neutral—or more neutral—criteria whose obtaining does not strictly imply the presence of the psychiatric syndrome for which they are supposed to be signs.

An alternative view of diagnostic criteria, drawing on McDowell's account and influenced by the empirical claims of Kraus, Maj, and Parnas, would stress the specific schizophrenic colouring of particular delusions, for example. It may seem that this carries the risk that identifying that a patient or client is experiencing such a delusion is riskier than making the vaguer claim that he or she is experiencing some sort of delusion or other. But this may not be so in context. In particular cases, the justification for thinking that the delusion carries a specific schizophrenic colouring may be what warrants the more general claim that the patient in question is thus experiencing some more general category of delusion.

This view also helps address a suggestion in Kraus' and Parnas' description mentioned earlier: that the connection between symptoms and psychopathological state is more direct than a mere evidential or causally indicating relation. The state is expressed directly in signs and symptoms, at least for those with the skill to see it. On the view developed above, skilled clinicians do not merely infer the diagnostic state of their patients and clients from signs and symptoms that are independent of or distinct from them. Rather they see (or hear), in what their patients say and do, the expression of a diagnostic condition.

It is natural to object to such a view (as the editors of this book did) that clinicians are fallible beings too, and so the shortcoming of the criteriological approach cannot be that criteria do not strictly imply the presence of what they are criteria for. But, on the view sketched, this objection presupposes the wrong account of the fallibility of such judgements. If criteria for mental illnesses were both general and defeasible, that would explain how knowledge claims could fail; but it would also fail to explain how knowledge is ever possible. On the alternative view sketched above, when all goes well, a skilled clinician is able to respond to the expressions of, say, schizophrenia that do indeed necessitate that the patient has schizophrenia. Fallibility is explained by the fact that some apparent criteria for schizophrenia are not in fact such criteria. But it is a mistake to assume that the best that even a skilled clinician can rely on is a description of the signs and symptoms that merely indicates that it is likely that someone has that syndrome.

6 Conclusions

I have considered the charge, made against criteriological models of diagnosis, that, by comparison with the gestalt judgement of a skilled clinician, criteriological descriptions of symptoms are essentially vague. I have argued that two independently plausible considerations help explain how this could be so. Epistemologically, diagnosis based on gestalt judgement could be akin to the kind of context-dependent practical skill that underpins one model of tacit knowledge. Such skill resists codification in general context-independent terms akin to the *DSM*'s and the ICD's diagnostic criteria, but is nevertheless a form of conceptually structured knowledge. Ontologically, the diagnostic criteria of the *DSM* and ICD may be more or less behavioural abstractions from underlying psychological reality. Skilled clinicians need not rely on neutral criteria, but on the direct expression of complex psychological wholes.

Acknowledgement

This chapter was written while I was a fellow of the Institute for Advanced Study (IAS), University of Durham. My thanks both to the IAS and to the University of Central Lancashire for granting me research leave.

References

APA (American Psychiatric Association). 2013. *Diagnostic and Statistical Manual of Mental Disorders, Fifth Edition: DSM-5*. Washington, DC: American Psychiatric Association.

Bridgman, P. W. 1927. *The Logic of Modern Physics*. New York, NY: Macmillan.

Fulford, K. W. M., Thornton, T., and Graham, G. 2006. *The Oxford Textbook of Philosophy and Psychiatry*. Oxford: Oxford University Press.

Hacker, P. M. S. 1995. 'Criterion'. In *Oxford Companion to Philosophy*, edited by T. Honderich, p. 171. Oxford: Oxford University Press.

Hempel, C. G. 1994. 'Fundamentals of taxonomy'. In *Philosophical Perspectives on Psychiatric Diagnostic Classification*, edited by J. S. Sadler, O. P. Wiggins, and M. A. Schwartz, pp. 315–31. Baltimore, MD: Johns Hopkins University Press.

Kraus, A. 1994. 'Phenomenological and criteriological diagnosis: Different or complementary?'. In *Philosophical Perspectives on Psychiatric Diagnostic Classification*, edited by J. S. Sadler, O. P. Wiggins, and M. A. Schwartz, pp. 148–62. Baltimore, MD: Johns Hopkins University Press.

McDowell, J. 1982. 'Criteria, defeasibility and knowledge'. *Proceedings of the British Academy* 68: 455–79.

Maj, M. 1998. 'Critique of the DSM-IV operational diagnostic criteria for schizophrenia'. *The British Journal of Psychiatry* 172: 458–60.

Parnas, J. 2011. 'A disappearing heritage: The clinical core of schizophrenia'. *Schizophrenia Bulletin* 37: 1121–30.

Polanyi, M. 1962. *Personal Knowledge*. Chicago, IL: University of Chicago Press.

Polanyi, M. 1967. *The Tacit Dimension*. Chicago, IL: University of Chicago Press.

Thornton, T. 2013. 'Clinical judgment, tacit knowledge, and recognition in psychiatric diagnosis'. In *The Oxford Handbook of Philosophy and Psychiatry*, edited by K. W. M. Fulford et al., pp. 1047–62. Oxford: Oxford University Press.

Wittgenstein, L. 1953. *Philosophical Investigations*. Oxford: Blackwell.

Chapter 7

Fuzzy boundaries and tough decisions in psychiatry

Hanfried Helmchen

1 Introduction

Physicians are constantly confronted with fuzzy boundaries. Their recognition of the need for sharp boundaries in making their decisions is often all the greater, the higher the pressures and the broader the boundary zones they face in their work. I will illustrate this using specific examples of diagnostic and therapeutic situations in my own field of psychiatry, problematize the respective and necessary boundary determinations, and finally draw some conclusions about those determinations.

2 Diagnostics

2.1 Recognizing an illness

When people feel unwell, some attribute it to fluctuations in the conditions of normal life, while others take it as a sign of illness and feel sick. People will come to feel sick that much sooner, the longer the condition persists and the less they are able to find an obvious explanation for it in the circumstances of their lives. People who feel sick go to the doctor. And, if a doctor's findings deviate from the physical or mental norm in a way that explains the discomfort, they will speak of an illness. Even in this most basic form, the process of recognizing an illness is characterized by a number of imprecisions, such as:

1. Individuals experience and value discomfort in different ways.

2. Their subjective interpretation is partly influenced by the intensity, changing duration, and inexplicability of the discomfort.

3. The individually specific intensity of suffering and the availability of a doctor determine when medical assistance will be sought.

4. The doctor's examination reveals, to some degree, a deviation from the norm; assessing that deviation will be that much more difficult, the less intensely

and the more slowly it evolves, that is, the less distinctly it contrasts with its context.

5. As soon as this deviation from the norm, as assessed by the physician, crosses a certain threshold and thereby satisfies an established disease criterion, the doctor can make a diagnosis.

It is worth noting that this assessment is as valid for psychiatry as it is for radiology, although radiology involves the use of apparently unequivocal and objective images, whereas psychiatry deals with what seems to be less stringent phenomena that extend across the threshold of normalcy, such as depressed mood.

This fundamental vagueness of diagnostic practice is complicated by the conceptual vagueness of disease concepts, as illustrated by the following questions:

1. Is a condition that deviates from the norm a disease or just a process that leads to this deviation? Specifically, are people with stable deviations from the norm, such as a congenital physical handicap or residual conditions of traumatic injury or illness, sick?

2. Are people who experience no discomfort sick if they have high blood pressure, or if they are taking preventative anti-hypertension medication for hypertonic secondary diseases, or if they are taking long-term, symptom-suppressing medication for schizophrenia or manic relapses?

3. Are people sick if they have neither symptoms nor complaints, but do have a preclinically or even prenatally determined pathogenic gene, such as a Huntington gene?

4. Are people whose indisposition cannot be explained in terms of an abnormal somatic process mentally ill? Are we dealing with simple discontent about the misery of life or with depression?

In spite of the ambiguity and vagueness evoked by these questions, doctors must determine whether an illness is present or not. For that determination establishes not just whether and how treatment will be administered, but also whether the patient is eligible for receiving public assistance. In arriving at their determination, doctors rely on certain signs of illness that, on the basis of experience, have been established as criteria for specific diseases and associated with specific diagnoses. But this involves established conventions that, by definition, remove the phenomena from their contexts. The following examples are intended to illustrate these fuzzy boundaries of lifeworld phenomena and how their resolution through clearer boundary demarcation facilitates decision-making.

2.2 **Reaching a diagnosis**

Contemporary diagnostic systems—either the international ICD-10 (International Statistical Classification of Diseases and Related Health

Problems) or the American *DSM-IV/DSM-5* (*Diagnostic and Statistical Manual of Mental Disorders*; see APA 2013)—link every diagnosis to diagnostic criteria. Based as it is on scientific and empirically grounded evidence, this link captures a substantial portion of the morbidity, but not all of it. The remaining morbidity, which cannot be grasped by operationalized methodologies, is labeled 'subthreshold'. In the literature, it is also termed 'subdiagnostic', 'subclinical' (i.e. mainly outpatient), 'subsyndromal' (because it can arise during the course of an explicit syndrome), and, in ICD-10 and *DSM-IV*, 'not otherwise specified' (NOS). We turn briefly to some of the problems in this diagnostically vague boundary space between health and sickness.

2.2.1 Definition of subthreshold mental illnesses

Subthreshold mental illnesses can be defined as illnesses that are too *mild* and/or too *short-term* to cross the commonly accepted threshold of diagnoses operationalized on the basis of the *number* and *duration* of symptoms (i.e. on the basis of diagnostic criteria); in other words they are illnesses that lie *below* this threshold.

And so, for example in *DSM-IV*, a case of relapsing, brief, depressive episodes is still classified as an 'unspecified depressive disorder' (APA 2000, 311), that is, as subthreshold, because with a duration of less than two weeks it does not fulfil the temporal criteria for depressive episodes. But because these short episodes can attain the same intensity and, depending on their frequency, cause the same degree of incapacitation and loss of quality of life as cases of depression of longer duration (Angst et al. 2006), they have been ranked as a specific diagnosis (F 38.10) within ICD-10 and hence have become 'suprathreshold'.

Subthreshold mental illnesses manifest prodromal, intermittent, and residual conditions of well-known mental illnesses or accompanying ('comorbid') syndromes of other mental or physical illnesses. They appear to be fairly common[1]

---

[1] Epidemiological studies have shown that subthreshold mental illnesses, especially in the realm of affective disorders (depression, anxiety, phobia), occur across all age groups and are between twice and four times more common than illnesses with specific diagnoses. For example, the Berlin Aging Study (BASE) found subthreshold depression in 17.8% of the sample and suprathreshold depression in 9.1% (Helmchen et al. 1999). The tendency of subthreshold depression to appear before and after major depressive episodes reflects the cross-sectional character of spectrum disorders. They often arise in combination with somatic illnesses, comprising 20–50% of older patients hospitalized for such conditions, and above all, it seems, when these illnesses compromise their ability to function physically and socially (see Angst 2007; Angst, Sellaro, and Merikangas 2000; Angst et al. 2006; Helmchen 2001; Wittchen, Nelson, and Lachner 1998).

and have serious consequences in terms of individual suffering and economic wherewithal.

2.2.2. Problems with the threshold

The diagnostic threshold described in 2.2.1 is clearly defined and therefore reliable in both ICD-10 and *DSM-IV*, but it is hardly valid, as illustrated by the discrepancies between the two diagnostic systems at the margins: for example, the diagnosis of neurasthenia remains in the ICD-10 but no longer features in *DSM-IV*.

Differences in the diagnostic thresholds used for individual diagnoses arise because their determination depends on the relationship between sensitivity and specificity—a relationship that professional organizations have judged to be optimal in minimizing both false positive and false negative cases. High thresholds result in high specificity, but also in many false negative cases. Low thresholds lead to higher sensitivity, but also to many false positive cases.

Summing up the symptomatology of neurasthenia, Simon Wessely remarked that 'in general . . . neurasthenic subjects experience more psychiatric distress than normal subjects, but less than those with well-defined psychiatric disorders such as depression. On the other hand, they usually score as highly, and occasionally higher, on measures of somatic symptoms' (Wessely 2001, 124–5). Although neurasthenia, given the relatively modest expression and specificity of its symptoms, is often deemed to be merely a subthreshold mental disorder, the level of suffering and functional constriction is often so great that people suffering from it insist on intervention, that is, frequently use medical services and hence cover increased costs.

The specific diagnostic assessment of neurasthenia is perhaps influenced more strongly by the cultural context. The influence of a zeitgeist can be clearly detected in neurasthenia's prominence in the early Soviet Union and in Mao's China, perhaps because these cultures allowed mental disorders to be socially accepted as somatic illnesses (Lee 1998). The effects of sociocultural influences can also be witnessed in the fact that the symptoms of Chinese Americans in Los Angeles who were diagnosed with neurasthenia could not be distinguished from the chronic fatigue syndrome diagnosed in Caucasian Angelinos/as, although the explanations given by each group for their illness were very different (Lin et al. 1996).

2.2.3. Problems with the concept of 'disease'

The threshold we have been considering can also be understood as a boundary between sickness and questionable sickness. But it is more important and difficult to determine a second threshold between subthreshold morbidity and non-morbid discomfort, namely the threshold between sickness and health. Determining this threshold remains a vexing problem. And this problem is embedded in an ongoing debate over the term 'disease' that is characterized by the dualities of natural versus normative implications, of objectifiable disease versus subjective illness, of statistical versus individual norms, of general versus specific concepts of disease (Helmchen 2006).

It is not possible to delve more deeply into these extensive, complex, and unresolved issues. What is clear, however, is that a general, comprehensive definition of either 'disease' or 'health' is problematic and that, as an aid to decision-making, no definition is practical, scientifically grounded, and non-tautological. We can be certain, however, that there often exists a broad threshold between sickness and health and that on this threshold the boundary between them cannot be definitively established, either on the basis of biomedical facts or on the basis of fundamental values shared by patients, doctors, and society. Ultimately we need to hone our criteria so that, in the diagnostic boundaryzone between sickness and health, we may be able to distinguish the early or late stages of a disease from discomforts and day-to-day problems that should not be assessed as diseases (Helmchen 2001). The criterion of 'inability' [*Nichtkönnen*] is especially significant here. In cases of socially (or in the broadest sense biologically) abnormal behaviour, one's inability will ultimately be accepted as grounds for medical (and financial) assistance only if at the very least it can be attributed to a specific (psychiatric) disease.

The inherent danger of circular reasoning can be avoided by understanding the inability to do otherwise as an indicator of potential illness that prompts one to search for specific symptoms of disease. For in modern welfare states, identifying a disease is a prerequisite for legitimate claims to support from the public health system. For this reason, the term 'disease' could acquire greater significance in contemporary reform debates, once the growing burden on social safety nets forces governments to impose greater restrictions on access to public assistance by insisting that disorders meet the criteria for being a disease.

The importance of these evaluations is especially evident in cases where patients' (neurotic) unwillingness [*Nichtwollen*] remains hidden to them and is experienced as inability [*Nichtkönnen*]. From the perspective of 'asylum psychiatry' in Germany, milder forms of mental illness were, traditionally, not a priority; for a long time psychiatrists were loath to recognize them as diseases (Kendell 1975), and above all tended to reject psychodynamic interpretations of them as 'neuroses'. But today psychiatrists assess these behavioural and experience-based disorders as diseases. However, psychologists like Eysenck viewed them not so much as diseases, but rather as behavioural disorders[2]

---

[2] This is one reason why one should be sceptical about applying the term 'disorder' to all mental illnesses, as seems to be the case in the term's use in contemporary diagnostic classification systems such as ICD-10 and *DSM-IV/DSM 5*.

acquired through a learning process and therefore better understood and treated by psychologists than by physicians (Eysenck 1960). Accordingly, in the German Bundestag hearings on the first draft of a psychotherapist law in 1980, health insurance agencies still refused to cover psychotherapeutic interventions, arguing that it was impossible to do this as long as no criteria existed for distinguishing between an illness and life's daily challenges. Today 'neuroses' are recognized in law as illnesses, patients have a right to be treated for them, and health insurance agencies have provisions for their treatment. With passage of the Psychotherapist Law in 1998, psychotherapeutic psychologists were recognized as an independent class of therapists. The recognition of 'neuroses' as curable illnesses enabled treatment to be paid for by the national health insurance agencies (Helmchen 2003).

2.2.4. The necessity of physicians' decisions

In spite of this unsatisfactory state of the theoretical basis for disease concepts, the practitioner must decide whether or not the individual patient is sick. To this end, the doctor uses an empirically tested, pragmatic procedure. Anamnesis and catamnesis allow for an initial assessment of intraindividual changes; in most cases of qualitatively abnormal symptoms, such as the hallucinations or delusions of people with psychosis, the commonly used categorical evaluation (yes/no) will suffice. But this approach is less successful in cases that exhibit constantly fluctuating variables such as mood and impulses, for example in 'neuroses' or personality disorders; hence a dimensional assessment (more/less) is advisable. This assessment uses thresholds (cut-off values) of expressed intensity, in an attempt to translate quantitative findings into qualitative categories. Finally, doctors employ traditional methods of clinical assessment (see Table 7.1).

Table 7.1 Criteria for the clinical evaluation of subthreshold mental illnesses

---

- ◆ Anamnesis: with episodes of specific 'supra'threshold mental illnesses
- ◆ Findings: with symptoms of specific 'supra'threshold mental illnesses
- ◆ Symptoms (*objective* meaning): with consequences for
  1. Performance
  2. Ability to work (absenteeism)
  3. Social relationships
  4. Quality of life
- ◆ Suffering (*subjective* meaning)
- ◆ Therapeutic need: for example according to the Global Assessment of Functioning Scale (GAF)

2.3 **Consequences of diagnostic decisions**

Here we must consider both the medical and the health policy consequences.

In *medical* terms, drawing diagnostic boundaries too narrowly does not adequately reflect significant aspects of medical treatment and care, because subthreshold mental disorders complicate other mental and somatic illnesses: they tend to lengthen the duration of somatic illnesses through complications and delayed remission; and they also increase the risk of chronicity, disability, and unemployability. But, even in the absence of other somatic diseases, mental illnesses themselves compromise our quality of life by reducing productivity, debasing our sense of self, isolating us from our social communities, and exposing us to the risk of suicide.

In terms of *heathcare policy*, subthreshold mental illnesses contribute to higher financial costs (as much as 35 percent) due to longer hospital stays (Levenson, Hamer, and Rossiter 1990) and greater demand for medical services.

For example, English researchers found that the risk of becoming unable to work was 4.8 times higher among clear-cut cases of depression and 1.5 times higher among cases of subthreshold depression. But because cases of subthreshold depression are much more common, they cause 51 percent more days of sick leave (Broadhead et al. 1990). Furthermore, these patients take relatively more time to treat: the researchers estimated that, although comprising only about 15 percent of general practitioners' caseload, they occupied between 25 and 30 percent of their time.

These higher costs include the costs of not recognizing and treating subthreshold morbidity, that is, the costs of early, residual, and attending (co-morbid) illnesses. At the same time, however, it is likely that the development, implementation, and improvement of prophylactic and early detection procedures, as well as the treatment of subthreshold morbidity, will also contribute to higher costs. And it is unclear which costs will be higher. Therefore further research on this question is needed.

But, in terms of healthcare policy, we must consider not just the financial costs, but also the potential social costs, especially of too broadly defined diagnoses, such as it was to be feared for some diagnoses by the introduction of *DSM* 5 (Frances 2013; see also Chapter 8). Heightened awareness of subthreshold (mental) illnesses runs the risk of unwarranted concerns about illness, of psychiatrization, and of stigmatization (Magruder and Calderone 2000; Sartorius 2007), such as when normal grieving is too quickly interpreted as depression, an occasional 'benign' forgetfulness as 'Alzheimer's', turbid or contradictory thoughts as schizophrenia.

Thus doctors and society are confronted by the uncertainty of whether recognizing subliminal morbidity or failing to recognize it—let alone refusing to recognize it—will impose more substantial costs on society.

3 **Therapy**

3.1 **Treating the sick**

Like the diagnostic process, the physician's therapeutic actions are impeded by vagueness. And this vagueness is comprised of

1. the merely partial fitness of a specific therapy for a specific illness, that is, the only approximately specific clarity of the indication; and

2. the evaluation of the effectiveness of the therapy for each individual patient.

In spite of considerable success in reducing this vagueness through standardized procedures that involve the evidence-based acquisition and algorithmic application of knowledge, at the individual level this vagueness can only be reduced, not eliminated. For it is the doctor who selects a therapy and assesses its results. That selection is based on

1. the doctor's awareness of *state-of-the-art knowledge* about the specific effectiveness of the treatment;

2. the doctor's experience and acquaintance with the *individual* patient;

3. and, not least today—especially given alternative forms of treatment—the *patient's decisions*.

Therapy must therefore remain individualized, because only doctors sufficiently familiar with their patients are in a position to choose the appropriate therapy. Likewise, the assessment of any specific treatment rests on an understanding of the effects of treatment on the individual patient. And those effects are influenced by the subjective perceptions of both the patient and the doctor. Maintaining individualized therapies is also necessary because vagueness, in spite of our best efforts to reduce it, cannot be completely eliminated. We can illustrate this by considering the most important methods used by doctors to reduce vagueness, namely evidence-based intervention and algorithmization.

3.1.1. Evidence-based intervention

Evidence-based intervention means that the potential usefulness or harmfulness of any given medical procedure will be evaluated according to standardized techniques adopted from the current scientific literature. Such an evaluation draws only on publications that qualitatively satisfy established criteria. The evaluation produces different categories regarding the reliability of assertions and the articulation of advantages and disadvantages. The categories are distinguished by different criteria: for example,[3] the reliability of an assertion is categorized on the basis of 'evidence', 'sign', 'no sign', 'to little data', or the degree of effectiveness is categorized quantitatively, on the basis of effective intensity or scaled scores. Definitions of such criteria, for example setting a specific scalar value as a threshold, are determinations that can be changed in order to account for different stages of a continually changing phenomenon, for example the slow remission of a depressive mood. Assessing effectiveness—in other words, the therapeutic response or results—is difficult if the effects are small. Moreover, the boundary into therapeutic ineffectiveness or non-response is often rather imprecise. Ultimately it all becomes a matter of assessing improvement, that is, a more or less continual change in the desired direction between the poles of 'healthy again' (or at least symptom-free) and 'still sick' or unimproved, or even deteriorated (Gaebel 2004). In this regard, determining a threshold is at once influenced by implicit normativity (Strech 2007) and dependent on the use to which that threshold is put: to establish the effectiveness of a new drug, a 50 percent reduction of the symptom score can suffice; but, for patients, only the absence of discomfort and a 100 percent symptom reduction is likely to be satisfactory.

3.1.2. Algorithmization

By algorithmization I mean the standardization of procedures. For example, in the hospital, I implemented a multistep plan for the treatment of depression once the doctors who treated the patients believed they had noticed improvements that I could not observe, given that I saw these patients only once every two weeks. For doctors on the wards, who work with their patients on a daily basis, the frustrating ineffectiveness of their therapeutic efforts can be especially difficult to bear and the impression that patients have improved can sometimes be wishful thinking.

The multistep plan therefore involves a qualitative, scaled evaluation of the depression's severity at regular intervals and a change in therapy if a predefined threshold is maintained (Adli et al. 2002; Bauer et al. 2009; Helmchen 1990). But such operationalization of therapeutic procedures encounters resistance from doctors on the wards who see their therapeutic autonomy—their application of general knowledge to the specific situation of their respective individual patients—as being threatened.

In response to these concerns, it should be noted that one can, and indeed must, deviate from the specifications of the multistep plan at any time if this

---

[3] This according to the methodological arsenal of the Institute for Quality and Efficiency in Health Care (IQWIG 2013).

is rationally and plausibly justifiable. But resistance to the algorithms of so-called disease management programs—which health insurance agencies are increasingly offering for chronic diseases—also have other origins: for example, patients participating in a disease management program and for whom an alternative therapy becomes necessary have no legal recourse to ensuring coverage of the program's costs.

Furthermore, criteria designed to reduce vagueness—especially the complex terms used in social security law, such as 'medical usefulness, necessity, and economy'—are themselves ambiguous and frequently subject to interpretive discrepancies.

3.2 Therapeutic interventions in healthy individuals

Finally, we can also consider the fact that in medicine clear boundaries can also become less sharp and more porous, as seen in the growing trend towards applying medical procedures to healthy individuals in order to improve what is perceived to be their inadequate or detrimental selves. I am talking here about the boundary between treating an illness and enhancing perceived deficits in otherwise healthy people. Three examples can help illustrate the difficulties that arise along this boundary:

1. The psychostimulant drug Methylphenidat (Ritalin™) has been used very successfully to treat mainly school children suffering from attention deficit/hyperactivity disorder (ADHD). It has now come to be applied broadly to school-age children without ADHD who are restless or performing poorly; reports indicate that between 10 and 15 percent of healthy US college students take this stimulant in order to enhance their performance (Farah et al. 2004), (Schöne-Seifert and Talbot 2010). These different uses of Ritalin have sparked debate about the boundary between the clear-cut treatment of an illness and the likewise unequivocal misuse of medical therapies, in this case cognitive doping. Indeed, the ethical implications of how we draw this boundary are as varied as the ethical implications of public funding for healthcare are unambiguous (Helmchen 2005).

2. Such boundary questions are also important in surgery. The ability of plastic surgeons to relieve personal suffering by operating in order to correct a bodily defect is certainly impressive. At the same time, however, the surgical aesthetization of the body surface of a healthy individual is highly problematic, in particular if used to mimic what may turn out to be fleeting aesthetic norms, such as lip or breast enlargement and facelifts.

3. Finally, a clear transgression of boundaries from a European perspective is the ritual genital mutilation of healthy girls in some African cultures (Meyer

2007). These operations, which normally have been undertaken by non-professionals, are now increasingly being performed by doctors because parents wish to avoid the complications associated with unqualified practice. But, pressured by cultural norms, parents also believe that they cannot avoid circumcising their daughters without stigmatizing them for a deviation from cultural norms and traditions. One can interpret this as an example of culture determining the boundaries of medical intervention. This boundary is also permeable, as shown by the recent case of the so-called Ashley treatments: American parents wanted to have their severely disabled daughter operated on many times, in order to keep her in a child-like state and hence be able to continue to care for her at home (Gerste 2007).

3.3 The existential meaning of the boundary between health and sickness

Differences between individuals manifest themselves above all in one's personal experience and association with illness, in other words in one's own definition of discomfort as illness: 'It would be much more appropriate [than to follow the WHO definition] to understand human health as the capacity to live with sickness, disability, and death'(Engelhardt 2005). Even though this idea seems to be basically correct—namely that the potential to live a fulfilling and 'good' life in spite of all limitations is one element of being healthy—any definition of health that also incorporates illness is effectively useless. Or at least this is the case in many tangible situations of the modern world, especially when it comes to the right to enjoy solidarity and the support of one's colleagues and compatriots: a person will continue to receive paid sick leave only if a doctor affirms his or her inability to work; only a sick person will have his or her medical bills paid for by national health insurance programs (Helmchen 2003). But in other respects a concept of health that includes illness—and vice versa—is by all means important. This is specifically so with regard to public education's responsibility to ensure that modern people are aware of the vagaries of life and contingent nature of existence and are thereby enabled to cope with sickness, disability, dying, and death on their own terms. Thus the remaining healthy portion of a psychiatric patient's personality is an important point of departure for therapeutic intervention (see Simon 1929).

4 Conclusions

1. There is a wide boundary zone separating what is clearly healthy and what is clearly sick. The transition from health to sickness (and back!) is usually

vague, often slow, and characterized by varying degrees of intensity. The perception of this gradual transition is often diffuse, both from one's own (subjective) and from others' (objective) point of view. Mild signs of illness are often ambiguous, and ambiguity provokes evaluations.

2. And thus, in this boundary zone, prior individual experience as well as normative assumptions determine a demarcation—which, for many reasons, is often necessarily clear-cut. These normative assumptions should be understood as prejudgements, in other words as prior and conventional—that is, automated or fixed—assessments. The demarcation is further determined by 'natural' medical findings and their sociocultural context, including patients' perceptions of those findings and their social consequences (perception of others, claims on public services); in a sociocultural context, the demarcation becomes a convention mutually agreed upon. Our diagnoses are also suppositions or conventions (Vollmöller 1998). Some examples of more or less distinct demarcations are criteria-based diagnostic schemata such as those in the ICD or in the *DSM*, standardized knowledge acquisition in evidence-based medicine, and standardized medical intervention using algorithms, such as disease management programs.

3. Demarcations are the norming of capriciousness, they target arbitrariness. But one must remain cognizant of the fact that norms have been set—and hence of their implicit arbitrariness—in order to avoid the dangers of reification. Here arbitrariness means assessing reality's diversity according to one's own current ideas. This might be optimal in terms of actual behaviour in a specific situation, but inadequate for longer term, less situation-dependent, more or less appropriate and useful assessments.

Establishing norms is a precondition for comparisons that, in turn, relate to issues of quality and justice. Ultimately we require norms for the purpose of orienting our evaluations. But they must not be located so far from reality that they fail to develop sufficient effectiveness. In other words they must apply to a sufficiently large portion of affected people's reality in order to be accepted and adhered to by their majority. Norms must therefore change when the realities of life change. The rate of change must correspond to people's ability to change: if the rate is too slow, that is, if the norms are too rigid, then they lose their ability to influence behaviour; and the same is true if the rate of change is too rapid, because people can then no longer internalize the norms and hence those norms cannot be introjected to influence behaviour. Using normative interventions in human ability in order to adjust the rate at which norms change is an essential function of the law.

Translated from the German by Eric J. Engstrom

Acknowledgement

This chapter is based on the following publication: H. Helmchen. 2007. 'Unscharfe Grenzen und scharfe Grenzsetzungen in der Psychiatrie'. *Die Psychiatrie* 4 (4): 201–8.

References

Adli, M. et al. 2002. 'Effectiveness and feasibility of a standardized stepwise drug treatment regimen algorithm for inpatients with depressive disorders: Results of a 2-year observational algorithm study'. *Journal of Clinical Psychiatry* **63** (9): 782–90.

Angst, J. 2007. 'The bipolar spectrum'. *The British Journal of Psychiatry* **190**: 189–91.

Angst, J., Sellaro, R., and Merikangas, K. R. 2000. 'Depressive spectrum diagnosis'. *Comprehensive Psychiatry* **41** (Suppl. 1): 39–47.

Angst, J. et al. 2006. 'Atypical depressive syndromes in varying definitions'. *European Archives of Psychiatry and Clinical Neuroscience* **256**: 44–54.

APA (American Psychiatric Association). 2000. *Diagnostic and Statistical Manual of Mental Disorders, Fourth Edition, Text Revision: DSM-IV TR*. Washington, DC: American Psychiatric Association.

APA (American Psychiatric Association). 2013. *Diagnostic and Statistical Manual of Mental Disorders, Fifth Edition: DSM-5*. Washington, DC: American Psychiatric Association.

Bauer, M. et al. 2009. 'Efficacy of an algorithm-guided treatment compared with treatment as usual: A randomized, controlled study of inpatients with depression'. *Journal of Clinical Psychopharmacology* **29**: 327–33.

Broadhead, W. E. et al. 1990. 'Depression, disability days, and days lost from work in a prospective epidemiologic study'. *Journal of the American Medical Association* **264**: 2524–8.

Engelhardt, D. v. 2005. 'Schillers Leben mit der Krankheit im Kontext der Pathologie und Therapie um 1800'. In *Schillers Natur. Leben, Denken und literarisches Schaffen*, edited by G. Braungart and B. Greiner, pp. 57–73. Hamburg: Felix Meiner.

Eysenck, H. J. 1960. 'Classification and the problem of diagnosis'. In *Handbook of Abnormal Psychology*, edited by H. J. Eysenck, pp. 1–31. London: Pitman.

Farah, M. J. et al. 2004. 'Neurocognitive enhancement: What can we do and what should we do?' *Nature Reviews Neuroscience* **5**: 421–25.

Frances, A. 2013. 'The new somatic symptom disorder in DSM-5 risks mislabeling many people as mentally ill'. *BMJ* 346. doi: 10.1136/bmj.f1580.

Gaebel, W. 2004. 'Course typologies, treatment principles, and research concepts'. *Pharmacopsychiatry* **37**: 90–7.

Gerste, R. D. 2007. 'Fall Ashley: Ein ethisches Dilemma'. *Deutsches Ärzteblatt* **104**: C84–C85.

Helmchen, H. 1990. 'Gestuftes Vorgehen bei Resistenz gegen Antidepressiva-Therapie'. In *Therapieresistenz unter Antidepressiva-Behandlung*, edited by H. J. Möller, pp. 237–50. Berlin: Springer.

Helmchen, H. 2001. 'Unterschwellige psychische Störungen'. *Der Nervenarzt* **72**: 181–9.

Helmchen, H. 2003. 'Krankheitsbegriff und Anspruch auf medizinische Leistungen'. *Der Nervenarzt* **74**: 395–7.

Helmchen, H. 2005. 'Ethische Herausforderungen der Psychiatrie'. *Journal für Neurologie, Neurochirurgie und Psychiatrie* **6**: 22–8.

Helmchen, H. 2006. 'Zum Krankheitsbegriff in der Psychiatrie'. *Der Nervenarzt* **77**: 271–5.

Helmchen, H. 2007. 'Unscharfe Grenzen und scharfe Grenzsetzungen in der Psychiatrie'. *Die Psychiatrie* **4** (4): 201–8.

Helmchen, H., and Linden, M. 2000. 'Subthreshold disorders in psychiatry: Clinical reality, methodological artifact, and the double-threshold problem'. *Comprehensive Psychiatry* **41** (Suppl. 1): 1–7.

Helmchen, H. et al. 1999. 'Psychiatric illnesses in old age'. In *The Berlin Aging Study. Aging from 70 to 100*, edited by P. B. Baltes and K. U. Mayer, pp. 167–96. Cambridge: Cambridge University Press.

IQWiG (Institut für Qualität und Wirtschaftlichkeit im Gesundheitswesen). 2013. *Allgemeine Methoden*. https://www.iqwig.de/download/IQWiG_Methoden_Version_4-1.pdf (accessed 27 May 2016).

Kendell, R. E. 1975. *The Role of Diagnosis in Psychiatry*. Oxford: Blackwell.

Lee, S. 1998. 'Estranged bodies, simulated harmony, and misplaced cultures: Neurasthenia in contemporary Chinese society'. *Psychosomatic Medicine* **60**: 448–57.

Levenson, J. I., Hamer, R. M., and Rossiter, L. F. 1990. 'Relation of psychopathology in general medical inpatients to use and costs of services'. *The American Journal of Psychiatry* **147**: 1498–503.

Lin, K. et al. 1999. 'A cross cultural study of neurasthenia and CFS in LA'. In *Xth World Congress of Psychiatry, Madrid, 23–28 August 1996*, edited by J. J. Lopez-Ibor et al., pp. 184. Göttingen: Hogrefe & Huber.

Magruder, K. M., and Calderone, G. E. 2000. 'Public health consequences of different thresholds for the diagnosis of mental disorders'. *Comprehensive Psychiatry* **41** (Suppl. 1): 14–18.

Meyer, P. 2007. 'Weibliche Genitalverstümmelung'. *Deutsches Ärzteblatt* **104**, C14–C15.

Sartorius, N. 2007. 'Stigma and mental health'. *The Lancet* **370**: 810–11.

Schöne-Seifert, B., and Talbot, D. 2010. '(Neuro-)enhancement'. In *Ethics in Psychiatry. European Contributions*, edited by H. Helmchen and N. Sartorius, pp. 509–30. Dordrecht: Springer.

Simon, H. 1929. *Aktivere Krankenbehandlung in der Irrenanstalt*. Berlin: De Gruyter.

Strech, D. 2007. 'Vier Ebenen von Werturteilen in der medizinischen Nutzenevaluation: Eine Systematik zur impliziten Normativität in der Evidenz-basierten Medizin'. *Zeitschrift für ärztliche Fortbildung und Qualität im Gesundheitswesen* **101**: 473–80.

Vollmöller, W. 1998. *Was heißt psychisch krank? Der Krankheitsbegriff in Psychiatrie, Psychotherapie und Forensik*. Stuttgart: Kohlhammer.

Wessely, S. 2001. 'Neurasthenia'. In *Contemporary Psychiatry*, edited by F. A. Henn et al., pp. 1935–43. Berlin: Springer.

Wittchen, H. U., Nelson, C. B., and Lachner, G. 1998. 'Prevalence of mental disorders and psychosocial impairments in adolescents and young adults'. *Psychological Medicine* **28**: 109–26.

Chapter 8

Reflections on what is normal, what is not, and fuzzy boundaries in psychiatric classifications

Lara Keuck and Allen Frances

1 Introduction

Diagnostic categories are ubiquitously used. The *Diagnostic and Statistical Manual of Mental Disorders* (*DSM*) provides an authoritative list for diagnosing and labelling mental disorders. In the United States, *DSM* categories can be found in epidemiological statistics, forensics, and research funding applications; doctors are required to use *DSM* classifications when documenting cases and submitting claims for remuneration to medical insurance companies. *DSM* labels have a long life. Having once been diagnosed with a mental disorder can prevent people from acquiring life insurance, adopting a child, or becoming a pilot.

The current re-edition of the *Diagnostic and Statistical Manual of Mental Disorders*, *DSM-5* (APA 2013), has expanded the definition of some of the most widely used psychiatric diagnostic categories, including major depressive disorder and attention deficit hyperactivity disorder, and has introduced new categories that further blur the line between normal and mentally ill, including minor neurocognitive impairment and disruptive mood dysregulation disorder. The experience with expansions of diagnostic categories (autism, attention deficit disorder, bipolar disorder) in *DSM-IV* has shown that definitional changes—and, very importantly, the way diagnostic labels are marketed, enacted, and (mis)used—redefine not only what being mentally ill means but also what remains accepted as normal behaviour. This displacement of normal behaviour can be described as diagnostic inflation (Frances 2013).

The expanded *DSM-IV* definitions have enabled doctors to include people who have heretofore been left out. For many of these new patients, the psychiatric label presumably did more harm than good, with respect to both their immediate reactions to medication and the mediate consequences that psychiatric diagnosis and treatment had on them. The pharmaceutical industry has profited from an enormous increase in sales, while at the same time the monetary and non-monetary public health costs as well as the often adverse societal and individual consequences have multiplied (see e.g. Moynihan and Henry 2006).

Using the lens of *DSM* definitional changes and their major impact on personal lives, psychiatry, and society, we want to revisit the question of what is normal and what is not. We provide examples from psychiatric practice and arguments from the philosophy of medicine to show what functions are served by reflection on what should and what should not be the target of psychiatric classifications. In doing so, we acknowledge that diagnostic labels unfold a reality of their own and that a critical examination of how this reality maps onto the world we want to live in is not only an issue of academic discourse in and about psychiatry, but also one relevant to society at large.

Therefore, when we argue that 'psychiatry' should be aware of the implications that concepts of the normal, the not normal, and the in-between have, we are addressing not only people within the institutionalized profession of clinical psychiatry and its societies, such as the American Psychiatric Association (APA), funding agencies like the National Institute of Mental Health, and *DSM* task forces, but also therapists and primary care physicians, public and corporate researchers, insurance companies, policy makers, other users and makers of psychiatric diagnoses, and beyond.

Against this backdrop, the main part of the chapter is devoted to reflections on 'the normal' (section 2), the 'not normal' (section 3), the 'in-between' (section 4), and 'diagnostic inflation' (section 5). We conclude with some suggestions on how the present use(s) of classification systems and the processes involved in their future revision might be enhanced in terms of doing more good than harm (section 5).

2 Reflections on the normal

Saving the normal and saving psychiatry are two sides of the same coin (Frances 2013). This implies a normative answer to a normative question. Psychiatry *should* care about the normal, because psychiatry's goal *should* be to help those who require treatment and to do no harm by exposing the worried well to the unwanted side effects of psychiatric diagnosis and treatment. These harms include, for instance, addiction, misuse or even lethal overdosing of prescription drugs, and misallocation of human and monetary resources. These harms have created considerable public health problems. For instance, in 2011, the Centers for Disease Control and Prevention noted that there were more deaths in the US due to prescription painkillers than to heroin and cocaine combined (CDC 2011).

The crucial point is that the toolkit of psychiatry is not per se good or bad. It can be of great help in some circumstances and of great harm in others. Just as a knife can be used to cut bread or to cut a throat, a diagnosis and treatment of major depressive disorder can save a life or can lead to unnecessary and chronic prescription drug use. The 'saving psychiatry' argument points out that, for one, there will be repercussions for the whole profession if psychiatric diagnosis and treatment are overused in instances in which they do more harm than good. For another, the argument adheres to a seemingly paradoxical consequence of the overuse, and thereby watering down, of psychiatric diagnoses: those who suffer from a condition that can indeed be bettered with the toolkit of psychiatry do not get the help they need. Psychiatric diagnosis and therapy can be very expensive and, if the available money and time are divided between few sick and many worried well, there will be fewer resources available for the sick. The conclusion of the 'saving psychiatry' argument is that it is in the interest of the psychiatric profession, of the patients in need of help, and of society at large to delineate more exactly between the circumstances in which psychiatric diagnosis and treatment are of use and those in which they do more harm than good. This brings us to the epistemological dimension of the problem of delineation.

Concepts of the normal and the mentally ill are interdependent. At first, this may seem circular: to understand what is normal, you need to know what is not normal, and vice versa. Yet there is a way out of this circle: being mentally ill can be construed as being (mentally) not normal. But the reverse is not necessarily true. One might well be (mentally) not normal in some way, yet not qualify as being mentally ill. The emphasis here is on not *necessarily* true and (mentally) not normal in *some* way.

First, not all kinds of being 'not normal' are (or should be treated as) medical problems. We will elaborate on this issue in the next section.

Second, even if we look only at those instances of being 'not normal' that include some biological abnormality, not all variation is pathological. Biologists have explained this phenomenon in terms of 'plasticity' and 'redundancy'. For instance, deficient calcium-signalling is thought to play an important role in many cases of mental disorders (Cross-Disorder Group of the Psychiatric Genomics Consortium 2013). But it has proven difficult to link the occurrence of specific genetic mutations to manifestations of the disease, because there seem to be several genes involved that may, at least partially, replicate one another's functions (see Rizzuto and Possan 2003). Individuals with mutations in the calcium-signalling pathway can be seen to exhibit a genetic abnormality. At the functional level, however, redundancy can pay off, and other genes that influence the calcium-signalling pathway can restore the biological function to what is considered normal.

Third, laboratory pathology is not equivalent to clinical disease. The French philosopher Georges Canguilhem articulated this conceptual issue—which acquires practical significance in translational medicine—in his study on 'The Normal and the Pathological':

> First of all, it should be pointed out that the physiologist, like the physicist and chemist, sets up experiments whose results he compares using this fundamental reservation that these data are valid 'all other things being equal' . . . . Having admitted that some conditions are normal, the physiologist studies the relations which actually define the corresponding phenomena, but he does not really objectively define which conditions are normal. (Canguilhem 1989, 145)

This argument alludes to the fact that, outside the ideal laboratory, in the real world (and the clinic), we never encounter situations in which all things are equal. However, in these circumstances we want to know whether a condition should be treated as a psychiatric problem or whether the behaviour in question should instead be considered as 'normal enough'. This theoretical consideration plays an important role in practice, especially in the evaluation of neuropsychological performance: children may perform significantly better in tests when comforted by their parents than when they are isolated from them (see Frances 2013, 248–50 for a case study on how isolated testing fostered a misdiagnosis of autism). But to view the comforting role of parents as a disturbance of the experimental situation mistakes the undisturbed experimental setting for a normal setting. A child with a similar condition in a less favourable environment may (or may not) have qualified for a diagnosis. If a performance or a condition is not harmful in the relevant environment, why should it be considered a disorder? Control conditions are defined for experimental purposes, so as to achieve comparability; this does not make them 'normal' for every test subject.

This brings us to a third dimension of the question of why reflection on the normal is important for psychiatry. Call it the evaluative dimension: to help ill people (re)turn to normal (ways of living) is an important aim of psychiatric work. The multiple brackets in the sentence indicate that this aim is not easily operationalized. First and foremost, what is considered a good outcome in clinical trial design need not be ideal for every human being. Also, society might want to embrace diverse ways of living. Assessing the success of a psychiatric intervention is perhaps as complicated as ascertaining the psychiatric diagnosis itself. The general directive—to help people who suffer from mental disorders—is clear, but questions about how to define mental disorders, how to anticipate suffering, and how to ensure that the intended help is actually helping have all elicited contentious debates within psychiatry and beyond.

This point becomes practically important not least with respect to risk–benefit analyses. Take for example therapeutic intervention in the case of mild symptoms of bipolar disorder: whether the side effects of antipsychotic treatment are worth risking depends on the therapeutic profile of the drug, the validity of the applied diagnostic category, and the judgement that, on balance, the symptoms are a bigger problem for patients (and their relatives) than the problems arising from possible side effects. For instance, substantive weight gain, a common side effect of antipsychotics, might not just give rise to metabolic and endocarditic diseases (see De Hert et al. 2011 and Harrison, Cluxton-Keller, and Gross 2012 for an evaluation of prescription drug use for 'emotional and behavioural disorders' in children), but also have adverse psychological consequences for patients. The amount of weight gain that can have negative effects on mental health (for instance due to loss of self-esteem and greater social isolation) varies not only culturally, but also individually. And this variance is a challenge for global risk–benefit assessments: to be truly meaningful, risk–benefit analyses need to complement the assessment of net weight gain with an assessment of the psychological effects of the physiological change. The latter assessment will, however, most probably have limited reach with respect to cross-context extrapolation.

The same is true for the potential benefits of antipsychotic treatment of 'emotional and behavioural problems' in children: the very concept of 'normal' child behaviour as a desired outcome of medical intervention depends on how a given society, community, school, or family addresses the need to manage, and thereby normalize, children's lives. In fact, that psychiatric professionals care about 'what is normal' is very much a sign of the times we live in: modern medicine has introduced concepts of the normal and the pathological into its hospitals and, over time, the normal has become an object of concern. This concern has been spurred by the use of the category of 'the normal' and by normalizing practices that make human conditions comparable and extend to contexts such as schools—where, for instance, IQ tests were first applied (see Gould 1996). It is beyond the scope of this chapter to historicize the normal more fully, but it should be noted that 'to save the normal' is a call for a broader construal of the normal, which should allow for a diversity of non-pathologized ways of living.

Taken together, concepts of normality serve at least three purposes in and for psychiatry: the normal marks what should not be treated as an illness; the normal provides a basis for scrutinizing the pathological, although it does not define normalcy outside the experimental setting; and, in the same vein, the normal acts as an ideal of optimal therapeutic outcome.

3 Reflections on the not normal

We could think that the not normal marks the target, the whole *raison d'être* of psychiatry. Yet our assessment of the normal and the pathological provides us with a very different approach. If being not normal is not identical to being (mentally) ill, and if psychiatry aims to treat only the mentally ill (in order to do as little harm as possible), then the not normal does not mark the target, but acts as another class of comparison—just as the normal does.

Some behaviour that qualifies as being 'not normal' or 'abnormal'—on whatever socially and culturally dependent terms—is treated as a psychiatric problem. And some 'not normal' behaviour is explicitly regarded as being attributable not to a disease (for which the patient would bear no responsibility), but instead to a wilful act. In this sense, the mentally ill can be understood as a subclass of the broader category of the abnormal. Indeed, the concept of the abnormal has been in use in psychiatric, legal, and pedagogical discourses on crime and punishment, on sexuality and morality, and on special needs and education at least since the nineteenth century (see Foucault 2003). At times still drawing on this interdisciplinary genealogy of the not normal, recent debates on the introduction or omission of diagnostic categories in the *DSM* pay much attention to the (potential) use of psychiatric categories in forensics, in regulating sexuality, and in obtaining special (school) services. One example involves the question whether sexual attraction to adolescents is pathological or illicit (see Frances' critical discussion about hebephilia in Frances 2013, 200–3).

Reflecting on the relationship between what is not normal and what is mentally ill demonstrates that psychiatry is practiced in a political world. What is mad and what is bad is not just a question of psychopathology, it is also a question about what society we want to live in. If criminal behaviour is medicalized, this renders responsible citizens as sick patients, and punishment is replaced by (involuntary) treatment. There are multiple entanglements between the medicalization of crime and the criminalization of mental illness, as nicely illustrated in the discussion on preventive detentions (see Chapter 11). Besides societal and political consequences, the fear is, again, that the overuse of psychiatric diagnosis to explain criminal behaviour impacts on the image of psychiatry as a profession as well as on the question of access to psychiatric help for those who need it. The argument is that a strong association between crime and psychiatric diagnosis may prevent people who suffer from mental illness from receiving diagnosis and treatment that could actually help them, because they do not want others to be afraid of them. This effect has been analysed in terms of the 'fear of stigma as a barrier to using health services' (see Rüsch, Angermeyer, and

Corrigan 2005). To save psychiatry (in the above mentioned sense), it therefore seems necessary not only to 'save the normal', but also to prevent all human behaviours that a given society considers to be not normal from being appropriated by psychiatry.

Like the normal, the 'not normal' is no given—there is no single, straightforward (biological, statistical, psychological, conceptual) way to delineate between the normal and the not normal or between different kinds of 'abnormal' behaviour. In the language of *DSM-5*, passions can be expressed as behavioural addictions, gluttony as binge-eating disorder, and temper tantrums as disruptive mood dysregulation disorder (see Frances 2013, 170–205). There may well be explanatory schemes that are drawn from such divergent perspectives as psychoanalysis and evolutionary theory and that can be used to argue that everyone is 'not normal' to some degree. But what degrees and kinds of 'not normal' should be included in the *DSM* depends on what is at stake. Today, what is at stake in most debates seems to be the personal and societal risks and costs of overusing prescription drugs, the freedom to be bad, eccentric, unruly, or undisciplined, and the acceptance that life is frequently accompanied by transformative pain that afflicts one or one's surrounding, including juvenile insubordination or grief after the loss of a loved one. This relates to the question: not normal with respect to what?

In neuropsychological testing, this question is translated into the methodological problem of defining the 'right' phenomenon and the 'right' so-called normative sample: for instance, in demarcating cognitive decline from diminished executive functioning, should cognitive performance be compared to one's own previous test results; to the average performance of a study population of the same gender, age range, and education (however defined); or to the best performing 25-year-olds in order to capture age-related cognitive decline? Another facet of the question 'Not normal with respect to what?' is, again, the gap between the laboratory and life: bad test results on cognitive performance often have significant consequences in everyday life (see Salthouse 2012).

Taken together, the not normal is a broader category that contains, but is not limited to, the mentally ill. There are several overlapping zones that link psychopathological concepts, transient life problems (see next section), and psychological reactions to severe, chronic somatic diseases. Moreover, social and cultural norms and legal policies regarding, for instance, sexual behaviour and substance use impact on what is presented as a potential psychiatric problem.

Within most contexts, the boundaries of the category 'not normal' as well as the boundaries between the different subclasses are not clear-cut. The categories of 'psychopathological', 'transient life problems', 'psychological reactions', and cognates are vague in that they give rise to borderline cases, that is, cases that could fall in either category. This vagueness is a feature of the language we use to describe the phenomena in question. This does not mean that the difficulty in deciding whether a given behaviour is a problem that should be subjected to psychiatric diagnosis and treatment—both with respect to individual cases and with respect to the introduction or revision of a category in the *DSM*—is due solely to a lack of more precise terminology. Rather, at least part of the fuzziness of types of 'abnormality' and of concepts of the 'normal' and 'abnormal' is due to features of the phenomena—features that are nowadays framed as functional redundancy, psychological resilience, or socio-environmental embeddedness—and the way they are evaluated. This brings us to the literal core of the problem of the normal and the not normal: the in-between.

4 Reflections on the in-between

In the previous sections we have argued that concepts of the normal have been used to characterize the pathological. We stressed that the not normal should, however, not be mistaken as automatically equating a medical or psychiatric condition. Indeed, the very question of how to delineate all of what is considered biologically or behaviourally not normal from problems that should fall into the psychiatric realm has been a crucial issue in the making of psychiatric classification. In this reading, we can say that both the normal and the not normal have functioned as comparative classes in relation to mental illness. Let us now turn to so-called in-between states that are denoted as risk conditions, mild symptoms, preclinical stages of disease, or to other notions that refer to some kind of condition that seems to fall within the medical domain but that is not considered a full-blown disease entity. These in-between notions mostly exhibit a certain degree of ambiguity because they can function as both a comparative class, namely *not* yet diseased, and a prodromal stage, namely not *yet* diseased. This double character of the in-between can be found in branches of somatic medicine as well. For instance, the historian Ilana Löwy described the ambiguity of oncological classification:

> The term *stage 0* had two distinct meanings. For some specialists, the main reason for the establishment of this classificatory category was the exclusion of results of the treatment of noninvasive lesions from statistics of cancer cures . . . . According to this interpretation, the meaning of 'stage 0' was 'not a true cancer', and the main accent was on '0' not on 'stage'. However, other experts viewed noninvasive cervical lesions as preinvasive ones and assumed that given sufficient time all such lesions would become malignant . . . . For these specialists, the meaning of 'stage 0' was 'a very early cancer', and the main accent was on 'stage', not on '0'. (Löwy 2010, 51–2)

The current discussion of psychosis risk exhibits a similar situation (see Frances 2013, 196–9): the diagnosis of 'psychosis risk syndrome' or 'attenuated psychotic symptoms syndrome'—as discussed in the first and second draft of *DSM-5*, but omitted in the final publication of *DSM-5*—were aiming at adolescents who were not *yet* psychotic (Maxmen 2012). Researchers have criticized that the diagnosis has been overused in teenagers that were *not* psychotic and will probably never be eligible for a diagnosis of full-fledged schizophrenia (Weiden 2012). The debate surrounding such diagnoses shows that the grey area between cases that clearly qualify for a psychiatric diagnosis and cases that clearly do not is of great relevance for psychiatry. On the one hand, the argument is put forward that much treatment comes too late, because processes of neurodegeneration have already damaged too many brain cells in cases of Alzheimer's disease or because antidepressants take too long to be effective in acute situations. It follows that the identification of a need for early diagnosis of dangerous conditions appears as a promising solution. The backlash of this strategy is that the risk of developing a mental disorder and the manifestation of clinical symptoms move closer together. Because many more people qualify for mild symptoms of borderline categories such as 'psychosis risk syndrome' or 'mild neurocognitive disorder' than for severe clinical manifestations of 'schizophrenia' or 'major neurocognitive disorder', more people become patients or are confronted with the fear of soon suffering from a severe, possibly untreatable mental illness. Therefore the argument is put forward that this development of conflating risk with disease should be critically analysed in light of the current (and not some future ideal) state of diagnosis and treatment. This strategy is itself laced with epistemological and methodological problems. For instance, it is difficult to assess whether mild symptoms are transient. Sadness is seen as a common reaction to various unfavourable situations in life, but persistent and overwhelming sadness can be a sign of depression. However, most people who have encountered debilitating emotions as a reaction to difficult life situations get better with time and return to normal without pharmacological intervention. 'Normality' in this sense appears to be both resilient and fragile. It is fragile because a 'normal' state of health is constantly at risk of being damaged. It is resilient because there are several ways to restore 'normality' even in the wake of damage. If pharmacological intervention sets in early, it is difficult to evaluate—especially in the primary care context in which most patients are diagnosed and drugs prescribed—why a person got better. This issue is an advantage for drug manufacturers: the effectiveness of drugs in medical practice (as perceived by the doctors who prescribe them and by the people who take them) can seem higher than in clinical trials because the spontaneous remedies attributable to the placebo effect count among the subjective and objective positive effects of taking the drugs.

One consequence of merging risk and prodromal stages with disease is that the boundaries of what is regarded to being normal are redefined: ever more conditions are regarded as potentially pathological rather than still normal. Shifting boundaries provide us with subtle test cases. Many people show mild symptoms for a limited period of their lives. Borderline cases point to conceptual problems of temporality: when does a mental illness start? What is the role of irreversibility? What are prodromal stages? When should or shouldn't we intervene?

Borderline cases play a huge role in psychopharmacological research and development, not just because of disease-mongering (see next section) but also on the grounds that it may be pharmacologically necessary to intervene early enough to prevent potentially irreversible and damaging symptoms. This argument has been put forward, for instance, as one of the prime reasons why clinical trials for Alzheimer's disease focus more on people at risk than on patients with severe dementia. Another reason is that patients with severe dementia are not able to provide informed consent to participate in the study. Ethics committees have therefore embraced only research that involves mildly cognitively impaired people with no certain diagnosis of Alzheimer's disease instead of testing drugs on people with an established diagnosis of what is nowadays called 'major neurocognitive disorder' (Nuffield Council on Bioethics 2009). There are good neurobiological reasons for intervening early enough in the degeneration process, and there are good ethical reasons against experimenting with humans who are unable to provide informed consent. But this practice has the side effect of promoting diagnostic expansion. Advertisements and calls for participations in clinical trials have helped to create diagnostic needs—needs that can now be satisfied with the *DSM-5* label 'mild neurocognitive disorder' (see Keuck 2012).

Taken together, in-between states generate research opportunities and clinical dilemmas. The opportunities entail the identification of prodromal or risk stages that can help us not just develop more effective and possibly prophylactic tools but also elicit more aetiological knowledge. The dilemma is that, although this strategy should (given the normative constraints on psychiatry sketched above) be implemented to help more people avoid mental disorders, the framing of in-between stages as psychiatric (research) categories tends at first to increase the number of people who qualify for a diagnosis of mental disorder. Given that there are no effective preventive treatments yet available, early and possibly uncertain diagnosis may itself cause harm.

For most in-between states, such as 'mild cognitive impairment' or 'psychosis risk', the categories denoting these states allow for two grey areas: one is between being normal and being at risk or exhibiting mild symptoms and the other is between this in-between state and the ascertained clinical diagnosis of dementia or schizophrenia. This doubling of borderline cases can be described as 'higher order vagueness': introducing categories to denote the grey area creates two new boundaries (see Chapter 3). Mild cognitive impairment, as discussed in terms of 'not normal, not demented' (Petersen et al. 1999), is a case in point: before, there was a grey area between normal and demented; then there were grey areas both between normal and mild cognitive impairment and between mild cognitive impairment and dementia. A category is vague if it allows for borderline cases that could or could not fall into it; higher order vagueness says that the categories used to denote the borderline cases have themselves borderline cases. In other words, no matter how many subcategories are introduced, the problem of vagueness does not go away. We see this in concepts that suppose a gradual transition between the normal and the not normal.

However, grey areas need not necessarily double; sometimes they only shift their location. In some cases, qualitative differences between healthy people who are and who are not at risk could be identified, for instance, because only those who exhibit a particular microbial infection or a genetic mutation may develop the given disorder (like syphilis or Huntington's disease). In these cases, there is only one grey area that has wandered from marking the boundary between 'normal and sick' into an area of 'being at risk and exhibiting clinical symptoms'. This in-between state can be particularly terrifying, especially if clinical symptoms set in gradually and no treatment is available. Clinicians and researchers are not the only ones to wonder when a disease begins; the people who are affected continuously ask themselves whether a mishap may already be a first sign of the disorder. The fear that arises from being in such a certified in-between state can lead to depression and has prompted relatives of people with Huntington's disease to refuse genetic testing (see Wexler 1995).

This example shows that in-between states provide psychiatry with difficult cases that can be used to reflect upon the normative power of psychiatric research and upon the consequences of knowing or not knowing. Such cases have also served as key examples in discussions about diagnostic inflation.

5 Reflections on diagnostic inflation

Diagnostic inflation describes, first, the numeric increase in incidents of psychiatric diagnosis. For instance, the rise in the prevalence of autism from 3–4 cases per 10,000 persons in the 1970s to estimates of 60 and more today could be described as 'diagnostic inflation'. However, as with all epidemiological trends that are assessed over time and across multiple sites, there are several methodological caveats when it comes to interpreting prevalence rates (see Fombonne

2003): the classification of autistic spectrum disorder that is applied nowadays is much broader than the concept of autism was in the 1970s; diagnostic practices have changed; the availability of services and the public's awareness of autism spectrum disorders have expanded; moreover, epidemiological surveys have developed new methods of case finding. In any event, independently of whether increasing prevalence rates are due to changes in conceptualizing and identifying the disorder in question or to some biological cause, such rates capture and unfold a social reality of their own.

Notably, diagnostic inflation can be due to the inclusion of either more cases that were formerly regarded as normal or more cases that were formerly regarded as not normal but not mentally ill. Increases in psychiatric diagnoses could be (and frequently are) explained as being true to nature. Such explanations include the idea that our stressful societies drive more people crazy, either because urban areas such as Midtown Manhattan increase human isolation (Srole et al. 1962) or because environmental toxins, directly or via somatic diseases, compromise mental health. Another explanation that is brought forward is that our awareness of mental health problems has increased and the diagnostic methods we use to detect them have become better, so that the increase in diagnostic rates reflects scientific progress.

In addition to its descriptive meaning and contrary to the idea that it signifies a valid trend, diagnostic inflation is also a negative evaluative term (see Frances 2013, 77–113). Just as monetary inflation is in most cases undesired, so is diagnostic inflation: in this understanding, it signals the risk of a possible epidemic—and not one due to a cause that can be treated by the medical system (e.g. due to an infectious agent like a virus). Rather the inflation and the possible epidemic are caused by the medical system itself. Hence the worry is that this sort of diagnostic hyperinflation does much more harm than good, because overly sensitive psychiatric diagnoses lack specificity: for the sake of delivering right a few early diagnoses that were missed beforehand, they capture too many people who do not profit (enough) from a diagnosis. This may be in the interest of some expert psychiatrist-researchers—who often head the *DSM* task forces and wish to promote their 'pet diagnoses'. For primary care physicians who acquire much of their psychiatric education from sales representatives of the pharmaceutical industry, the prescription of a seemingly easy and safe to use drug for low-threshold diagnoses offers a billable and, given their time limitations, quick way to comfort their patients. In the United States primary care physicians are the ones responsible for most psychiatric diagnoses and psychopharmacological prescriptions. Direct-to-consumer advertising of prescription drugs and so-called disease awareness campaigns have fostered this development: patients who 'asked their doctor', as seen on television, were

17 times more likely to receive medication than patients who did not ask for drugs (see Smith 2012). This has been criticized, because overtreatment has adverse effects on both individuals and societies. The detection of diagnostic inflation should therefore be particularly worrisome in psychiatry, as it puts the whole system at risk. Diagnostic hyperinflation is, in this reading, an indicator of system failure.

There are some stakeholders within the system that profit from such 'psychiatry gone wrong' developments, at least in the short term. Most critics have pointed in particular to the pharmaceutical industry, where marketing costs usually double the total costs for research and development of new therapeutics (see Gagnon and Lexchin 2008). Sales numbers for a drug increase in proportion to the number of people diagnosed with a disorder (or relevant symptoms) for which the drug in question has a Food and Drugs Administration (FDA) approval or is used off label.

Against this backdrop, one can suggest a third reading of diagnostic inflation, which has been debated in terms of 'disease-mongering': diagnostic inflation as an active marketing strategy designed to increase the sales of the pharmaceutical industry. This reading points out that the pharmaceutical industry profits directly from a larger market and from consumers who start early with potentially lifelong medication. The increase in prescription rates for antipsychotic drugs has acted as an illustrious example. A recent study from Canada—which is known to have significantly lower prescription rates than the United States—has shown that even in British Columbia rates for children and adolescents have increased 3.8-fold (including a 18.1-fold increase in prescriptions for second-generation antipsychotic drugs) from 1996 to 2011 (Ronsley et al. 2013).

Of particular interest is that this diagnostic inflation affects children and adolescents. In their case the potentially harmful effects of premature diagnostic labelling and psychotherapeutic treatment are unforeseeable, given that the long-term risks of pharmacological interventions for brain (and personality) development cannot be assessed within the limited time frame of phase 3 clinical trials. Furthermore, children are in a unique situation because they are dependent on parents and other adults.

In general, diagnostic inflation may also have reverse consequences: initiatives such as 'neurodiversity societies' and 'mad pride' parades indicate that diagnostic inflation might have some positive effect on the societal acceptance of hitherto stigmatized diagnoses.

This being said, it remains true that diagnostic inflation has been introduced chiefly as a neologism intended to capture the ill state of psychiatry, which is due to conflicts of interest, profit orientation dogmas, biased risk–benefit analyses, opaque *DSM* revision processes, and meagre psychiatric education of primary care physicians, to name just a few deficiencies (see Frances 2013). The normative undertone of 'diagnostic inflation' acts as a provocation launched against reified readings of epidemiological statistics. It may not apply in all situations, but it reminds us that readings of current diagnostic trends should always be done with care and suspicion.

6 **Conclusion and outlook**

In this chapter we have taken a closer look at the functions that notions of the normal, the not normal, and the in-between have served within psychiatry and at how they have been issues of concern in current discussions about diagnostic inflation. There is much more to say and historicize about these issues than we could sketch in this essay, but we hope to have pointed out some nuclei of further debate. Drawing on existing scholarship, we have emphasized that normal conditions have been a basis for scrutinizing the pathological in experimental settings. This might have impacted on, but should not be misunderstood as automatically defining, what is considered to be normal in everyday life. Similarly, the aim of returning to normal has influenced the definition of the measures we use to assess the outcome of psychiatric intervention. But this should not cloud the fact that what is ideal for a clinical trial need not be ideal for everyone's life or for society. This becomes even clearer when we look at how notions of the not normal have been used within debates on the order of mental disorders. A broader category than the mentally ill, the not normal has been put forward to remind us that psychiatry is practiced in a political world. The matter of what is evaluated as not normal behaviour or biology and what is seen as a particular psychiatric problem is connected not only to scientific theories of pathology, but also to societal evaluations of deviation. Against this background, it seems that it has been a crucial legitimization strategy of modern psychiatry to ensure that psychiatric diagnoses are not overinclusive with respect to either the normal or the not normal.

This strategy faces particular challenges when it encounters the grey area between what is considered normal and what is considered mentally ill. This area has been of particular interest in the context of research and pharmaceutical marketing strategies. In many cases, 'the not yet diseased' and 'the worried well' are indistinguishable. In some of these cases, it might mark a welcome breakthrough if people at risk could be clearly identified and effectively helped. However, given the current state of psychiatric diagnosis and treatment, this is mostly pie in the sky. The adverse effects of expanding diagnostic categories are, however, already very real. It is another legitimizing strategy of psychiatry to navigate between promising futures and a critical acknowledgement of current limitations.

Against this background, critical psychiatry frames the directive for further developments in psychiatric diagnosis and treatment as an imperative: 'do less harm'. This slogan acknowledges that it is probably impossible to eliminate all harm, not least because 'harm' is a volatile target, dependent on changing societal and cultural values. It is, however, also acknowledged that it is very well and without much sophistication possible to reduce much of the harm that is caused by present-day diagnostic inflation and overtreatment (Frances 2013, 209–27; Batstra and Frances 2012). Harm, in this case, includes the deterioration of individual lives through the effects of diagnostic labelling; disabilities and deaths due to prescription drugs and polypharmacy; and the misallocation of healthcare and educational resources, together with the immense costs incurred for the use of ineffective drugs in the treatment of mild, transitory, short-term forms of disorders. Less harm can be expressed in a series of practical recommendations (see Frances 2013, 209–27): prescriptions and polypharmacy should be monitored and equipped with an alarm system. All branches of government should work to prevent the pharmaceutical industry from promoting overtreatment. The *DSM* revision process should be restructured and possibly put under new auspices, in order to ensure a transparent and critical revision (see also Frances and Widiger 2012). School services should be decoupled from a clinical diagnosis of, for instance, autism. The allocation of extra help should be based on school needs rather than on the attribution of a diagnostic label that has been defined for medical needs (Frances 2013, 147–9). Furthermore, the extensive use of the *DSM* in forensics should be reconsidered and *DSM* labels should be supplemented by forensic-specific classifications. Diagnostic labels should in general be attributed much more carefully, and watchful waiting should be accepted as a diagnostic and therapeutic strategy that is refundable through medical insurance. Mild or prodromal forms of mental disorders should not be incorporated into broadly applied diagnostic manuals such as the *DSM* unless there are valid diagnostics and effective treatments that clearly outweigh the risks of misapplication. Finally, the *DSM*'s revisers and users—as well as any risk–benefit analysts—should be sensitive to the intricate interplay between concepts of normalcy, politics of the not normal, aetiological theories of disease generation, and effects of diagnostic inflation.

If the aim of a critical psychiatry is, as Frances' book *Saving Normal* argues in greater detail, 'to save psychiatry', then our reflections in this chapter show that this aim might also involve accepting that psychiatric knowledge and action will always provide us with difficult cases, which transgress and defy any simple model of mental illness.

References

APA (American Psychiatric Association). 2013. *Diagnostic and Statistical Manual of Mental Disorders, Fifth Edition: DSM-5*. Washington, DC: American Psychiatric Association.

Batstra, L., and Frances, A. 2012. 'Diagnostic inflation: Causes and a suggested cure'. *The Journal of Nervous and Mental Disease* **200**: 474–9.

Canguilhem, G. 1989. *The Normal and the Pathological*. New York, NY: Zone Books.

CDC (Centers for Disease Control and Prevention). 2011. Prescription Painkiller Overdoses at Epidemic Levels. Press release. http://www.cdc.gov/media/releases/2011/p1101_flu_pain_killer_overdose.html (accessed 28 May 2016).

Cross-Disorder Group of the Psychiatric Genomics Consortium. 2013. 'Identification of risk loci with shared effects on five major psychiatric disorders: A genome-wide analysis'. *The Lancet* **381**: 1371–9.

De Hert, M. et al. 2011. 'Metabolic and endocrine adverse effects of second-generation antipsychotics in children and adolescents: A systematic review of randomized, placebo-controlled trials and guidelines for clinical practice'. *European Psychiatry* **26**: 144–58.

Frances, A. 2013. *Saving Normal: An Insider's Revolt against Out-of-Control Psychiatric Diagnosis, DSM-5, Big Pharma, and the Medicalization of Ordinary Life*. New York, NY: William Morrow.

Frances, A., and Widiger, T. 2012. 'Psychiatric diagnosis: Lessons from the DSM-IV past and cautions for the DSM-5 future'. *Annual Reviews of Clinical Psychology* **8**: 109–30.

Fombonne, E. 2003. 'The prevalence of autism'. *Journal of the American Medical Association* **289**: 87–9.

Foucault, M. 2003. *Abnormal: Lectures at the Collège de France (1974–1975)*. New York, NY: Picador.

Gagnon, M.-A., and Lexchin, J. 2008. 'The cost of pushing pills: A new estimate of pharmaceutical promotion expenditures in the United States'. *PLoS Medicine* **5**: e1. http://dx.doi.org/10.1371/journal.pmed.0050001 (accessed 27 May 2016)

Gould, S. J. 1996. *The Mismeasure of Man* (2nd edn). New York, NY: W. W. Norton.

Harrison, J. N., Cluxton-Keller, F., and Gross, D. 2012. 'Antipsychotic medication prescribing trends in children and adolescents'. *Journal of Pediatric Health Care* **26**: 139–45.

Keuck, L. K. 2012. 'Diagnostic misconceptions? A closer look at clinical research on Alzheimer's disease'. *Journal of Medical Ethics* **38**: 57–9. [Published as Lara K. Kutschenko.]

Löwy, I. 2010. *Preventive Strikes: Women, Precancer, and Prophylactic Surgery*. Baltimore, MD: Johns Hopkins University Press.

Maxmen, A. 2012. Psychosis risk syndrome excluded from DSM-5. *Nature News*. doi: 10.1038/nature.2012.10610.

Moynihan, R., and Henry, D. 2006. 'The fight against disease mongering: Generating knowledge for action'. *PLoS Med* **3**(4): e191. doi: 10.1371/journal.pmed.0030191.

Nuffield Council on Bioethics. 2009. 'Research'. Chapter 8 in *Nuffield Council on Bioethics Dementia: Ethical Issues*, pp. 128–42. Cambridge: Cambridge Publishers LTD.

Petersen, R. C. et al. 1999. 'Mild cognitive impairment: Clinical characterization and outcome'. *Archives of Neurology* **56**: 303–8.

Rizzuto, R., and Pozzan, T. 2003. 'When calcium goes wrong: Genetic alterations of a ubiquitous signaling route'. *Nature Genetics* **34**: 135–41.

Ronsley, R. et al. 2013. 'A population-based study of antipsychotic prescription trends in children and adolescents in British Columbia, from 1996 to 2011'. *Canadian Journal of Psychiatry* **58**: 361–9.

Rüsch, N., Angermeyer, M. C., and Corrigan, P. W., 2005. 'Mental illness stigma: Concepts, consequences, and initiatives to reduce stigma'. *European Psychiatry* **20**: 529–39.

Salthouse, T. 2012. 'Consequences of age-related cognitive declines'. *Annual Reviews in Psychology* **63**: 201–26.

Smith, B. L. 2012. 'Inappropriate prescribing'. *Monitor on Psychology* **43** (6), 36–40. http://www.apa.org/monitor/2012/06/prescribing.aspx (accessed October 10, 2014).

Srole, L. et al. 1962. *Mental Health in the Metropolis: The Midtown Manhattan Study.* New York, NY: McGraw-Hill.

Weiden, P. J. 2012. 'The Risk That DSM-5 Will Promote Even More Inappropriate Antipsychotic Exposure in Children and Teenagers'. *Current Psychiatry Reviews* **8**: 271–6.

Wexler, A. 1995. *Mapping Fate: A Memoir of Family, Risk, and Genetic Research.* Berkeley, CA: University of California Press.

Chapter 9

Vagueness, the sorites paradox, and posttraumatic stress disorder

Peter Zachar and Richard J. McNally

1 Introduction: Vagueness

Let's see now, Who is on first base, What is on second, I Don't Know is on third.
Are you the guy that knows the names of the baseball players?
Why certainly.
So who's on first?
Yes.
Are you going to tell me the name of the guy on first base?
Who.
What are you asking me for?
I'm not asking you, I'm telling you. Who is on first.
I'm asking you who's on first!
That's the man's name.
Who's name?
Yes.

The vaudeville sketch *Who's on First?*, made famous by Bud Abbott and Lou Costello, trades upon ambiguity in the meaning of the term "who." The two meanings can be distinguished and ambiguity eliminated by offering definitions. For instance, in the sketch, Abbott uses Who as a proper name, as in Doctor Who or Cindy Lou Who, while Costello understands "who" as a pronoun such as "you" or "we."

A key difference between ambiguity and vagueness is that disambiguation cannot eliminate vagueness once and for all. Introduced into philosophy with the paradox of the heap (also called, after its Greek name, the sorites paradox; Hyde 2014), vagueness is a property of concepts that produce borderline cases. If we start with a few grains of sand scattered on the floor and gradually add one grain of sand at a time, at what point does the sand become a heap? Most thinkers conclude that there is no precise point at which adding one grain will transform the sand into a heap. As gradual changes are made, the sand begins to approximate a heap.

There are clear cases of non-heaps and heaps, but also a borderline or transitional region where boundaries are fuzzy and malleable. If you have a heap and start removing one grain of sand at a time, every new pile is perceptually indistinguishable from what came before. As you create smaller but successively hard to distinguish collections of sand, it is likely that smaller and smaller collections will be called heaps.

Scientists define concepts as precisely as circumstances allow. Psychopathologists are no exception. Indeed, the *Diagnostic and Statistical Manual of Mental Disorders* (*DSM*; see APA 2013) defines mental disorders in terms of their signs and symptoms, specifying the precise number of them needed to qualify for the diagnosis. For example, a diagnosis of major depression requires that one must have five out of nine symptoms that persist for at least two weeks and cause marked distress or impairment in social or occupational functioning. Explicit definitions of mental disorders reduce ambiguity and foster the reliability of diagnosis.

What often remains after explicit definitions eliminate ambiguity is vagueness—and there is no shortage of borderline cases in psychiatric nosology. In *DSM-IV* many borderline cases were assigned a diagnosis of *not otherwise specified* (NOS). So "depressive disorder not otherwise specified" referred to cases that did not satisfy formal criteria for a diagnosis but were similar enough to major depression to be considered part of a broader depression spectrum.

In some settings, vagueness may signify ignorance. Consider emergency rooms. It is not always possible to acquire enough information to make a definitive psychiatric diagnosis in an emergency room, but one can make an approximate diagnosis. An example of approximate diagnosis in *DSM-5* is *unspecified depressive disorder*. This is called *epistemic vagueness* by some, and the expectation is that more information will increase diagnostic clarity (Sorensen 2001; Williamson 1994).

Many psychiatrists and psychologists believe that much of the vagueness in psychiatry is epistemic. Their hope is that yet to be discovered information involving biomarkers, endophenotypes, and underlying mechanisms will lead to increased diagnostic clarity (Cuthbert and Kozak 2013; Hyman 2010; Insel et al. 2010; Sanislow et al. 2010). For instance, the presence of a particular biomarker may reliably indicate an incipient depression for a person with a history of depression. Lacking such biomarkers, the distinction between a depressive disorder and normal anhedonia is vague.

However, not all vagueness in psychiatry can be eliminated through the discovery of new facts. Biomarkers and mechanisms may exist in *degrees*. Different *combinations* of endophenotypes may produce transitional regions where there is still no fact of the matter as to where exactly the normal becomes abnormal. In other words, not all vagueness is epistemic.

Much of the vagueness in psychiatry is a consequence of our reliance on general concepts such as "abnormal," "distress," and "disorder." For some uses these concepts do what we ask of them, for others they fail. Vagueness emerges in those instances where a general concept such as abnormal applies more or less, but there is a transitional region where a clear distinction between appropriately applied (a psychiatric heap) and misapplied (a false positive) is difficult to make.

2 **Psychological trauma**

In World War II and in the Korean War, American psychiatrists were aware that many soldiers experienced debilitating reactions to combat stress, but they expected that those reactions would dissipate once the stressor was no longer present. The diagnoses psychiatrists used for these cases included war neurosis, traumatic syndrome, and gross stress reaction (Kardiner 1959; Scott 1990). Persistence of symptoms, they thought, implied preexisting psychological problems or vulnerabilities (Jones and Wessely 2001).

In the early 1970s psychiatrists encountered a new pattern of symptoms among veterans of the Vietnam War that involved haunting memories of their combat experiences. The new feature was that the symptoms were delayed, appearing only months or years after the soldiers returned home. In some cases the symptoms were so debilitating that the veterans sought disability benefits, but without a formal diagnostic label for their problems these veterans could not access mental health services from the Veterans Administration (VA), nor could they be eligible for psychiatric disability compensation.

The delayed emergence of a war-related stress syndrome in Vietnam veterans in the early and mid-1970s was surprising for several reasons. First, psychiatric breakdown in World War I and World War II occurred during the war itself rather than years later (Jones and Wessely 2001). The phenomenon of soldiers finishing their tour of duty without mental health problems only to break down years later was unprecedented. Second, psychiatric casualties were relatively rare in Vietnam by comparison to previous wars. The rate of psychiatric breakdown was 12 per 1,000 men in Vietnam, whereas the rate varied between 28 and 101 per 1,000 men during World War II for American troops (Dean 1997, 40). Third, among the psychiatric cases diagnosed in Vietnam itself, only

3.5 percent of them received the diagnosis of "combat exhaustion" (Marlowe 2001, 86). Most mental health problems in Vietnam involved other issues (e.g., drug use, conduct problems). Fourth, as Marlowe noted, "combat stress casualties were at their lowest for the years of the highest-intensity combat" (ibid., 85; i.e., during the mid- to late 1960s), and only 3.5 percent of all psychiatric casualties diagnosed in Vietnam itself were combat exhaustion cases (ibid., 86). An inverse relation between combat intensity, defined as the rate of soldiers killed or wounded, and combat stress reactions was historically unprecedented (Jones and Wessely 2001).

According to Scott (1990), another factor that complicated the acceptance of post-Vietnam syndrome was that its advocates, Robert Lifton (1973) and Chaim Shatan (1973), were outspoken opponents of the war. The disorder, they believed, was a result of the Vietnam War being conducted as a counterinsurgency operation. To speak of any predisposition to chronic mental disorders, they believed, would amount to unjustly blaming veterans for their suffering (Blank 1985).

Because post-Vietnam syndrome was introduced about the same time that the protests against the war were becoming widespread, it became highly politicized. To depoliticize the issue, the advocates broadened the scope of the disorder beyond the politics of the war and began arguing that a similar symptom pattern occurs in survivors of concentration camps. Noticing this similarity allowed a new reading of the literature on psychic trauma (Chodoff 1963; Freud 1961 [1920]; Furst 1967; Titchener and Ross 1974), drawing attention to a shared cluster of symptoms seen among survivors of catastrophic experiences such as rape and natural disasters (Burgess and Holmstrom 1974).

As originally formulated, the post-Vietnam syndrome emphasized guilt, alienation, and emotional numbing. The more general syndrome retained numbing but added intrusive reexperiencing of the trauma, avoidance of things that remind one of the trauma, and exaggerated startle response.

After psychiatrists began work on the third edition of the *DSM*, Lifton and Shatan succeeded in securing appointments to a *DSM-III* advisory committee on reactive disorders. From this position, they were able to convince the other members of the committee to include the syndrome—now renamed posttraumatic stress disorder (PTSD)—in the new manual. As classified in the *DSM-III* of 1980, PTSD referred to a cluster of symptoms that develop after a traumatic event that falls outside the range of usual human experience and that would invoke significant distress in almost everyone.

In medicine *trauma* refers to an injury to the body caused by an external agent. So a blow to the body with a blunt instrument and breaking the skin with a sharp instrument both cause traumas. Applied to psychiatry, a psychological trauma is an injury to the mind caused by an external agent. Over time, this metaphor has become literalized. For most people, the primary meaning of trauma has become psychological trauma.

In the transition from general medicine to psychiatry, however, there has been a shift in the meaning of the concept. In medicine, a pinprick and being stabbed with a knife are both traumas. In psychiatry, the analogue of a pinprick would be considered normal stress, whereas "traumatized" refers to severe stress reactions. With the concept of severity we enter the realm of vagueness.

3 Symptoms of posttraumatic stress disorder

The diagnostic criteria for PTSD have evolved over the past three decades. *DSM-5*, the current edition of the manual, appeared in May 2013 (APA 2013). One thing that has not changed is that PTSD remains unusual in psychiatric nosology for having an aetiological event as one of its criteria (criterion A). To assign the diagnosis, an assessor must first establish that a person has experienced a traumatic stressor. Few diagnoses are like this. For example, assessors can assign a diagnosis of major depressive disorder if the person has symptoms for at least two weeks and those symptoms impair everyday functioning or provoke clinically significant distress. Although major stressors often precede the onset of depression, assessors need not establish exposure to a stressor to assign the diagnosis. Yet they may not diagnose PTSD unless an identified stressor surmounts a threshold of severity to qualify as *traumatic*, regardless of the presence of PTSD symptoms.

PTSD comprises four clusters of symptoms in *DSM-5*. The *intrusion* cluster (B criteria) denotes manifestations of memory for the trauma. Unbidden memories of the experience emerge as intrusive thoughts, nightmares, and sensory images ("flashbacks") of the trauma, plus psychological and physiological reactivity upon encountering reminders of the experience. The *avoidance* cluster (C criteria) covers efforts to avoid thoughts, feelings, and reminders of the trauma. The cluster concerning *negative alterations in cognitions and mood* (D criteria) includes emotional numbing (e.g., difficulty feeling positive emotions), distorted blame of oneself or others, and pervasive negative emotions (e.g., anger and shame). The cluster denoting *alterations in arousal and reactivity* (E criteria) includes aggression, recklessness, exaggerated startle, and hypervigilance.

Many people experience acute symptoms in the days following a trauma (see, e.g., Rothbaum et al. 1992). To distinguish normal distress from PTSD, the authors of *DSM-5* ask that the requisite number of symptoms in each cluster persist for at least one month and produce marked distress or impairment in social, occupational, or other important areas of functioning before the diagnosis can be assigned.

4 **Vagueness and posttraumatic stress disorder**

Consider the following case. A woman is in an accident in which her car rolls over several times. Soon after the accident she is dazed and emotionally numb. Over the next few weeks she has intrusive memories of the event and is afraid to drive anywhere. In which cell of Table 9.1 do her reactions belong? Do they represent normal and expectable reactions or abnormal, maladaptive reactions to a catastrophic event?

When a mammal such as a gazelle is caught by a predator, before being killed it sometimes becomes limp and immobile—and silent. Its eyes go blank, which is analogous to a dissociative and numbing response. This is likely a normal reaction. If the gazelle's response is normal and adaptive, perhaps the woman's numbing response was also normal. What if, after being caught, the gazelle luckily escapes? Having a heightened hypervigilance about life-threatening events in the future would seem very adaptive for gazelles—and humans.

Consider these cases as well. Two men are alone in their firm's office early in the morning when the building begins to rattle and shake. Objects fall off desks and shelves onto the floor. It is an earthquake. When asked about the event soon after, each man states that he was startled, but the quake began and ended so quickly that neither was sure what was happening.

It also turns out that during the quake the load-bearing pillars at the back of building were damaged. Later that morning, the part of the building the two men had been in collapsed into rubble.

Six months later they are interviewed again. The first man is coping reasonably well. He occasionally has some frightening dreams about the earthquake, but they are, he says, "just dreams." Despite having some symptoms, he is resilient. The second person has experienced a significant decline in functioning associated with symptoms of PTSD. He has intrusive thoughts about being caught in collapsing buildings and is also having panic attacks. He remembers the earthquake as terrifying.

In our final case, the wife of the first man is horrified when she learns of the building's collapse. After the quake her husband intended to stay at work

Table 9.1 Response quality to stressor severity

	Normal stress	Subtraumatic stress	Traumatic stress
Resilient response			
Normal response			
Abnormal response			

despite an evacuation order and only left because she insisted he do so. She soon starts having intrusive thoughts about her husband's being caught in the collapsing buildings and is also having panic attacks.

When the degree of stress varies on a continuum and the response severity varies on a continuum, borderline cases are generated. In theory, there will be borderline cases between every cell in Table 9.1. However, the transitional regions that bedevil the classification of PTSD are between subtraumatic versus traumatic events and normal versus abnormal responses.

In terms of the narrow *DSM-III* notion of traumatic stressor, only the woman in the car accident would be a case of PTSD —and only if the symptoms cause her to experience a significant decline in functioning. Also, if "a few weeks" is only three weeks, watchful waiting would still be an option. The problem is that the second person in the earthquake seems more traumatized than the woman who had the car accident.

The case of the wife is similar enough to the case of the second person to begin to look like a case of PTSD too. As this gradual extension continues, what would have been considered a borderline case becomes PTSD. Eventually cases that previously would not have been candidates for a PTSD diagnosis might become borderline cases—such as the case of someone seeing the death and destruction caused by an earthquake on television.

The problem with a gradual extension is that, although similar cases are successively placed next to one another, eventually we come to a point where the beginning of the chain and the end of the chain are very different from each other. This is why a diagnostic category that includes under its scope being a survivor of the World Trade Center bombings on September 11, 2001 and watching the buildings collapse on television is ludicrous (McNally 2009; Shephard 2004). It is a classic sorites situation.

5 Vagueness and the severity of the traumatic stressor

As noted, the original *DSM-III* formulation defined a traumatic event as one that lies outside the range of usual human experience and would evoke significant symptoms of distress in almost anyone. The manual furnished canonical examples of traumatic events. Combat, natural disasters, rape, and torture were among these examples. The manual also ruled out ordinary stressors that fall outside the perimeter of the traumatic. These included business losses, marital conflict, and chronic illness.

Accordingly, the original diagnosis of PTSD presupposed that anyone exposed to traumatic stressors was liable to develop the disorder. Conversely, stressors falling short of the threshold for trauma presumably lacked the capacity to produce the symptomatic profile of PTSD.

Yet we cannot establish by fiat whether a stressor can cause PTSD. The issue is empirical, not conceptual or definitional—and empirical findings soon surfaced that violated the original formulation. First, epidemiologists found that exposure to criterion A traumatic stressors is not sufficient to produce PTSD because not everyone exposed develops symptoms (Breslau et al. 1991). This implied that vulnerability factors affect whether trauma-exposed people develop the disorder.

Second, other studies revealed that people who were not directly exposed to *DSM-III* criterion A stressors could still develop the PTSD symptom configuration. Some individuals exhibited the full range of PTSD symptoms even though they had neither directly experienced trauma nor personally witnessed the trauma of other people. For example, receiving news about the violent death of a loved one—without directly witnessing it—resulted in apparent PTSD (Saigh 1991). Other reports showed that directly experiencing subtraumatic stressors could also cause PTSD symptoms (for a review, see Dohrenwend 2010). For example, people exposed to obnoxious jokes at work (McDonald 2003), giving birth to a healthy baby after an uncomplicated delivery (Olde et al. 2006), and having a wisdom tooth extracted (de Jongh et al. 2008) all succumbed to PTSD or to approximative PTSD.

In response to the issue of indirect exposure, the *DSM-IV* PTSD committee worried that people who developed genuine symptoms after learning about threats to others would be denied the diagnosis and reimbursable treatment. Accordingly, the definition of trauma underwent a *conceptual bracket creep* (McNally 2003) whereby people who were not present at the scene of the trauma became eligible as trauma survivors themselves as long as they experienced extreme fear, helplessness, or horror at learning about threats to other people. This subtly shifted the emphasis from the external stressor to the person's emotional reaction.

If the development of symptoms is causally mediated by the person's reaction, then in theory symptoms could develop in response to a wide range of stressors as long as the person reacted with terror. In other words, once intrusive thoughts, numbing, and avoidance are identified as symptoms *of* a trauma syndrome, if that symptom configuration appears, according to some, this confirms the traumatic character of the event for that person (Kraemer et al. 2009).

The conceptual bracket creep promulgated by the *DSM-IV* definition of trauma wherein what was previously borderline cases came to be considered cases of PTSD had consequences for epidemiology. Rather than being a rare event falling outside the boundary of everyday experience, trauma suddenly became common. Indeed, nearly everyone became a trauma survivor under *DSM-IV*, as Breslau and Kessler (2001) discovered. Interviewing adults living in Southeastern Michigan, they found that 89.6 percent of them had been exposed to the *DSM-IV* expanded notion of a criterion A stressor. Other epidemiologists reported that 4 percent of American adults living far from the sites of the September 11 terrorist attacks succumbed to apparent PTSD, seemingly from viewing the attacks on television (Schlenger et al. 2002). Not only could one now qualify as a "trauma survivor" without having been at the scene of the trauma, the people whose physical integrity was actually imperiled by trauma could be strangers to some of the "trauma survivors" (McNally and Breslau 2008).

What should we make of those whose apparent PTSD eruptions in response to events that the authors of *DSM-III* never envisioned possessed this capacity? One interpretation is that people often misinterpret queries about PTSD symptoms, especially when completing questionnaires in the absence of a clinician capable of clarifying ambiguous items. Another interpretation is that these individuals really do have PTSD, but its cause lies as much with preexisting risk factors as with the nominal stressor itself. Perhaps these people carry a heavy burden of vulnerability, which renders them especially sensitive to minor stressors. In such cases the stressor recedes into the causal background as the risk factors move into the causal foreground.

McNally and Robinaugh (2011) reported findings consistent with this *background–foreground inversion*. They found that lower cognitive ability was a better predictor of PTSD for women whose childhood sexual abuse was mild in severity than it was for women whose abuse was moderate in severity. That is, the vulnerability factor of lower cognitive ability increased PTSD risk more for the less severe stressor.

McNally and Robinaugh tested this hypothesis within a stressor category (i.e., childhood sexual abuse). In contrast, Breslau, Troost, Bohnert, and Luo (Breslau et al. 2013) tested it across stressor categories, capitalizing on the fact that interpersonal stressors such as rape are usually more predictive of PTSD than are impersonal stressors such as industrial accidents.

Using a large epidemiological sample, Breslau et al. (2013) found that the importance of risk factors (e.g., preexisting depression, parental alcohol abuse) did not differ between more severe categories of trauma (sexual assault) and less severe categories of trauma (accidents). Moreover, in another epidemiological study, Breslau, Chen, and Lou (2013) found that lower intelligence was not more predictive of PTSD for people exposed to assaultive violence than for people exposed to less severe trauma (i.e., disasters, accidents). Hence the epidemiological data indicate that vulnerability factors increase PTSD risk regardless of the severity of the stressor.

The conceptual bracket creep in the *DSM-IV* definition of trauma reflects psychiatry's acknowledgment that people report suffering from the full range of PTSD symptoms after experiencing stressful events that fall far short of the original *DSM-III* threshold for trauma. Indeed, some studies have shown that subtraumatic stressors are more provocative of PTSD symptoms than are stressors that clearly qualify for criterion A (Gold et al. 2005; Long et al. 2008; Mol et al. 2005). These studies indicate that the relation between the kind of stressor and the likelihood of developing PTSD symptoms or PTSD is vastly more complicated than most of us have realized.

Underscoring this complexity is a series of four studies designed to develop a generic, objective measure of stressor severity applicable to diverse trauma type. Assessment of criterion A requires a clinician to judge whether the stressor surpasses the threshold for qualifying as traumatic. In these studies Rubin and Feeling (2013) discovered that different measures of event severity intercorrelated strongly, but none predicted the severity of PTSD symptoms or probable PTSD diagnosis. Such findings suggest that a generic severity dimension does not exist; rather, "trauma" is the result of an interaction between subjective reactions and events.

5.1 Working with vagueness

As we have just seen, one of the most challenging sources of vagueness in diagnosing PTSD concerns whether a stressor qualifies as *traumatic*. One way of avoiding this source of vagueness would be to abolish criterion A altogether. If exposure to a traumatic event were not requisite for the diagnosis, then assessors would not have to worry whether the inciting event qualified as traumatic. Indeed, some clinical scholars have called for the abolition of criterion A, arguing that PTSD should be placed on the same footing as major depression, panic disorder, and other *DSM* syndromes that often arise following exposure to diverse stressors but whose criteria set does not include exposure to a specific stressor (Maier 2006).

On the other hand, there are several reasons why this proposal is problematic (McNally 2009). First, key PTSD symptoms, such as intrusive thoughts, nightmares, and avoidance, possess *intentionality* in Brentano's sense (Brentano 1984 [1899]). Intentionality denotes "aboutness"—whenever one has intrusive thoughts, the thoughts have referential content; they are about something, and that something is the traumatic event. Likewise, to exhibit avoidance, one must avoid something, and that something is a set of reminders of the traumatic event. These symptoms are not merely *caused* by the trauma, they are *about* the trauma.

Second, as clinical scholars have observed (Spitzer, First, and Wakefield 2007), many symptoms of PTSD are nonspecific in the sense that they overlap with symptoms of other disorders. For example, difficulty sleeping, loss of interest in previously enjoyed activities, and irritability occur in other disorders as well, and it is the memory of the traumatic event that unifies them into a PTSD syndrome (Young 1995, 5). As Breslau, Chase, and Anthony (2002) put it, "[i]t is their connection to a specific stressor that transforms the list of PTSD symptoms into a distinct *DSM* disorder" (574). If we were to dispense with criterion A, the syndrome would unravel.

To increase diagnostic clarity, the *DSM-5* committee responsible for revising the criteria for PTSD modified criterion A in two ways. First, although *DSM-IV* certified that learning about threats to other people can be "traumatic," the *DSM-5* version of criterion A requires that the threatened individuals must be friends or family, in keeping with the intent, but not the words, of criterion A in *DSM-IV*. Accordingly, hearing news about the murder of a stranger does not qualify as traumatic for the recipient of this news, whereas hearing that one's child has been killed by a drunk driver does. The committee also excluded trauma exposure via media as qualifying for criterion A (except for people for whom such exposure is part of their vocational role).

Second, criterion A in *DSM-IV* also specified that the person's reaction to the stressor had to involve extreme fear, horror, or helplessness. In the language of behavioural psychology, including the person's reaction to the stressor in the definition of trauma conflates the response with the stimulus. In the language of medicine, it conflates the host with the toxin (McNally 2009). Accordingly, the *DSM-5* committee deleted the extreme emotional reaction requirement from criterion A.

6 Vagueness and degree of impairment

As reviewed earlier, to distinguish normal distress from disorder, the *DSM* committees have specified that disorders must produce clinically significant distress or significant impairment in social, occupational, and other key areas of functioning. Vagueness surfaces as the clinician must determine how much distress qualifies as clinically significant. Complicating matters is the ambiguity of the notion of clinically significant distress. Does it imply "metadistress"— that is, marked distress about one's symptoms; does it refer to the experience of intense suffering alone; or is it redundant—in other words equivalent with impairment whereby anyone who experiences numerous, frequent, and severe symptoms that interfere with functioning has clinically significant distress?

The concept of impairment is vague without being ambiguous. That is, how much social impairment counts as clinically significant? Here normative issues slip invariably into the seemingly objective diagnostic process. For instance, expectations for normal functioning can vary across cultures and over time.

Moreover, judgments about impairment are far from trivial. For example, according to the National Vietnam Veterans Readjustment Study (NVVRS; Kulka et al. 1990), 30.9 percent of all men who served in Vietnam suffered from PTSD at some point in their lives and 15.2 percent still had the disorder in the late 1980s, when this epidemiological survey was conducted. These data puzzled military historians (Jones and Wessely 2001, 133–134; Shephard 2004, 392). They wondered how 30.9 percent of the men met criteria for PTSD when only 12.5 to 15 percent of them served in combat units (Dean 1997; King and King 1991). Indeed, as Ben Shephard told the second author, "the real problem with the NVVRS" is that its equation of symptoms with genuine psychopathology results in "numbers which in any other context are patently absurd" (McNally 2007a, 193).

One possible explanation for these extraordinarily high prevalence estimates was that the *DSM-III-R* criteria that were used in the late 1980s did not require impairment (or marked distress) for diagnosing PTSD. Accordingly, many people diagnosed with PTSD in this study may not have qualified for the disorder, had impairment been required.

To investigate these issues, Dohrenwend et al. (2006) reanalyzed data from the NVVRS. To classify someone as a case of PTSD, the researchers had to (1) corroborate trauma exposure via military and other archival records; (2) ensure that the veteran's PTSD was related to the war (e.g., did not occur prior to serving in Vietnam); and (3) ensure that the veteran's symptoms had to result in more than mild impairment.

For the majority of the cases diagnosed with PTSD in the original survey, there was archival corroboration of both trauma exposure and the war-related onset of symptoms. However, the prevalence estimates dropped dramatically when Dohrenwend and colleagues required more than mild impairment. Because the *DSM-III-R* criteria for PTSD lacked an impairment criterion, Dohrenwend and colleagues cleverly consulted data from the Global Assessment of Functioning (GAF) scale administered by the clinical interviewers in the NVVRS in order to gauge impairment. This version of the GAF ranged from 1 (extreme impairment) to 9 (very high level of functioning). Dohrenwend and colleagues classified veterans as impaired if the clinical interviewer had assigned a rating of 7 or less to signify a veteran's level of functioning. After these adjustments, the lifetime prevalence rate of PTSD dropped from 30.9 percent to 18.7 percent and the current prevalence rate dropped from 15.2 percent to 9.1 percent, respectively. That is, the prevalence rates dropped by 40 percent.

The modal PTSD case in the NVVRS, however, had a GAF rating of 7. The description for a 7 reads: "Some difficulty in social, occupational, or school functioning, but generally functioning pretty well, has some meaningful interpersonal relationships OR some mild symptoms (e.g., depressed mood and mild insomnia, occasional truancy, or theft within the household)" (Kulka et al. 1990, 2). McNally (2007b) noted that someone who is "functioning pretty well" does not seem impaired. What about using a slightly more stringent definition of impairment? For instance, a rating of 6 signifies "[m]oderate difficulty in social, occupational, or school functioning OR moderate symptoms (e.g., few friends and conflicts with peers, flat affect and circumstantial speech, occasional panic attacks)" (Kulka et al. 1990, 2). Had Dohrenwend and colleagues defined impairment as a rating of 6 or less, the estimate of current prevalence would have dropped by 65 percent, not 40 percent.

Nor is this the last word on gradualism and impairment. Depending on whether and how one defines impairment, the current (late 1980s) prevalence rate of PTSD in Vietnam veterans is 15.2 percent (original estimate), 9.1 percent (Dohrenwend et al. 2006), or 5.4 percent (McNally 2007b). The prevalence would have dropped further had impairment been defined as a rating of 5 or less, where 5 signifies "unable to keep a job" (Kulka et al. 1990, 2)—which is a criterion for being awarded a disability pension of 100 percent.

7 Posttraumatic stress disorder and combinatorial vagueness

The sorites paradox refers to the vagueness inherent in continua, which is also called *degree vagueness*. Degree vagueness depends on there being more or less of the same thing, such as trauma severity and impairment. A different source of vagueness is termed *combinatorial vagueness*. Combinatorial vagueness depends on two or more things possessing many of the same parts, but the match is not identical.

One of the standard complaints about *DSM* categories is that they are polythetic—in other words are defined by a menu of diagnostic criteria none of which is necessary or sufficient. Take PTSD. In order to be diagnosed with PTSD in *DSM-5*, one must have a six-symptom pattern drawn from a list of 20 symptoms. In fact two people can both be diagnosed with PTSD and have no symptoms in common.

To suggest that two people who share no symptoms do not have the same disorder would represent a strong diagnostic literalism (Kendler and Zachar 2008; Zachar 2014a). Such literalism is not consistent with the traditional classification perspectives of psychiatry and psychology. Whether conceptualized using the infectious disease model or the latent variables of factor-analytic psychology, the symptoms of PTSD are considered to be fallible indicators of a pathological condition. Symptoms are surface features. The underlying pathology represents the *essential reality* behind the appearances.

What is attractive about this essentialist view of psychopathology is that, if one discovers the nature of the underlying pathology, one can distinguish valid cases of a disorder from apparent cases. The psychiatrist Steven Hyman (2010) explicitly defined validity as referring to whether a diagnosis picks out a *natural kind* on the basis of aetiology or pathophysiology. The most committed natural kind perspective on PTSD would view it as category that exists whether or not we include it in our classification model. According to this view, the traumatic syndrome is a psychic wound caused by extreme stress and whose basic nature is the same between individuals, across cultures, and over time. So railway spine in the nineteenth century, shell shock in World War I, and PTSD are all the same thing—and the way in which they are the same is potentially an empirical question.

The concept of a natural kind defined by an underlying causal essence, however, is deserving of critical scrutiny (Boyd 1991; Hacking 2007; Kendler, Zachar, and Craver 2011; Zachar 2014b). One recently proposed alternative to essentialist models of psychiatric disorders emphasizes causal networks (Borsboom 2008; Cramer et al. 2010; McNally 2012). A causal network approach still classifies syndromes, but views them as homeostatic property clusters. Homeostatic property clusters are causally produced, but the causal work is distributed. Instead of possessing causal essences that play privileged roles, property clusters are the result of multiple and dynamic causal packages.

How does a causal network approach to PTSD differ from the traditional approach? In the causal network approach, PTSD is considered to be a cluster of shared properties. These properties cohere as a result of a variety of causal influences such as internal causes (such as biological processes), external causes (the trauma event), and direct relationships between the symptoms themselves.

Underlying causes of both a biological and a psychological nature may unite some symptoms, but they are not the only factors holding the cluster together. For instance, recent research by McNally et al. (2015) suggests that a symptom such as hypervigilance may serve as a causal factor in the development of other PTSD symptoms, such as being easily startled and feeling that the future is foreshortened. The feeling of a foreshortened future might in turn be a bridge between hypervigilance and emotional numbing and, more remotely, a pathway to social disconnection.

From this perspective, rather than being surface properties that supervene on an underlying reality, the PTSD cluster is in some sense constituted by its symptoms. Symptoms are parts of PTSD. They can also be combined together in different ways, in a variety of part–whole relationships. For example, although two people can be diagnosed with PTSD and not share any symptoms, each must have at least one symptom from an intrusive symptom cluster—namely intrusive memories, distressing dreams, flashbacks—one symptom from the avoidance cluster, and so on. For mereological structures such as this one, *similarity relations at multiple levels of analysis* rather than a *shared underlying essence* make two things be of the same kind.

Another feature of the network model is that the PTSD cluster is a part of a larger psychiatric symptom domain that includes depressions, anxieties, somatic problems, obsessions, personality traits, and even psychoses. Many property clusters can occur in this domain, only a few of which are recognized and named.

Because clusters occupy a shared symptom space, they can also enter into mutual relationships. For instance, the PTSD cluster and the depression cluster share symptoms such as anhedonia and concentration problems. Those symptoms can function as bridges between clusters. From this perspective, when someone is *comorbid* for PTSD and depression, comorbidity, instead of referring to *the co-occurrence of two separate disease entities*, refers to a complicated symptom pattern (a greater whole) that includes within its scope two or more clusters that happen to be officially recognized in the classification system.

When the construct of post-Vietnam syndrome was first proposed, the psychiatrists who resisted it did so in part because they believed that the symptom pattern could be adequately subsumed under others disorders already listed in the manual, such as depression, hysteria, and substance abuse (Helzer, Robins, and Davis 1976). According to this view, what came to be called PTSD is itself a borderline case of these other disorders, perhaps even a hybrid of two or more. *DSM-III* made PTSD a whole unto itself. In fact, the current popularity of the PTSD construct raises the specter of diagnostic overshadowing, in which symptom clusters that are largely depressive or anxious in constitution are labelled PTSD as long as the person has a trauma history.

With respect to vagueness, the network model offers another way of understanding the nature of transitional regions. Symptom clusters can emerge and spread through the psychiatric domain. The number of symptoms (parts) can vary, the frequency of the symptoms' occurrence can vary, and the duration of symptoms can vary. As the number of symptoms grows and their occurrence and/or duration increases, the chance that they will be associated with suffering or will interfere with functioning is greater. But, given that number, rate of occurrence, and duration can vary, there must be transitional regions that lie somewhere in between the category of low symptomatic, functional (sand scattered on the floor), and highly symptomatic, dysfunctional (a psychiatric heap).

There is also one potentially important difference between the degree and the combinatorial models of vagueness. In a pure degree or dimensional model differences are only quantitative. Transitions are gradual and linear. In a combinatorial system there can be gradual exchanges of parts, but new configurations can also be established rapidly due to *critical tipping points*. These involve sudden shifts of state than cannot be modelled simply as additions of more of the same thing (Gladwell 2002; van de Leemput et al. 2014). With respect to PTSD, cases that seem to involve significant changes in personality (without a history of brain injury) might be considered to have made it to, and then passed, a tipping point. They may result from a major event or an accumulation of many smaller events, but the empirical possibility of sudden transitions to new states is an issue for consideration.

8 Conclusions

What is the bottomline importance of vagueness and of the sorites paradox for psychiatry and clinical psychology? To better answer that question, let us examine the paradoxical part of the sorites paradox. If we begin with one grain of sand and add a second, the second grain does not make a heap. If we add a third, the third grain does not make heap, nor does a fourth, nor a fifth. Adding one grain of sand cannot transform something into a heap. Therefore, it is claimed, one can never make a heap by adding grains of sand one at a time. That is the paradox.

What makes it a paradox is that it seems like an absurd conclusion. Of course we can construct a heap by adding grains of sand to a pile one at a time. And if we start with a heap and take away one grain of sand, at some point we will end up with scattered sand as well. When dealing with vague predicates like 'heap', it does not make sense to ask—using one grain of sand as the unit of measurement—what the threshold is where one grain makes the difference between being and not being a heap. We would be asking for a degree of clarity and precision that is not appropriate for that concept.

It is easy to see this with pile of sand, but not always so easy with other vague concepts. How many symptoms does one need in order to have a valid case of PTSD? Which symptoms count? Once we stipulate criteria, we can ask how many new cases of PTSD can be expected to develop in the United States in a single year, or how many people in the United States can be expected to have PTSD in their lifetime. Because the *DSM* specifies precise diagnostic thresholds, we expect PTSD to be crisp and countable in these ways, but expecting such questions to have definitive answers is a bit like expecting that we can discover how many grains of sand one needs in order to have a genuine heap.

If one is educated about the nature of vague concepts, such questions are misplaced. With respect to vagueness, the goal for the science of psychopathology and for clinical practice should be not to discover the correct diagnostic algorithm for distinguishing valid cases of PTSD from false positives, but rather to know how to think about and deal with those transitional regions where neither "normal" nor "disordered" clearly applies.

References

APA (American Psychiatric Association). 2013. *Diagnostic and Statistical Manual of Mental Disorders, Fifth Edition: DSM-5*. Washington, DC: American Psychiatric Publishing.

Blank, A. S. Jr. 1985. "Irrational reactions to post-traumatic stress disorder and Vietnam veterans." In *The Trauma of War: Stress and Recovery in Vietnam Veterans*, edited by S. S. Sonnenberg, A. S. Blank, Jr., and J. A. Talbott, pp. 69–98. Washington, DC: American Psychiatric Press.

Borsboom, D. 2008. "Psychometric perspectives on diagnostic systems." *Journal of Clinical Psychology* **64**: 1089–1108.

Boyd, R. 1991. "Realism, anti-foundationalism and the enthusiasm for natural kinds." *Philosophical studies* **61**: 127–148.

Brentano, F. 1984 [1899]. "On the origin of our knowledge of right and wrong." In *What Is an Emotion?* edited by C. Calhoun and R. C. Solomon, pp. 205–214. New York, NY: Oxford University Press.

Breslau, N., and Kessler, R. C. 2001. "The stressor criterion in DSM-IV posttraumatic stress disorder: An empirical investigation." *Biological Psychiatry* **50** (9): 699–704.

Breslau, N., Chase, G. A., and Anthony, J. C. 2002. "The uniqueness of the DSM definition of post-traumatic stress disorder: Implications for research." *Psychological Medicine* **32** (4): 573–576.

Breslau, N., Chen, Q., and Luo, Z. 2013. "The role of intelligence in posttraumatic stress disorder: Does it vary by trauma severity?" *PLoS One* **8** (6): e65391. doi: 10.1371/journal. pone.0065391.

Breslau, N. et al. 1991. "Traumatic events and posttraumatic stress disorder in an urban population of young adults." *Archives of General Psychiatry* **48** (3): 216–222.

Breslau, N. et al. 2013. "Influence of predispositions on post-traumatic stress disorder: Does it vary by trauma severity?" *Psychological Medicine* **43** (2): 381–390.

Burgess, A. W., and Holmstrom, L. L. 1974. "Rape trauma syndrome." *The American Journal of Psychiatry* **131** (9): 981–986.

Chodoff, P. 1963. "Late effects of the concentration camp syndrome." *Archives of General Psychiatry* **8** (4): 323–333.

Cramer, A. O. J. et al. 2010. "Comorbidity: A network perspective." *Behavioral and Brain Sciences* **33** (2–3): 137–150.

Cuthbert, B. N., and Kozak, M. J. 2013. "Constructing constructs for psychopathology: The NIMH research domain criteria." *Journal of Abnormal Psychology* **122** (3): 928–937.

de Jongh, A. et al. 2008. "Anxiety and post-traumatic stress symptoms following wisdom tooth removal." *Behaviour Research and Therapy* **46** (12): 1305–1310.

Dean, E. T., Jr. 1997. *Shook over Hell: Post-Traumatic Stress, Vietnam, and the Civil War.* Cambridge, MA: Harvard University Press.

Dohrenwend, B. P. 2010. "Toward a typology of high-risk major stressful events and situations in posttraumatic stress disorder and related psychopathology." *Psychological Injury and Law* **3** (2): 89–99.

Dohrenwend, B. P. et al. 2006. "The psychological risks of Vietnam for US veterans: A revisit with new data and methods." *Science* **313** (5789): 979–982.

Freud, S. 1961 [1920]. *Beyond the Pleasure Principle*, translated by J. Strachey. New York, NY: W. W. Norton.

Furst, S. S. (ed.). 1967. *Psychic Trauma*, New York, NY: Basic Books.

Gladwell, M. 2002. *The Tipping Point: How Little Things Can Make a Big Difference.* New York, NY: Little, Brown.

Gold, S. D. et al. 2005. "Is life stress more traumatic than traumatic stress?". *Journal of Anxiety Disorders* **19** (6): 687–698.

Hacking, I. 2007. "Natural kinds: Rosy dawn, scholastic twilight." *Royal Institute of Philosophy* **61** (Suppl. 82): 203–239.

Helzer, J. E., Robins, L. N., and Davis, D. H. 1976. "Depressive disorders in Vietnam returnees." *Journal of Nervous and Mental Disease* **163** (3): 177–185.

Hyde, D. 2014. "Sorites paradox." In *The Stanford Encyclopedia of Philosophy*, edited by E. N. Zalta. http://plato.stanford.edu/entries/sorites-paradox (accessed May 28, 2016).

Hyman, S. E. 2010. "The diagnosis of mental disorders: The problem of reification." *Annual Review of Clinical Psychology* **6**: 155–179.

Insel, T. et al. 2010. "Research domain criteria (RDoC): Toward a new classification framework for research on mental disorders." *American Journal of Psychiatry* **167**: 748–751.

Jones, E., and Wessely, S. 2001. "Psychiatric battle casualties: An intra- and interwar comparison." *The British Journal of Psychiatry* **178**: 242–247.

Kardiner, A. 1959. "Traumatic neuroses of war." In *Handbook of Psychiatry*, edited by A. Arieti, pp. 245–257. New York, NY: Basic Books.

Kendler, K. S., and Zachar, P. 2008. "The incredible insecurity of psychiatric nosology." In *Philosophical issues in psychiatry: Explanation, phenomenology, and nosology*, edited by K. S. Kendler and J. Parnas, pp. 368–385. Baltimore, MD: Johns Hopkins University Press.

Kendler, K. S., Zachar, P., and Craver, C. 2011. "What kinds of things are psychiatric disorders?' *Psychological Medicine* **41**: 1143–1150.

King, D. W., and King, L. A. 1991. "Validity issues in research on Vietnam veteran adjustment." *Psychological Bulletin* **109** (1): 107–124.

Kraemer, B. et al. 2009. "Is the stressor criterion dispensable? A contribution to the criterion: A debate from a Swiss sample of survivors of the 2004 tsunami." *Psychopathology* **42** (5): 333–336.

Kulka, R. A. et al. 1990. *Trauma and the Vietnam War Generation: Report of Findings from the National Vietnam Veterans Readjustment Study* (Brunner/Mazel Psychosocial Stress series, 18). New York, NY: Routledge.

Lifton, R. J. 1973. *Home from the War: Vietnam Veterans—neither Victims nor Executioners.* Oxford: Simon & Schuster.

Long, M. E. et al. 2008. "Differences in posttraumatic stress disorder diagnostic rates and symptom severity between criterion A1 and non-criterion A1 stressors." *Journal of Anxiety Disorders* **22** (7): 1255–1263.

Maier, T. 2006. "Post-traumatic stress disorder revisited: Deconstructing the A-criterion." *Medical Hypotheses* **66** (1): 103–106.

Marlowe, D. H. 2001. *Psychological and Psychosocial Consequences of Combat and Deployment with Special Emphasis on the Guld War.* Santa Monica, CA: RAND.

McDonald, J. J. Jr. 2003. "Posttraumatic stress dishonesty." *Employee Relations Law Journal* **28**: 93–111.

McNally, R. J. 2003. *Remembering Trauma.* Cambridge, MA: Harvard University Press.

McNally, R. J. 2007a. "Can we solve the mysteries of the National Vietnam Veterans Readjustment Study?" *Journal of Anxiety Disorders* **21** (2): 192–200.

McNally, R. J. 2007b. "Revisiting Dohrenwend et al.'s revisit of the National Vietnam Veterans Readjustment Study." *Journal of Traumatic Stress* **20** (4): 481–486.

McNally, R. J. 2009. "Can we fix PTSD in DSM-V?" *Depression and Anxiety* **26** (7): 597–600.

McNally, R. J. 2012. "The ontology of posttraumatic stress disorder: Natural kind, social construction, or causal system?" *Clinical Psychology: Science and Practice* **19** (3): 220–228.

McNally, R. J., and Breslau, N. 2008. "Does virtual trauma cause posttraumatic stress disorder?" *American Psychologist* **63** (4): 282–283.

McNally, R. J., and Robinaugh, D. J. 2011. "Risk factors and posttraumatic stress disorder: Are they especially predictive following exposure to less severe stressors?" *Depression and Anxiety* **28** (12): 1091–1096.

McNally, R. J. et al. (2015). "Mental disorders as causal systems: A network approach to posttraumatic stress disorder." *Clinical Psychological Science* **3** (6), 836–849.

Mol, S. S. L. et al. 2005. "Symptoms of post-traumatic stress disorder after non-traumatic events: Evidence from an open population study." *The British Journal of Psychiatry* **186** (6): 494–499.

Olde, E. et al. 2006. "Posttraumatic stress following childbirth: A review." *Clinical Psychology Review* **26** (1): 1–16.

Rothbaum, B. O. et al. 1992. "A prospective examination of post-traumatic stress disorder in rape victims." *Journal of Traumatic Stress* **5** (3): 455–475.

Rubin, D. C., and Feeling, N. 2013. "Measuring the severity of negative and traumatic events." *Clinical Psychological Science* **1** (4): 375–389.

Saigh, P. A. 1991. "The development of posttraumatic stress disorder following four different types of traumatization." *Behaviour Research and Therapy* **29** (3): 213–216.

Sanislow, C. A. et al. 2010. "Developing constructs for psychopathology research: Research domain critera." *Journal of Abnormal Psychology* **119**: 631–639.

Schlenger, W. E. et al. 2002. "Psychological reactions to terrorist attacks: Findings from the National Study of Americans' Reactions to September 11." *Journal of the American Medical Association* **288** (5): 581–588.

Scott, W. J. 1990. "PTSD in DSM-III: A case in the politics of diagnosis and disease." *Social Problems* **37** (3): 294–310.

Shatan, C. F. 1973. "The grief of soldiers: Vietnam combat veterans' self-help movement." *American Journal of Orthopsychiatry* **43** (4): 640–653.

Shephard, B. 2004. "Risk factors and PTSD: A historian's perspective." In *Posttraumatic Stress Disorder: Issues and Controversies*, edited by G. M. Rosen, pp. 39–61. Chichester: Wiley & Sons, Ltd.

Sorensen, R. 2001. *Vagueness and Contradiction*, Oxford: Oxford University Press.

Spitzer, R., First, M. B., and Wakefield, J. C. 2007. "Saving PTSD from itself in DSM-V." *Journal of Anxiety Disorders* 21: 233–241.

Titchener, J. L., and Ross, W. D. 1974. "Acutre or chronic stress as determinents of behavior, character, and neurosis." In *American Handbook of Psychiatry: Adult Clinical Psychiatry* (2nd edn.), edited by S. Arieti and E. B. Brody, pp. 39–60. New York, NY: Basic Books.

van de Leemput, I. A. et al. 2014. "Critical slowing down as early warning for the onset and termination of depression." *Proceedings of the National Academy of Sciences of the United States of America* 111 (1): 87–92.

Young, A. 1995. *The Harmony of Illusions: Inventing Post-Traumatic Stress Disorder*. Princeton, NJ: Princeton University Press.

Williamson, T. 1994. *Vagueness*, London: Routledge.

Zachar, P. 2014a. *A metaphysics of psychopathology*, Cambridge, MA: MIT Press.

Zachar, P. 2014b. "Beyond natural kinds: Toward a relevant psychiatric taxonomy." In *Classifying Psychopathology: Mental Kinds and Natural Kinds*, edited by H. Kincaid and J. S. Sullevin, pp. 75–104. Cambridge, MA: MIT Press.

Part IV

Social, moral, and legal implications

Chapter 10

Moral and legal implications of the continuity between delusional and non-delusional beliefs

Ema Sullivan-Bissett, Lisa Bortolotti,
Matthew Broome, and Matteo Mameli

1 Introduction

In this chapter we explore two aspects of gradualism about mental illness by arguing that it is difficult to distinguish pathological and non-pathological beliefs on the basis of their epistemic features, and by examining and ultimately defending the claim that there is no *categorical* difference between delusional and other epistemically faulty beliefs (what we shall call *the continuity thesis*). In section 2 we argue that no effective demarcation between pathological and non-pathological beliefs can be achieved on the basis of mere epistemic criteria and we appeal to considerations about the factors that influence belief formation. This supports the continuity thesis. In section 3 we consider some of the moral and legal implications of the continuity thesis, focusing in particular on the role of epistemically faulty beliefs in the attribution of moral responsibility and legal accountability for criminal actions that are motivated by those beliefs.

2 Delusional and non-delusional belief

Belief is an attitude with a standard of correctness according to which true beliefs are correct and false beliefs are incorrect. We might say that it is 'part of the "job description" of belief as a distinctive propositional attitude that beliefs are correct or incorrect depending upon the state of the world' (Railton 1994, 74). While other cognitive states can have contents that are true or false, truth and falsehood are a 'dimension of assessment of beliefs as opposed to many other psychological states or dispositions' (Williams 1970, 136). Correctness conditions then follow not only from the propositional content of a state, but also from the state itself. We also evaluate beliefs with respect to epistemic values other than truth; they are appropriate targets for claims about whether they are *rational* or *justified*. Epistemic norms—including norms of evidence ('a belief is correct if it rests upon sufficient evidence'), knowledge ('a belief is correct if and only if it aims at knowledge'), and rationality ('a belief is correct if and only if it is rational')—are thought to be ones that govern belief (Engel 2007, 181). These norms govern *only* belief: it would be inappropriate to say of my imaginings or supposings that they are rational, irrational, justified, unjustified, and so on.

Many philosophers have taken such features of belief to highlight something necessary about the nature of belief and have sought to explain the conditions under which beliefs are formed and the norms to which we seem to respond in forming a belief. Some philosophers do this by appeal to belief's having an *aim* (McHugh 2011 and 2012; Steglich-Petersen 2006 and 2009; Velleman 2000). Belief, it is suggested, is something that *aims* at the truth, such that, *as believers*, we aim to believe that *p* only if *p* is true.[1]

These teleological accounts explains belief's standard of correctness by pointing out that 'believing *p* is correct only if *p* is true because only true beliefs achieve the aim involved with believing' (Steglich-Petersen 2009, 395). The other epistemic norms we highlighted earlier—those of evidence, knowledge, and rationality—are explained by appeal to the claim that 'following them promotes the aim of believing truly' (ibid., 396). If aims have rules or standards associated with achieving them, then epistemic norms might be considered the rules or standards conducive to achieving belief's aim (McHugh 2011, 371).

Others have claimed that belief is norm-governed, though there has been considerable debate over what the norms governing belief might be. Where normative theorists agree is on the claim that belief is constitutively normative, and it is by appeal to this that we can explain why beliefs have a standard of correctness and are governed by norms regarding their formation (see, for example, Shah 2003; Shah and Velleman 2005; Wedgwood 2002).[2]

---

[1] At least one other aim of belief has been put forward by Conor McHugh: the aim of knowledge (McHugh 2011). It is beyond the scope of this chapter to discuss the various formulations of the aim account; we only mention it here to make salient the idea that ordinary beliefs are idealized in certain respects. This omission is also acceptable since, as Timothy Chan has pointed out, '[g]iven that knowledge entails truth, if belief aims at knowledge, it also aims at truth' (Chan 2013, 10).

[2] These are not views that all of the present authors endorse, but they do demonstrate how we might think about non-delusional beliefs, their link with truth, and the conditions under which they are formed (see Sullivan-Bissett under review; and Sullivan-Bissett and Noordhof under review, for objections to these accounts).

The teleological and the normative accounts of belief offer explanations of our doxastic behaviours (such as focusing on the truth when we think about what to believe, gathering evidence, revising beliefs upon the presentation of new evidence, and so on). The explanations offered involve the claims that belief is constitutively aimed at truth, or constitutively normative. It is consistent with such accounts that there can be a break between truth and other epistemic features (there can be a rational false belief or a justified false belief, for example). But, even in cases in which we come to believe something false, we are guided by the aim of belief, or manifest our commitment to a norm of belief, and these aims or norms are said to be explanatory of our doxastic practice.

Delusions fail to meet many epistemic standards. It might look as if they are not beliefs aimed at truth or governed by a norm of truth, as if they are not responsive to evidence in the ways in which ordinary beliefs typically are. They might be considered as less responsive or even non-responsive to the epistemic norms outlined earlier, which we think other beliefs are responsive to. Differences between delusional and non-delusional beliefs have led some philosophers to argue that delusions are not beliefs at all, but are rather, for example, misidentified imaginings (Currie 2000) or empty speech acts (Berrios 1991).[3] The *Diagnostic and Statistical Manual of Mental Disorders (DSM)-5* describes delusions as follows:

> Fixed beliefs that are not amenable to change in light of conflicting evidence. Their content may include a variety of themes (e.g. persecutory, referential, somatic, religious, grandiose) . . . . Delusions are deemed bizarre if they are clearly implausible and not understandable to same-culture peers and do not derive from ordinary life experiences . . . . The distinction between a delusion and a strongly held idea is sometimes difficult to make and depends in part on the degree of conviction with which the belief is held despite clear or reasonable contradictory evidence regarding its veracity. (APA 2013)

Like all definitions of delusions, the *DSM-5* definition is controversial; but, if we compare it with another influential definition, we cannot but notice that the focus is on the epistemic surface features of delusions:

> A person is deluded when they have come to hold a particular belief with a degree of firmness that is both utterly unwarranted by the evidence at hand, and that jeopardises their day-to-day functioning. (McKay, Langdon, and Coltheart 2005, 315)

Delusional beliefs are formed on the basis of insufficient evidence and may also be incompatible or badly integrated with the person's other beliefs (Bortolotti and Broome 2008, 822). This characterization of delusions as *fixed* beliefs that are *not amenable to change in the light of evidence* and as held *with a*

---

[3] We will assume a doxastic approach to delusions in this chapter (for a defence of doxasticism, see Bayne and Pacherie 2005 and Bortolotti 2009, 2012).

degree of firmness that is utterly unwarranted by the evidence at hand implies that non-delusional ordinary beliefs are 'constantly modified by their experiential validation or refutation' (Maher 1988, 32) and that, in consequence, people with delusions are failing to do something that people without delusions routinely do.

Given that teleological and normative accounts of belief are seeking to explain the constraints under which people believe (that is, why they focus on evidence, why truth is their guide, and why they are responsive to norms of evidence, knowledge, and rationality in their belief formation), if delusions are not subject to such constraints, this may mark them out as different from ordinary beliefs. On the basis of their considerable epistemic faults, delusional beliefs may look different from ordinary, non-delusional beliefs in that they exhibit a difference in kind, and not just in degree. This is precisely the conclusion we seek to resist in this chapter.

2.1 Non-delusional epistemically faulty belief

Here we suggest that non-delusional beliefs are idealized in the psychological and, especially, in the philosophical literature. We do this by considering two kinds of epistemically faulty belief as they appear in the non-clinical population: beliefs from doxastic biases and beliefs from self-deception. We shall show that these beliefs also exhibit failures of rationality and depart from epistemically ideal practices of belief formation and belief maintenance.

2.1.1. Doxastic biases

A practice is a *doxastic bias* if it is an unreliable doxastic practice in terms of truth (Hazlett 2013, 41). The self-enhancement bias is one example of a widespread doxastic bias, and this encompasses 'overly positive self-evaluation, unrealistic optimism, illusions of control, self-serving causal attributions, valence biases in recall and processing speeds, biased attention to evidence, [and] biased self-focused attention' (ibid., 52). In an oft-cited study that looked into the self-perceptions of people with and without depression, participants' self-ratings across various dimensions were compared with ratings given by other people about those same participants. It was found that the 'initial self-perceptions of the depressed subjects were less discrepant with observer ratings' than were those of controls (Lewinsohn et al. 1980, 210). The self-ratings of people with depression 'did not differ significantly' from those of their observers, whereas controls rated themselves 'significantly more positively' than did their observers. People with depression, then, were the 'most realistic' with regard to their self-perceptions, whereas controls 'were engaged in self-enhancing distortions' (ibid., 211).

Several other studies have shown that most people are vulnerable to positive illusions, considering themselves (and sometimes their romantic partners) to be above average, or better than most others, when asked about positive traits and abilities. Moreover, people tend to exhibit unrealistic optimism about their future, underestimating the likelihood of their experiencing negative events and overestimating the likelihood of their experiencing positive events (for a review, see Hazlett 2013 and Bortolotti and Antrobus 2015). In the psychological literature, it has been suggested that positive illusions and unrealistic optimism are adaptive and contribute to mental health, making people happier, more productive and creative, more caring, and more resilient (Taylor 1989; Sharot 2011). In his discussion of the empirical studies, Peter Railton claims that '[i]t would appear to be part of the normal, healthy operation of one's self image that one discount negative evidence and defy the odds' (Railton 1994, 93).

The biases discussed here serve to modify the standards for sufficient evidence required for belief. People do not treat evidence the way they do on purely epistemic grounds; non-epistemic factors are involved when they form beliefs about themselves or make predictions about their future.

2.1.2. Self-deception

In self-deception, beliefs include a motivational element that can involve a process of misreading or ignoring evidence as one comes to a belief. The motivational element of the belief-forming process may be a pro-attitude towards a proposition's being *true* (wishful self-deception), a proposition's being *believed* (willful self-deception), or a proposition's being *false* (dreadful self-deception; see Van Leeuwen 2007, 423–5).

Let us give an example to demonstrate the non-epistemic factors involved in self-deceptive belief formation. Consider a person who has the false and motivated belief that his wife is faithful. There may be evidence available to him that his wife is unfaithful, insofar as certain features of her behaviour are *perceptually available* to him (he sees that she arrives home late, that she is uninterested in him, and so on). We might think, though, that the alternative, epistemically more worthy belief that his wife is unfaithful is unavailable in a weaker sense: it has a kind of *motivational unavailability*. The person, we can presume, is highly motivated for it to be the case that his wife is faithful (wishful self-deception), or at least is motivated for it to be the case that he *believes* that his wife is faithful (wilful self-deception). Consider another case: that of a person with anorexia nervosa who comes to believe that she is overweight, and she has a strong desire for this to be false (dreadful self-deception). Is the person in these cases aiming at the truth when she forms the belief (as the teleological account of belief would claim)? Or is she responding to a norm of belief (as the normative account of belief would claim)? It might be that she is doing either, but what makes it the case that these beliefs are aimed at the truth or governed by a norm of truth may be very different from what is going on in an epistemically ideal case, where motivational factors are not playing a significant role in the fixation of belief.

2.2 Non-epistemic factors in faulty belief

We outlined common instances of beliefs that fail to satisfy the same standards that delusions, too, fail to satisfy. Either the mechanisms responsible for belief production are not geared in all cases towards truth or, even when they are, they often miss that target. The cases of belief we have discussed above depart considerably from the idealized conception of beliefs as mental states that are responsive to evidence and revised in the light of counterevidence. The formation and maintenance of the beliefs we considered are paradigmatically influenced by non-epistemic factors.

To further explain what these cases have in common and how they can be regarded as instances of epistemically faulty belief, we can look at Yaacov Trope and Akiva Liberman's (1996) concept of *confidence thresholds* for belief. The idea here is that there is a correlation between a person's confidence threshold and the evidence that is required to reach the threshold: the lower the threshold, the less evidence is required to reach it. The *acceptance threshold* is 'the minimum confidence in the truth of a hypothesis that [one] requires before accepting it, rather than continuing to test it', while the *rejection threshold* is 'the minimum confidence in the untruth of a hypothesis that [one] requires before rejecting it and discontinuing the test' (Trope and Liberman 1996, 253, cited in Mele 2000, 34). What is meant by *cost of information* in this model is the resources and effort a person needs in order to acquire and process information relevant to the target proposition. What is meant by *cost of false acceptance* and *cost of false rejection* is the subjective importance a person attaches to avoiding falsely believing a proposition, and falsely believing the negation of a proposition, respectively (Trope and Liberman 1996, 252, cited in Mele 2000, 34). If this model is correct, our desires can influence our beliefs by functioning to change our confidence thresholds: (1) in several cases of doxastic bias, pro-attitudes play a role in belief formation; (2) in the case of self-deception, an attitude towards the target proposition plays a role in generating a belief in that proposition, a belief that would not be acquired were the attitude absent. So belief formation is often influenced by non-epistemic factors, which include motivational ones.[4]

---

[4] It might be that it is even justified to make justification standards and confidence thresholds context-relative. This kind of claim is not the one we are after in this chapter. We are not trying to give a normative account of how believers ought to behave; rather we are doing descriptive work. So we remain neutral on whether it is justified or rational to have lower evidence thresholds in some cases. We are just pointing out that, as a matter of fact, we *do* have lower thresholds.

Allan Hazlett suggests that there may be coping mechanisms in the form of self-deception, which would go some way towards offsetting the negative consequences of bad life events, and that such mechanisms may also give rise to 'less extreme' biases that could be 'useful as means of coping with the events of everyday life' (Hazlett 2013, 61). Ryan McKay and Daniel Dennett (2009) go as far as to argue for the presence of a doxastic shear pin, a mechanism that allows desires to influence belief formation when the person would be harmed by believing what she has evidence for and would struggle to manage negative emotions. In some of these cases, the epistemically faulty belief (they call it 'misbelief') can be biologically or psychologically adaptive. Interestingly, candidates for adaptive misbeliefs include positive illusions and delusions.

We saw that in many cases non-epistemic factors influence the fixation of belief, and this indicates that a different strength of regulation for truth, or responsiveness to evidence, and so on applies to different instances of believing. Hence it is difficult to group all beliefs together by appealing to their epistemic surface features. To be clear: we are not suggesting that the attitudes resulting from doxastic biases and self-deception are not beliefs; we think that they are. Rather our claim is that it is implausible to suggest that the reason why these cognitions are beliefs is that they share some good epistemic feature with other, non-delusional beliefs and *then* claim that delusional beliefs are different in kind because they are epistemically poor or lack some good epistemic feature.

Next we turn to delusions and argue that the way in which they are formed is continuous with the epistemic faults detected in the two cases discussed above, namely doxastic biases and self-deception.

2.3 **Delusional belief**

Let us turn now to epistemically faulty beliefs that are also delusional. In this section we shall argue for the continuity thesis in two steps. First, we notice how the most popular theories of delusion formation are compatible with, or actively support, the continuity thesis. Second, we observe that the epistemic faults that characterize delusional beliefs also characterize non-delusional beliefs, and in particular beliefs due to doxastic biases or self-deception.

2.3.1. Delusion formation

Here we cannot provide a detailed description of all the promising theories of delusion formation discussed in the literature, but by appealing to the most influential proposals we aim to show that delusions are best understood as beliefs, and as continuous with non-delusional beliefs. In particular, delusions are seen as understandable (sometimes even rational) responses to anomalous experience. The process by which people form delusions should not be understood as radically or categorically different from the process by which people form ordinary beliefs.

According to the one-factor account of delusion formation, people with delusions do not suffer from an *abnormal* deficit or bias in their mechanisms of belief formation or belief evaluation. The clinically significant difference between a person with delusions and a person without is in the kinds of experiences they have. Brendan Maher claimed that 'delusional beliefs are developed in much the same way that normal beliefs are' (Maher 1988, 22) and that the experiences of people with delusions are such as to distort the evidence available to them. This means that delusions are not held in the face of obvious counterevidence, as they are often characterized; rather they are held 'because of evidence strong enough to support [them]' (Maher 1974, 99). One-factor accounts do not deny that reasoning biases might be involved in the process by which people come to form delusional beliefs; they claim only that 'delusions occur when those biases are exaggerated or introduced by intractable anomalous experiences ... the delusion results from an anomalous experience rationalized by a mind whose divergence from ideal rationality is within the normal range of human psychology' (Gerrans 2002, 52).

One popular version of the one-factor theory is the prediction error theory proposed by Phil Corlett and colleagues.[5] When people experience something that does not match their current understanding of the world, a prediction error signal is produced and either the input is reinterpreted or the model of the world is revised to take into account the new experience. The hypothesis is that, in people with delusions, the excessive production of prediction error signals falsely suggests that a person's internal model of the world needs to be updated.

> Prediction error theories of delusion formation suggest that under the influence of inappropriate prediction error signal, possibly as a consequence of dopamine dysregulation, events that are insignificant and merely coincident seem to demand attention, feel important and relate to each other in meaningful ways. Delusions ultimately arise as a means of explaining these odd experiences. (Corlett et al. 2009, 1)

On this account, delusion formation differs from the formation of other beliefs only in so far as prediction error signalling is disrupted. The process of belief formation is the same in the case of delusional and non-delusional beliefs, but the signalling is disrupted in the case of delusions.

According to the two-factor account of delusion formation, we need to appeal to two factors in order to explain why a person comes to form a delusional belief. The first factor is the anomalous experience appealed to by one-factor

---

[5] For another account of delusion formation based on a prediction error model, see Hohwy (2013).

theorists, but two-factor theorists claim that this is not sufficient for the delusion to be formed or maintained, and so some clinically significant deficit or bias in belief-forming or maintaining mechanisms also needs to be posited. Philosophers and psychologists endorsing this view disagree on how to characterize the second factor. Some characterizations of the second factor provided so far indicate a difference in degree rather than in kind between delusional and non-delusional beliefs. According to the version of the two-factor theory recently proposed by Max Coltheart and colleagues, people with delusions form beliefs in line with a Bayesian model of abductive inference, according to which 'one hypothesis H_1 explains observations O better than another hypothesis H_2 just in case $P(O|H_1) > P(O|H_2)$' (Coltheart, Menzies, and Sutton 2010, 271, cf. McKay 2012). Considering a case of the Capgras delusion[6] where a man mistakes his wife for an impostor, the two hypotheses in play are the *stranger hypothesis* (the woman who looks like my wife is not my wife) and the *wife hypothesis* (the woman who looks like my wife is my wife). Coltheart and colleagues argue that

> the observed data are clearly much more likely under the stranger hypothesis than under the wife hypothesis. It would be highly improbable for the person to have the low autonomic response if the person really was his wife, but very probable indeed if the person were a stranger. (Coltheart, Menzies, and Sutton 2010, 277)

> [I]f the stranger hypothesis explains the observed data much better than the wife hypothesis, the fact that the stranger hypothesis has a lower prior probability than the wife hypothesis can be offset in the calculation of posterior probabilities. And indeed it seems reasonable to suppose that this is precisely the situation with the subject suffering from Capgras delusion. The delusional hypothesis provides a much more convincing explanation of the highly unusual data than the non-delusional hypothesis; and this fact swamps the general implausibility of the delusional hypothesis. (Ibid., 278)

On this view, the second factor explains the maintenance of the delusion. The person does not reject the delusional hypothesis once the disconfirming data start to come in, because he seems to be

> ignoring or disregarding any new evidence that cannot be explained by the stranger hypothesis. It is as though he is so convinced of the truth of the stranger hypothesis by its explanatory power that his conviction makes him either disregard or reject all evidence that is inconsistent with the hypothesis, or at least cannot be explained by the hypothesis. (Ibid., 279–80)

The account of delusion formation proposed by Philippa Garety and David Hemsley (1994) explicitly endorses the continuity thesis. The basic thought is that

---

[6] Capgras delusion is the '[b]elief that others, often related, have been replaced by identical or near identical others; variations exist in which objects or animals are believed changed; the symptoms may be chronic or permanent' (Ellis, Luaté, and Retterstøl 1994, 119).

delusions are formed due to a multiplicity of factors, including past experience, affect, self-esteem, motivation, and biases in reasoning (especially probabilistic reasoning) and perception. Some factors interact with one another, and some are more prominent in the formation of some delusions than others. There is no need to hypothesize a radical deviation from normal processes of belief formation and maintenance; some of the biases responsible for the epistemic faults of delusions— such as selective attention, confirmation bias, and jumping to conclusions—may affect people with delusions more than clinical and non-clinical controls, but they are not distinctive factors. The multifactorial view acknowledges that many of the biases responsible for the formation of delusional beliefs are biases that all people are prone to. This view explicitly characterizes the difference between delusional and non-delusional beliefs as a difference in degree.

2.3.2. Delusions and other epistemically faulty beliefs

Beliefs formed as a result of doxastic biases are continuous with delusional beliefs, as their epistemic faults can be described in terms of the subject's failing to take into account or respond to statistical evidence that is available to them. It has been claimed that in some cases, people who develop delusional beliefs have the same biases as the rest of the population, but are vulnerable to those biases to a greater extent. For instance, delusional and non-delusional beliefs can be due to the *attribution error*, whereby the person attributes positive events to herself and negative events to external factors or to other people. People who develop persecutory delusions may have an exaggerated tendency to fall prey to the attribution error and other similar biases (Freeman et al. 2002). In other cases, people who develop delusional beliefs have a different bias from the one that affects the rest of the population, but both groups are affected by biases that lead to the formation of epistemically faulty beliefs. For instance, when evaluating evidence for a statement, people tend to wait until they have more clues than they need before coming to a decision. This tendency is often called 'conservatism' (Stone and Young 1997; McKay 2012). Empirical evidence, it has been claimed, suggests that people who develop delusions have the opposite tendency and 'jump to conclusions', that is, come to a decision about whether a statement is true without having sufficient evidence (see Fine et al. 2007, but also Ross et al. 2015). This latter tendency is often called 'revisionism'. Both tendencies are epistemically problematic, but conservatism is more widespread in the non-clinical population.

Even the epistemic feature of delusions that is considered most distinctive— resistance to counterevidence—is actually a very common feature of non-delusional beliefs (Bortolotti 2009, ch. 2). Once they adopt a hypothesis, people are very reluctant to abandon it, even when copious and robust evidence against it becomes available. This is true of prejudiced and superstitious beliefs (see, for example, Rusche and Brewster 2008), but also of beliefs in scientific theories (see, for example, Chinn and Brewer 2001), a context in which responsiveness to evidence should be seen as highly important. Self-enhancing beliefs are especially resistant to counterevidence, and people continue to believe that they are skilled, talented, attractive, successful, and so on even when their life experiences repeatedly suggest otherwise. In order to maintain a positive image of themselves, they reinterpret negative feedback and focus on selected evidence that supports their self-enhancing beliefs (Hepper and Sedikides 2012).

Beliefs in the context of self-deception can be vulnerable to a number of doxastic biases and are also resistant to counterevidence. Indeed, non-clinical instances of self-deception have been compared to *motivated* delusions—that is, delusions that can be construed as playing a defensive function and delusions whose formation is affected by what the person desires to be true (McKay and Kinsbourne 2010). Motivated delusions can include erotomania, where a person believes that another is in love with her; grandiose delusions, where the person believes that she is, for example, a largely misunderstood genius; and anosognosia, where the person denies having a serious impairment.[7] In the formation of such delusions, just like in self-deception, motivational influences play a role in the adoption of a belief, and the resulting belief is not well supported by or responsive to the evidence.

These considerations are, obviously, not conclusive. We have considered how delusional and non-delusional beliefs are formed and what epistemic faults delusional and non-delusional beliefs are vulnerable to. We might look elsewhere for the difference between delusions and otherwise epistemically faulty beliefs. Considering how a person reacts when she is made aware of her cognitive biases and confronted with powerful arguments against her belief might introduce a significant difference between delusional and non-delusional beliefs. We might think that a person with delusional beliefs would reject alternative explanations of her beliefs or experiences offhand, whereas a person with non-delusional beliefs would be much more responsive to feedback.

As it happens, empirical evidence does not support discontinuity in this area. It is well known that people are very resistant to changing their beliefs, even when they are told what reasoning mistakes and biases affected the formation of those beliefs (Stalmeier, Wakker, and Bezembinder 1997; Lichtenstein and Slovic 1971; Tversky and Kahneman 1983), and we already saw that people ignore or reinterpret negative feedback on their own performance in order to protect self-enhancing beliefs. The claim that people with delusions are

---

[7] See Mele (2008), Davies (2008), and Bortolotti and Mameli (2012) for a discussion of how delusions relate to self-deception.

resistant to cognitive probing also needs to be qualified. There are strong indications that cognitive behavioural therapy is efficacious in reducing the rigidity of delusional states and the person's preoccupation with the topic of the delusion (Coltheart 2005; Kingdon, Ashcroft, and Turkington 2008). Although the evidence gathered so far does not suggest that cognitive behavioural therapy is effective in leading the person to abandon a delusion altogether, cognitive probing does contribute to the person's adoption of a more critical attitude towards the content of the delusion (Bortolotti 2009, ch. 2). Thus focusing on how people respond to challenges is not a promising way to argue for discontinuity between delusional and non-delusional beliefs.

2.4 Interim conclusion

So far we have argued that epistemically faulty delusional and non-delusional beliefs do not differ in kind. Delusions, like other beliefs, are resistant to counterevidence, and the formation of delusions, like the formation of other epistemically faulty beliefs, is influenced by non-epistemic factors. In the case of delusional and non-delusional beliefs alike, there can be considerable resistance to abandoning a belief once it has been adopted and biases and motivational factors may influence belief formation. Next we move to the moral and legal implications of this view.

3 Moral and legal implications of the continuity view

What factors should be taken into account when attributing criminal responsibility to perpetrators of severe crimes? Here we will discuss three cases of people with epistemically faulty beliefs who committed serious offences. Our purpose is to ask whether the presence of *delusional* as opposed to *non-delusional* beliefs is always a reason to doubt the responsibility people have for those actions that seem to be guided or motivated by their beliefs. If there is no categorical difference between delusions and other epistemically faulty beliefs, why is the presence of delusions regarded as a key factor in establishing criminal responsibility?

The first case we consider is that of Bill, who attacks a neighbour because he believes the neighbour is shouting insults at him and intends to harm him (Broome, Bortolotti, and Mameli 2010). The second case is that of Jeremiah Wright, who killed his son while believing that his son was a cardiopulmonary resuscitation (CPR) dummy (Kotz 2011). The third case is Anders Breivik's perpetration of mass murder in Norway (Bortolotti, Broome, and Mameli 2014).

The analysis of these cases puts some pressure on the view that the presence of delusions is sufficient to determine whether agents are morally responsible and legally accountable for their criminal actions.

3.1 **Three cases**

3.1.1. Bill

Matthew Broome and colleagues describe the case of a young man with a diagnosis of schizophrenia who attacked his neighbour after experiencing auditory hallucinations about that neighbour's making loud noise and insulting him repeatedly. Bill was convicted of assault but his sentence was affected by a preexisting diagnosis of schizophrenia. He was sentenced to two years' probation and his custodial sentence was suspended.

> [S]uppose Bill had actually had a very noisy neighbor. What kind of ascription of responsibility would we have made in relation to the harm inflicted on his neighbor in those circumstances? What kind of punishment would Bill have deserved for his attacking his truly noisy neighbor? Should the fact that the experiences were hallucinatory (and thereby that the neighbor was not in fact noisy) make a difference in relation to how we conceive of Bill's responsibility for what he did and of the punishment he deserves? It is true that Bill was hallucinating: He was hallucinating that his neighbor was making loud noises, and the content of the hallucination explains in part why he attacked his neighbor. Had he not hallucinated that his neighbor was making loud noises, Bill would have probably not attacked and harmed his neighbor. But it is also true that having noisy neighbors does not morally justify assaulting them. That is, had Bill's neighbor been truly noisy, Bill would have still been doing something blameable in assaulting his neighbor. If one has a noisy neighbor, then one should try to convince his neighbor to be less noisy, and, failing that, one should perhaps call the police. (Broome, Bortolotti, and Mameli 2010, 182)

We find here that the psychotic symptoms experienced by Bill help to *explain* but not necessarily *justify* his aggressive behaviour towards his neighbour. His experiences (auditory hallucinations) and delusional beliefs (the belief that his neighbour intended to harm him) help to explain why he assaulted his neighbour, but the assault was not inescapable or excusable on the grounds provided by such experiences and beliefs.

What we can draw from the case of Bill is that the presence of delusions is not sufficient for us to regard the person who committed a crime as unaccountable by reason of insanity, though of course the presence of delusions is relevant to the person's full psychological profile at the time when the crime was committed and thus should be taken into account. For instance, it is possible that the presence of the delusion signals the presence of reasoning impairments that affect the agent's decision-making capacities.

3.1.2. Jeremiah Wright

Our next case is different from the case of Bill in important ways. On 14 August 2011 Jeremiah Wright killed his seven-year-old son, Jori, who had cerebral palsy requiring full-time care (Kotz 2011). He beheaded and dismembered the child in the home he shared with the child's mother. Wright was charged with, and tried for, first-degree murder. Wright was suffering from a delusion at the time of the killing (as well as before and after the act). He believed that Jori was not his son, but a CPR dummy placed in his home as part of a government experiment. Wright was found not guilty on the grounds of insanity.

A police report stated that 'Wright said that he recently saw the way the dummy looked at him and there were signs and little things the dummy did to him that let him know that Jori was not his son, but a dummy' (Quigley 2013). Dr. Sarah DeLand, director at the mental facility in which Wright was housed, and George Seiden, a psychiatrist working with Wright, testified that Wright believed Jori was a CPR dummy. Wright told DeLand and Seiden that Jori was a government social experiment, claiming: 'I don't believe they can do anything to me because it wasn't a real person. His skull was made of plastic. He had foam in him' (ibid.).

Now let us suppose, as we did with the case of Bill, that Wright's beliefs were not delusional and their contents were true. Let us suppose, then, that Jori, the seven-year-old boy, was actually a CPR dummy. What ascription of responsibility would we make with respect to the 'harm' inflicted on Jori, and what kind of punishment would Wright deserve? In Bill's case, his belief that his neighbour was shouting at him would help to explain, but not to justify Bill's assault, as having noisy neighbours does not justify assaulting them. But if Wright had a CPR dummy in his home, then it would not be morally wrong to 'decapitate' and 'dismember' that dummy, given that it would not be a living being capable of feeling pain and suffering.

Wright's psychotic symptoms, like Bill's, help explain his behaviour. Bill feels threatened and frustrated because he believes his neighbour is causing him trouble and might intend to harm him. In addition, Bill might think that other courses of action are closed to him, given his history of mental illness—calling the police, for instance, may not be an attractive option if Bill suspects that the police will not believe him. Wright wants to prevent the government from spying on him, and thus wants to destroy the dummy. The difference between the two cases is that, in Wright's case, if the content of his belief were true, it would not be morally problematic to destroy the dummy, and the action could be justified by Wright's desire to stop the government's intrusion in his life. Wright's actions would be permitted, given his belief that Jori was a CPR dummy. Unlike in Bill's case, then, in Wright's case the presence of the belief is sufficient for us to regard the person who committed the crime as unaccountable, since what Wright did would not be morally problematic if his belief were true. Wright's actions were not *inescapable*: he could have done otherwise, given his beliefs. But his delusions offer both some explanation and justification for his actions.

From the first two cases alone it is obvious that the relationship between delusions and criminal responsibility is not a straightforward one. In Bill's case, the delusion went some way towards explaining his action, but it did not justify that action. In Wright's case, the delusion went some way towards explaining and justifying his action, as it relieved him of culpability. However, his action was not *inescapable*, given his delusional beliefs.

3.1.3. Anders Breivik

In July 2011 Anders Breivik killed 77 people in Norway. In August 2012 he was sentenced to 21 years in prison. As part of his first psychiatric evaluation, he was diagnosed with paranoid schizophrenia and some of his more implausible beliefs were regarded as persistent, systematized, and bizarre delusions. For instance, one belief he reported was that he was the leader of a Knights Templar organization that, according to the Norwegian police, does not exist. However, this first assessment that led to the diagnosis of schizophrenia was overruled by a second assessment, according to which Breivik's strange beliefs were not psychotic symptoms in the context of schizophrenia or of some other psychotic disorder, but could be explained by a personality disorder. On the basis of the fact that he never manifested hallucinations, the second pair of assessors described Breivik's behaviour as caused by a narcissistic personality disorder accompanied by pathological lying (Melle 2013).

If it had been shown that Breivik experienced psychotic symptoms at the time of his crime, then he would have faced trial with a diagnosis of psychosis and would not have been regarded as accountable for his actions. This is because, in the Norwegian Criminal Procedure Code, when one has psychotic symptoms, one cannot be attributed criminal responsibility for his or her action: 'a person is not criminally accountable if psychotic, unconscious, or severely mentally retarded at the time of the crime' (Melle 2013, 17). If Breivik's diagnosis of a psychotic disorder had been confirmed, he would have been regarded as 'criminally insane' and sentenced to compulsory psychiatric treatment (Måseide 2012). As a result of the second assessment and his new diagnosis of personality disorder, Breivik was held accountable for his actions, as he was thought not to have been psychotic at the time of his criminal act.

Some questions could be raised about the relation of Breivik's beliefs to his actions. Just as Bill could have attempted to talk to his neighbour or call the police instead of planning an assault and just as Wright could have removed the 'dummy' from his home or put it out of sight without destroying it, so too could Breivik have genuinely believed that multiculturalism was one of the greatest harms in Norwegian society without engaging in the actions that led him to kill 77 people. Breivik's thoughts could have been channelled into joining a political party in which such views were shared, or he could have campaigned against multiculturalism. That is, his beliefs go some way towards explaining his action but do not justify it and do not make it inescapable.

3.2 Does it matter whether the perpetrator's beliefs are delusional?

The cases we have looked at highlight that we cannot assume that the presence of delusions implies no or reduced responsibility for action. A more local and nuanced view of responsibility needs to be articulated. More precisely, further argument is needed to support the claim that the presence of delusions and other psychotic symptoms is an appropriate criterion for criminal insanity.

In all three of the cases we considered (each coming from a different legal jurisdiction: the United Kingdom, the United States, and Norway), one key question in the psychiatric assessment that led to sentencing was whether the person's system of beliefs was delusional. We saw that the presence of a diagnosis of schizophrenia was instrumental to Bill's lenient sentence. We saw that Wright was found not guilty for reasons of insanity and was committed to a psychiatric hospital for care. And we saw that the presence of delusions alone, if confirmed by the second psychiatric assessment, would have indicated Breivik's lack of responsibility for his mass murder in Norwegian law.

The continuity thesis we have defended in section 2 makes it problematic to rely so heavily on the presence of beliefs that are delusional when assessing responsibility. For claims about responsibility, the significance of the presence of delusional beliefs may derive from the following consideration. If poor reality testing (or some other relevant cognitive deficit associated with delusion formation) is affecting the beliefs a person is prepared to endorse to the extent that such beliefs are implausible even to members of the person's culture or subculture, then maybe such failure of reality testing (or other relevant cognitive deficit) is also implicated in some of the person's decision-making processes, including those processes that led the person to act criminally. But this link between the presence of psychotic symptoms and impaired decision-making is just a hypothesis that needs to be tested.

The assumption that people who have psychotic symptoms or who have received a diagnosis of schizophrenia lack responsibility or have reduced responsibility for their actions on the grounds that their decision-making capacities are impaired is especially problematic, because the behaviour of two people with psychosis or schizophrenia can differ almost entirely. Some people with schizophrenia are able to function well, both cognitively and socially, and to control their delusions to some extent. The presence of psychiatric symptoms and of a diagnosis of schizophrenia should be taken into account in the courtroom, but it should not be regarded as sufficient for determining responsibility.

4 Conclusions and implications

In section 2 we defended gradualism with respect to the distinction between delusional and non-delusional epistemically faulty beliefs. We argued that there is continuity between them: they can be resistant to counterevidence and their formation process may be influenced by biases and motivational factors. Reflecting on the recent psychological literature on delusions, we saw that the mechanisms posited to explain the adoption of delusional hypotheses are not radically different from, but are continuous with, standard mechanisms of belief formation.

In section 3 we turned to the implications of the continuity thesis for moral and legal issues concerning responsibility for action. How should we view the presence of delusions, which is often considered as a key criterion for criminal insanity, if there is no clear demarcation between delusional and non-delusional beliefs to be made on epistemic grounds? We argued that the role of delusional beliefs in motivating action does not seem to be different from the role of other epistemically faulty non-delusional beliefs, unless we assume that the presence of delusions also signals the presence of a cognitive deficit that impacts on the decision to commit a given crime.

Moreover, we suggested that having beliefs that are epistemically faulty, whether delusional or not, rarely provides a justification for criminal action. It may contribute to an explanation of the crime, but in most cases it does not make the criminal action inescapable or excusable.

Acknowledgements

Lisa Bortolotti, Matteo Mameli, and Matthew Broome acknowledge the support of the Wellcome Trust for a project entitled 'Moral Responsibility and Psychopathology' (WT099880MA). Lisa Bortolotti and Ema Sullivan-Bissett acknowledge the support of the Arts and Humanities Research Council for a project entitled 'Epistemic Innocence of Imperfect Cognitions' (AH/K003615/1) and of a European Research Council Consolidator Grant (grant agreement 616358) for a project entitled 'Pragmatic and Epistemic Role of Factually Erroneous Cognitions and Thoughts' (PERFECT). All four authors are grateful to Geert Keil for his helpful comments on an earlier draft of this chapter.

References

APA (American Psychiatric Association). 2013. *Diagnostic and Statistical Manual of Mental Disorders, Fifth Edition: DSM-5*. Washington, DC: American Psychiatric Association.

Bayne, T., and Pacherie, E. 2005. 'In defence of the doxastic conception of delusions'. *Mind and Language* 20 (2): 163–88.

Berrios, G. E. 1991. 'Delusions as 'wrong beliefs: A conceptual history'. *British Journal of Psychiatry* 159: 6–13.

Bortolotti, L. 2009. *Delusions and Other Irrational Beliefs*. Oxford: Oxford University Press.

Bortolotti, L. 2012. 'In defence of modest doxasticism about delusion'. *Neuroethics* **5**: 39–53.

Bortolotti, L., and Antrobus, M. 2015. 'Costs and benefits of realism and optimism'. *Current Opinion in Psychiatry* **28** (2): 194–8.

Bortolotti, L., and Broome, M. R. 2008. 'Delusional beliefs and reason giving'. *Philosophical Psychology* **21** (6): 821–41.

Bortolotti, L., Broome, M. R., and Mameli, M. 2014. 'Delusions and responsibility for action: Insights from the Breivik case'. *Neuroethics* **7**: 377–82.

Bortolotti, L., and Mameli, M. 2012. 'Self-deception, delusion and the boundaries of folk psychology'. *Humana Mente* **20**: 203–21.

Broome, M., Bortolotti, L., and Mameli, M. 2010. 'Moral responsibility and mental illness: A case study'. *Cambridge Quarterly of Healthcare Ethics* **19** (2): 179–87.

Chan, T. 2013. 'Introduction: Aiming at truth'. In *The Aim of Belief*, edited by T. Chan, pp. 1–16. Oxford: Oxford University Press.

Chinn, C. A., and Brewer, W. F. 2001. 'Models of data: A theory of how people evaluate data'. *Cognition and Instruction* **19** (3): 323–93.

Coltheart, M. 2005. 'Delusional belief'. *Australian Journal of Psychology* **57** (2): 72–6.

Coltheart, M., Menzies, P., and Sutton, J. 2010. 'Abductive inference and delusional belief'. *Cognitive Neuropsychiatry* **15** (1): 261–87.

Corlett, P. R. et al. 2009. 'Why do delusions persist?'. *Frontiers in Human Neuroscience* **3** (12): 1–9.

Currie, G. 2000. 'Imagination, delusion and hallucinations'. *Mind and Language* **15** (1): 168–83.

Davies, M. 2008. 'Delusion and motivationally biased belief: Self-deception in the two-factor framework'. In *Delusions and Self-Deception: Affective Influences on Belief Formation*, edited by T. Bayne and J. Fernández, pp. 71–86. Hove: Psychology Press.

Ellis, H. D., Luauté, J. P., and Retterstøl, N. 1994. 'Delusional misidentification syndromes'. *Psychopathology* **27**: 117–20.

Engel, P. 2007. 'Belief and normativity'. *Disputatio* **2** (23): 179–203.

Fine, C. et al. 2007. 'Hopping, skipping or jumping to conclusions? Clarifying the role of the JTC bias in delusions'. *Cognitive Neuropsychiatry* **12** (1): 46–77.

Freeman, D. et al. 2002. 'A cognitive model of persecutory delusions'. *British Journal of Clinical Psychology* **41**: 331–47.

Garety, P. A., and Hemsley, D. 1994. *Delusions: Investigations into the Psychology of Delusional Reasoning*. Oxford: Oxford University Press.

Gerrans, P. 2002. 'A one-stage explanation of the cotard delusion'. *Philosophy, Psychiatry, & Psychology* **9** (1): 47–53.

Hazlett, A. 2013. *A Luxury of the Understanding: On the Value of True Belief*. Oxford: Oxford University Press.

Hepper, E. G., and Sedikides, C. 2012. 'Self-enhancing feedback'. In *Feedback: The Handbook of Praise, Criticism, and Advice*, edited by R. Sutton, M. Hornsey, and K. Douglas, pp. 43–56. London: Peter Lang.

Hohwy, J. 2013. *The Predictive Mind*. New York, NY: Oxford University Press.

Kingdon, D., Ashcroft, K., and Turkington, D. 2008. 'Cognitive behavioural therapy for persecutory delusions: three case examples'. In *Persecutory Delusions: Assessment,*

Theory and Treatment, edited by D. Freeman, R. Bentall, and P. Garety, pp. 393–410. Oxford: Oxford University Press.

Kotz, P. 2011. 'Jori Lirette, 7, dismembered by Jeremiah Wright, his mom's boyfriend'. *True Crime Report*. 18 August 2011. http://www.truecrimereport.com/2011/08/jori_lirette_7_dismembered_by.php (accessed 15 May 2016).

Lewinsohn, P. M. et al. 1980. 'Self-competence and depression: The role of illusory self-perceptions'. *Journal of Abnormal Psychology* **89** (2): 203–12.

Lichtenstein, S., and Slovic, P. 1971. 'Reversals of preference between bids and choices in gambling decisions'. *Journal of Experimental Psychology* **89** (1): 46–55.

Maher, B. 1974. 'Delusional thinking and perceptual disorder'. *Journal of Individual Psychology* **30** (1): 98–113.

Maher, B. 1988. 'Anomalous experience and delusional thinking: The logic of explanations'. In *Delusional Beliefs*, edited by T. Oltmanns and B. Maher, pp. 15–33. Chichester: John Wiley & Sons Ltd.

Måseide, P. H. 2012. 'The battle about Breivik's mind'. *The Lancet* **379** (9835). doi: 10.1016/S0140-6736(12)61048-4

McHugh, C. 2011. 'What do we aim at when we believe?'. *Dialectica* **65** (3): 369–92.

McHugh, C. 2012. 'Belief and aims'. *Philosophical Studies* **160**: 425–39.

McKay, R. 2012. 'Delusional inference'. *Mind & Language* **27** (3): 330–55.

McKay, R., and Dennett, D. 2009. 'The evolution of misbelief'. *Behavioral and Brain Sciences* **32**: 492–510.

McKay, R., and Kinsbourne, M. 2010. 'Confabulation, delusion, and anosognosia: Motivational factors and false claims'. *Cognitive Neuropsychiatry* **15** (1): 288–318.

McKay, R., Langdon, R., and Coltheart, M. 2005. ' "Sleights of mind": Delusions, defences, and self-deception'. *Cognitive Neuropsychiatry* **10** (4): 305–26.

Mele, A. 2000. *Self-Deception Unmasked*. Princeton, NJ: Princeton University Press.

Mele, A. 2008. 'Self-deception and delusion'. In *Delusions and Self-Deception: Affective Influences on Belief Formation*, edited by T. Bayne and J. Fernandez, pp. 55–70. Hove: Psychology Press.

Melle, I. 2013. 'The Breivik case and what psychiatrists can learn from it'. *World Psychiatry* **12** (1): 16–21.

Quigley, R. 2013. 'Father "who hacked his disabled son's head off and left it by the road for his mom to see believed the boy, 7, was a dummy or robot" '. *The Daily Mail*, 31 January (updated version). http://www.dailymail.co.uk/news/article-2271394/Jeremiah-Wright-Father-hacked-disabled-sons-head-left-road-mom-believed-boy-7-dummy-robot.html (accessed 27 May 2016).

Railton, P. 1994. 'Truth, reason, and the regulation of belief'. *Philosophical Issues* **5**: 71–93.

Ross, R. M. et al.. 2015. 'Jumping to conclusions about the beads task? A meta-analysis of delusional ideation and data-gathering'. *Schizophrenia Bulletin* **41** (5), 1183–91.

Rusche, S. E., and Brewster, Z. W. 2008. ' "Because they tip for shit!" The social psychology of everyday racism in restaurants'. *Sociology Compass* **2** (6): 2008–29.

Shah, N. 2003. 'How truth governs belief'. *The Philosophical Review* **112** (4): 447–82.

Shah, N., and Velleman, J. D. 2005. 'Doxastic deliberation'. *The Philosophical Review* **114** (4): 497–534.

Sharot, T. 2011. *The Optimism Bias: A Tour of the Irrationally Positive Brain*. New York, NY: Pantheon Books.

Stalmeier, P. F. M., Wakker, P. P., and Bezembinder, T. G. 1997. 'Preference reversals: Violations of unidimensional procedure invariance'. *Journal of Experimental Psychology: Human Perception and Performance* **23** (4): 1196–205.

Steglich–Petersen, A. 2006. 'No norm needed: On the aim of belief'. *The Philosophical Quarterly* **56** (225): 499–516.

Steglich–Petersen, A. 2009. 'Weighing the aim of belief'. *Philosophical Studies* **145** (3): 395–405.

Stone, T., and Young, A. W. 1997. 'Delusions and brain injury: The philosophy and psychology of belief'. *Mind & Language* **2** (3/4): 327–64.

Sullivan-Bissett, E. under review. 'Explaining Doxastic Transparency: Aim, Norm, or Function?'

Sullivan-Bissett, E., and Noordhof, P. under review. 'Transparent Failure of Norms to Keep Up Standards of Belief'.

Taylor, S. E. 1989. *Positive Illusions: Creative Self-Deception and the Healthy Mind*. New York, NY: Basic Books.

Trope, Y., and Liberman, A. 1996. 'Social hypothesis testing: Cognitive and motivational mechanisms'. In *Social Psychology: Handbook of Basic Principles*, edited by E. Higgins and A. Kruglanski, pp. 239–70. New York, NY: Guildford Press.

Tversky, A., and Kahneman, D. 1983. 'Extensional vs intuitive reasoning: The conjunction fallacy in probability judgment'. *Psychological Review* **90** (4): 293–315.

Van Leeuwen, D. S. N. 2007. 'The product of self-deception'. *Erkenntnis* **67** (3): 419–37.

Velleman, D. J. 2000. *The Possibility of Practical Reason*. Oxford: Oxford University Press.

Wedgwood, R. 2002. 'The aim of belief'. *Philosophical Perspectives* **16**: 267–97.

Williams, B. 1970. 'Deciding to believe'. In B. Williams, *Problems of the Self*, pp. 136–51. Cambridge: Cambridge University Press.

Chapter 11

Mental illness versus mental disorder: Arguments and forensic implications

Hans-Ludwig Kröber

1 Introduction

The assumptions we make about the conceptual antagonism between sanity and insanity, about mental illness and mental normality, or simply about the gradual differences between these conditions have far-reaching social consequences. On the one hand, the range of normality can be stretched infinitely. Today this notion is evoked, for example, by the magic notion of "social inclusion," that is, by the non-discrimination of handicapped people: costly facilities for the deaf, the blind, and the mentally handicapped can be abolished and economized because these people are not categorically handicapped but rather partially sighted, partially able to hear, or partially able to learn. Thus, normal schools can accommodate of them. On the other hand, the deviating, the quantitatively dissimilar is conceptualized as a "disorder," a term that is equally expandable: even normality can be classified as "compulsive conformity" and thus as a disorder (which sometimes happens), not to mention common emotions such as sorrow, anger, or joy. Britons, it is said, have always known that every passion is a disorder. Expanding the concept of a mental disorder well into the realm of normality and sanity has led to several hundred new diagnoses in the fifth edition of the American *Diagnostic and Statistical Manual of Mental Disorders* (*DSM-V*: APA 2013; see Frances 2013) and has bestowed upon psychotherapists a plethora of desirable new and unproblematic patients. But this expansion has also led to truly sick patients having to wait for months to receive treatment and has had disastrous consequences in the context of forensic psychiatry. In 1951 the European Convention on Human Rights permitted the confinement of mentally ill persons who posed a threat to themselves or others. However, the Convention didn't use the term "illness" but relied instead—and rather unpsychiatrically—on the term "unsound mind." In 2011 the German legislature turned this category into "psychiatric disorders" that warranted the prophylactic and persistent detention of former convicts who have served their sentences.

Forensic psychiatrists must be concerned that a categorical difference exists between accountable and unaccountable agents, not only legally but also with regard to their mental condition. Legal responsibility is structured in the German criminal code of 1975 as follows:

> Any person who at the time of the commission of the offence is incapable of appreciating the unlawfulness of their actions or of acting in accordance with any such appreciation due to a pathological mental disorder, a profound consciousness disorder, debility or any other serious mental abnormality, shall be deemed to act without guilt. (Article 20)

In reality, "mental illness" is almost the only justification for deculpation [*Dekulpation*] or diminished responsibility—that is, for deciding that there is a lack of criminal responsibility—except for occasional cases of severe "mental retardation." Neither a "profound consciousness disorder" nor a "serious mental abnormality" (e.g., severe personality disorders, adjustment disorders, and sexual deviations) constitutes grounds for deculpation, although both lead to "diminished responsibility." German criminal law implicitly applies a concept of illness (whatever its name), be it a "legal" or a "criminal" one. What matters in this context is that, unlike the concept of illness applied by health insurance companies, the law demands that in relation to "sanity" there be a categorical difference and not just a gradual one ("mental aberration").

2 Antagonisms and transitions

Naturally the question arises as to whether insisting on the concept of illness is warranted or whether the "sane" transitions instead without friction into the "insane." Such a transition would imply that no categorical difference exists between the endpoints: between sea and land, day and night, poor and rich, sane and insane. The existence of a transient area poses problems of definition and diagnosis. Time poses another challenge: When does Achilles pass the turtle and when is he in front of instead of behind it? The basic question is: Are quantitative differences the only ones that exist in reality, or does quantity turn into quality at some point? This forensic–psychiatric chapter takes the view that illness is qualitatively different from a mere quantitatively altered mental state. A schizophrenic psychosis is not only gradually different, but categorically different from mental sanity. An IQ of 50, for mental handicap, is qualitatively different from an IQ of 90. The other quality arises not from the altered quantity of the IQ, but rather from the person's functional detriment, in other words from the opening or closing of entry points to one's surroundings. A mentally handicapped person with an IQ of 50 faces an entirely different, reduced world, which nonetheless remains highly complex and exceeds the person's capabilities to respond to it. This is not limited to the inability to perform simple arithmetic tasks, or even to read and write. The mentally handicapped person leads a fundamentally different life despite all well-intentioned efforts made by others to "include" him or her—efforts that often seem to deny reality. Having highly underdeveloped intellectual capabilities, as in this case, is not usually considered to be an illness; instead it is labelled a mental handicap. If these capabilities once existed and have deteriorated due to the neurological process called Alzheimer's disease, then we speak of an illness. Both states differ not only gradually but qualitatively from the state of normal intelligence and mental sanity. What is structured seamlessly is the measuring tool; what is structured in stages is the functional intellectual capacity.

In the context of medicine and psychiatry we clearly find such stages—stages that signal fundamental differences. Blood alcohol concentration can be measured along a continuum from 0.0 g/kg up to 6.0 g/kg (it seems no one ever wished to drink more). The differences in one's individual perception are not just gradual but categorical: at 0.0 per mill one is sober; at 1.0 per mill one is gradually altered, becoming reckless and silly and having slower reaction speeds and reduced fine motor skills; at 2.5 per mill fundamental cerebral functions are lost; and at 4 per mill an average consumer of alcohol is dead. At the very least, that must be acknowledged to be a categorical difference.

3 Mental disorder and illness

For the most part, modern psychiatry applies an a theoretical concept of "disorder": different impaired functions are described without distinguishing pathological disorders from non-pathological disorders, or even from disorders similar to an illness. Of course, that eliminates neither illnesses nor the subjective experience of being ill. For researchers, the dissolution of "illness" into one or multiple "disorders" is often useful, just as it is for the billing practices of health insurance companies. For legal purposes, however, it often suffices to establish that someone is "ill" as a result of one or multiple disorders. After all, even people with multiple functional mental detriments have only one single, individual, complex clinical picture. Illness is therefore not assessed according to the number of functional disorders but according to its quality and intensity in relation to intentional control, the preconditions of intent, and social interaction. In this respect, an "accumulation of multiple mental disorders" is primarily an expression of a certain inclination to differentiate; people examined in this way will probably not experience "multiple disorders" but rather feel disordered, or even overwhelmed in some diverse but coherent manner. The same is true when multiple personality disorder is diagnosed: such patients also have only one personality, albeit an imbalanced and particularly complex one.

Even when it is sane, our mental apparatus is not perfect. It can be deceived and disturbed, and it is prone to errors. Observing basic mental competences elucidates how illness differs from varieties of normality and how it tends to be associated with disculpation, and how non-pathological disorder tends to be associated with (potentially diminished) responsibility. In German psychiatry, Kurt Schneider's (1948) somatic postulate was significant. He claimed that illness exists (conceptually) only in the physical organism. Therefore, for illnesses such as schizophrenia, which in his day had not been adequately studied, a somatic cause was to be hypostatized. Today hardly any psychiatrist or psychologist denies the somatic foundations of mental illnesses; equally undisputed are non-somatic, psychological, and social factors that can lead to mental illnesses and, in turn, to an alteration of their somatic foundations.

But if everything—even emotional well-being, body height, athletic talent, and intelligence—is rooted in somatic functions and is correlated with biological processes, then what is illness and, in particular, what is mental illness? Illness is a fatefully descending, bodily mediated alteration of one's condition that the affected person cannot wilfully annul. It de facto renders her unfree. She is unfree because of the extensive or total suspension of important functions. Alexander Mitscherlich proposed to the German Society for Psychotherapy and Deep Psychology that deculpation should be defined as "a somatically or non-somatically induced pathological disorder that is beyond volitional control and that, as far as its causes are concerned, is invisible to the perpetrator" (Mitscherlich, as cited by Schild 1990, 665).

In psychiatric contexts, Häfner (1981), Blankenburg (1989), and Helmchen (2006) have dominated the discourse. They have indicated that the line between "illness" and "sanity" can be drawn differently according to the social function concerned (health insurance companies, criminal judges, spouses, etc.). According to Häfner (1981, 50), "the inability to fulfil social duties due to a functional deficit of the psycho-physical organism" lies at the core of a general concept of illness. Later he also emphasized the "involuntary and substantial impairment of vital functions"—mostly accompanied by reduced well-being (Häfner 1997, 159). Blankenburg (1989, 138) believed that the essential determinant of illness was "a certain inability, an incapacity to act (differently)."

According to Helmchen (2006, 272), "[t]his *involuntary* and substantial inability appears evident in severe manifestations." But in the majority of doubtful and mild disorders the identification of such an inability is problematic.

Furthermore, according to Helmchen, there will always be an unbridgeable gap between the inner experience of being ill and the objectifying glance of an outside observer (which can only capture the surface)—especially since mental illness can only be grasped through communication between patient and doctor. Not even reference to psychosocial impairment can bridge this gap. Despite the fact that it is usually open to external observation, it cannot be objectified so as to capture the same quality experienced by the ill individual. Neither can "social normality" serve as a benchmark, since it is nothing but a shifting convention. Helmchen points out that replacing the term "illness" with "disorder" in diagnostic manuals has rather aggravated the problem.

It should be added here that this dilemma also arises in the context of criminal law. Psychiatrists can hardly say whether there is any overall dogmatic position to be adopted regarding the question of which factors, as set out in Article 20 of the 1975 German criminal code, ought to eliminate or diminish legal and personal responsibility. If the aforementioned legal prerequisites for deculpation and diminished responsibility are connected to neither a psychiatric nor a legal concept of illness (with which they needn't be congruent), the evaluation will be adjourned until individual cases demand individual normative action. The factors that determine the legitimacy of individual normative actions are at times indistinguishable.

It is beyond dispute, however, that mental illness is the critical benchmark in the "psychopathological system of reference" (Saß 1991). According to this benchmark, other situations such as personality disorders, paraphilia, or mental handicaps are evaluated by asking whether they are comparable to mental illnesses in their impairment of perceptions, reasoning, affect regulation, and behavior (Kröber 2007b, 2009a). It is the knowledge of mental illness that makes the forensic evaluation of sociopathy and personality disorders accessible (Saß 1987).

4 Psychiatric reasoning on legal responsibility: Yes or no? Or a little bit?

In the German legal system, the forensic–psychiatric expert is an "assistant of the court." He or she is required to conduct a psychiatric examination of the accused person, arrive at a diagnosis, and write a forensic psychiatric report. Moreover, he or she has to draw conclusions about the defendant's legal responsibility. This work must be unbiased, fair-minded, and conducted in good faith.

There has always been a consensus among psychiatrists about the following: mental disorders that annul one's ability to perceive and test either reality or basic thought processes erase one's self-determination or free will. Dementia, paranoia, mania, and psychotic depression render the perpetrator of an illegal act free from legal responsibility. This was evidently true even before the establishment of psychiatry as a scientific discipline and the development of clinical institutions in the nineteenth century.

A forensic assessment and evaluation that included psychiatric questions existed long before the nineteenth century. The *Constitutio criminalis Carolina* of 1532 acknowledges mental disturbances as a general reason for mitigation. Starting with the *Practica nova imperialis Saxonia rerum criminalium* of Carpzow (1595–1666), medical faculty councils in the seventeenth and eighteenth century developed a practice of medical assessment. This in turn led to the establishment of diagnostic and assessment standards derived essentially from case histories.

These assessments found their way into German laws like the Bavarian Code of 1751, which absolved from punishment those who were only half demented, or like the Prussian General State Laws of 1794 (II, 20), especially its articles 16 ("If a person is unable to act free there is no crime and no penalty") and 18 ("Everything that increases or diminishes a person's ability to act freely and deliberately, increases or diminishes the degree of culpability.")

Psychiatric assessment only became part of an increasingly independent medical discipline in the nineteenth century. The professional journals published in the middle of the nineteenth century were always for general *and* forensic psychiatry.

Concerning questions of legal responsibility, psychiatry did not react merely to legal requirements. Psychiatrists developed their own ideas about freedom of will on the basis of their experiences with mentally ill patients. And they have long sought to influence both legislators and criminal law practices to their advantage. The founder of forensic psychiatry was Paolo Zacchia (1584–1659), the private physician of two popes and a consultant to the Vatican Supreme Court. In his *Quaestiones medico-legales* (1621), Zacchia defended the competence of physicians with the argument that "dementia" and similar diseases were known only to physicians (Janzarik 1972). In contrast, Immanuel Kant was skeptical about the capabilities of physicians. In his *Anthropology*, he explained that only someone raving in a feverish state suffers from a somatic disease. Someone talking mad without evident physical signs of disease must be considered crazy or disturbed and, if he commits a crime, should thus be referred to the philosophical and not to the medical faculty. Kant argued:

> For the question of whether the accused . . . was in possession of his natural faculties of understanding and judgment is a wholly psychological question; and although a physical oddity of the soul's organs might indeed sometimes be the cause of an unnatural transgression of the law of duty . . . physicians and physiologists in general are still not

advanced enough to see deeply into the mechanical element in the human being so that they could explain, in terms of it, the attack that led to the atrocity, or foresee it. (Kant 2006 [1798], 108 [§ 51])

In their discussions of legal responsibility, psychiatrists did not necessarily refer to the respective legal statutes but rather to terms in the philosophy of law. In Germany these terms were primarily defined by Kant's *Critique of Pure Reason* (Kant 1929 [1781], 464–5 (B 561–2)) and then Hegel's *Philosophy of Right* (Hegel 1970 [1821]).

Psychiatrists were convinced that they had to express their views on the *freedom* or *bondage* of the individual: "Is or was the individual in possession of psychic freedom or was he capable of psychic self-determination according to rational arguments?" (Friedreich 1835, 134). This was a direct reference to Kant.

For some psychiatrists, however, mental illness was not incompatible with individual responsibility and guilt. For example, Heinroth wrote: "Humans have only themselves to blame for becoming melancholic, crazy, demented, etc." (Heinroth 1825, 261). By virtue of his own guilt, the perpetrator acquires the diathesis to psychic illness.

> And, in turn, his guilt evokes the principle of psychic illness, the deprivation of reasoning, and thus his bondage . . . . Should he be excused, should he be released because he acted in a mentally confused and will-bound state? No! Both this confusion and this dependence are his work, his creation, the fruit of his deeds, his life and the pinnacle of his guilt. He may thus have made himself incapable of punishment, but he is not without guilt. (Heinroth 1833, 198)

There is another reference in Griesinger (1845), who argues that the lesson of accountability is better derived from the notion of level-headedness than from the notion of freedom. He pleads that physicians should state whether there was a disease. Then they should say whether it disturbed mental health at all and whether it specifically cancelled, limited, or *could* limit freedom of action. Later, some psychiatrists insisted on returning to purely medical statements. Thus Krafft-Ebing (1892, 22) explains that "[n]either accountability nor the freedom of will but rather the determination of mental health or illness" is the actual task of the medical evaluation.

The influential jurist Edmund Mezger argued that the ability to act lawfully lies in the rational structure of the individual, that is, in his ability to resist having his actions determined by momentary stimuli. "The individual is accountable when the ability to rationally determine his will is generally present; if this is lacking, we have to consider him unaccountable" (Mezger 1913, 43). If the lawyers are determinists, then they—like many psychiatrists—are usually also compatibilists: A person is responsible if she is able to act according to her reasons. (The meaning of "reason" in this context is not *causa*, but Kant's "reason": *Vernunftgründe, raison.*)

5 Gradual deviance: No disease but a personality disorder

Psychiatry, and especially forensic psychiatry, have had no difficulty making the concept of legal responsibility plausible to the public if the perpetrator is psychotic. But they have real problems conceptualizing personality disorder and diminished legal responsibility in forensically viable terms. The German imperial criminal code (*Reichsstrafgesetzbuch*) of 1871 codified legal *non-responsibility* in terms of a pathological disorder of mind. The term "pathological disorder" covered essentially psychotic illnesses and severe organic brain diseases. Forensic psychiatry is in fact quite capable of differentiating between mental illness in the strict sense of the word and mental health. Mental illness is a global qualitative alteration of psychic functions and of a person's overall ability to relate to her environment. In essence, this corresponds to the concept of "psychosis." A mentally ill person lives in a system of interactions with other people and with the world—a system in which meanings have been totally altered as a result of the illness. The mentally ill individual is not able to control this alteration. The schizophrenic is not responsible for his illness, since the disorder alters his social relations with compelling power; therefore the psychosocially disturbed schizophrenic bears no responsibility and no criminal guilt for his social conduct. This is the logical deduction of criminal non-responsibility. A modification of the German criminal code in 1975 allowed for the possibility of "deculpating" offenders suffering from personality disorders. "Deculpation" is a partial reduction in criminal responsibility; exculpation is a total cancelation of responsibility. Since 1975, the binding rule of law is this:

> Any person who at the time of the commission of the offence is incapable of appreciating the unlawfulness of their actions or of acting in accordance with any such appreciation due to a pathological mental disorder, a profound consciousness disorder, debility or any other serious mental abnormality, shall be deemed to act without guilt. (Article 20)

This last category pertains to severe personality disorders, adjustment disorders, and sexual deviations that, although they seldom justify exculpation, typically result in diminished responsibility and correspondingly diminished punishment according to Article 21 of the criminal code.

The law states that only *substantial* impairment of criminal responsibility can justify deculpation. Thus German forensic psychiatrists have tried to develop psychiatric criteria for diminished criminal responsibility in the case offenders with personality disorders (Kröber 1995). Most would agree that neither every conspicuous mental symptom nor every personality disorder substantially diminishes legal responsibility. An effort was made to discriminate between "minor" and "severe" forms of personality disorders. Additional difficulties arose from the fact that individuals with severe personality disorder are not necessarily severely affected in all their actions and therefore are not invariably deculpated (Kröber 2009b). For example, there is no reason for excusing an impulsive offender for a carefully planned and consciously committed offense.

The more closely one examines the issue, the more evident it becomes that the question of a defendant's ability to act in accordance with an understanding of the wrongfulness of his or her action can only be answered approximately and not definitively by psychiatric means. In fact, how much of the burden of presumed self-control and will power criminal law imposes upon a person is a normative question.

In practice, antisocial behavior patterns fall under the individual's responsibility; character traits, which are regarded as a part of an adult's own responsibilities, are considered to be the only criterion for antisocial personality disorder. Accordingly, Janzarik wrote that, unlike the process of a mental illness, a personality disorder allows for conflict and adaptation. "A person's responsibility for their development cannot be taken from them as long as the person's own decisions essentially formed that development" (Janzarik 1993, 432).

Considering the wide spectrum of antisocial personalities, this pragmatic position is justifiable (Kröber 1995; 2007a). Above all, sociological theories of criminality demonstrate that antisocial and criminal conduct can be explained in many different ways. German criminologists in particular have resisted the suggestion that criminal behavior can be understood in terms of psychopathological processes. If people with antisocial personalities, like anyone else, are subject to social influences and learning processes, they act as rational and competent citizens; their decision not to comply with the law should not be considered pathological. The fact that, because of their special mental strengths and weaknesses, they might be inclined to criminal behavior should not, from this point of view, be treated differently from the fact that somebody else is predisposed to become a psychiatrist or a hairdresser due to his strengths and weaknesses. It has been rightly noted that considering criminal behavior to be a psychiatric disorder creates a social option for state intervention and that this option is in fact being exercised in order to ensure unlimited confinement via indeterminate placement in forensic psychiatric facilities.

References

APA (American Psychiatric Association). 2013. *Diagnostic and Statistical Manual of Mental Disorders, Fifth Edition: DSM-5*. Washington, DC: American Psychiatric Association.

Blankenburg, W. 1989. "Der Krankheitsbegriff in der Psychiatrie." In *Psychiatrie der Gegenwart*, vol. 9: *Brennpunkte der Psychiatrie*, edited by K. P. Kisker et al., pp. 119–145. Berlin: Springer.

Frances, A. 2013. *Saving Normal: An Insider's Revolt against Out-of-Control Psychiatric Diagnosis*. New York, NY: William Morrow.

Friedreich, J. B. 1835. *Systematisches Handbuch der gerichtlichen Psychiatrie*. Leipzig: Wigand.

Griesinger, W. 1845. *Die Pathologie und Therapie der psychischen Krankheiten*. Stuttgart: Krabbe.

Häfner, H. 1981. "Der Krankheitsbegriff in der Psychiatrie." In *Zum umstrittenen psychiatrischen Krankheitsbegriff*, edited by R. Degkwitz and H. Siedow, pp. 16–54. Munich: Urban & Schwarzenberg.

Häfner, H. 1997. "Was tun mit Krankheiten, die keine sind?" *Münchner Medizinische Wochenschrift* 139: 158–160.

Hegel, G. W. F. 1970 [1821]. *Grundlinien der Philosophie des Rechts*, edited by E. Moldenhauer and K. M. Michel. Frankfurt: Suhrkamp.

Heinroth, J. C. A. 1825. *System der psychisch-gerichtlichen Medizin*. Leipzig: Hartmann.

Heinroth, J. C. A. 1833. *Grundzüge der Criminal-Psychologie, oder: Die Theorie des Bösen in ihrer Anwendung auf die Criminal-Rechtspflege*. Berlin: Dümmler.

Helmchen, H. 2006. "Zum Krankheitsbegriff in der Psychiatrie." *Nervenarzt* 77: 271–275.

Janzarik, W. 1972. "Forschungsrichtungen und Lehrmeinungen in der Psychiatrie: Geschichte, Gegenwart, forensische Bedeutung." In *Handbuch der Forensischen Psychiatrie*, vol. 1, edited by H. Göppinger and H. Witter, pp. 588–662. Berlin: Springer.

Janzarik, W. 1993. "Seelische Struktur als Ordnungsprinzip in der forensischen Anwendung." *Nervenarzt* 64: 427–433.

Kant, I. 1929 [1781]. *Critique of Pure Reason*, translated by Norman Kemp Smith. London: Macmillan.

Kant, I. 2006 [1798]. *Anthropology from a Pragmatic Point of View*, edited by R. B. Louden. Cambridge: Cambridge University Press.

Krafft-Ebing, R. v. 1892. *Lehrbuch der gerichtlichen Psychopathologie* (3rd edn). Stuttgart: Enke.

Kröber, H.-L. 1995. "Konzepte zur Beurteilung der 'schweren anderen seelischen Abartigkeit.'" *Nervenarzt* 66: 532–541.

Kröber, H.-L. 2007a. "The historical debate on brain and legal responsibility—revisited." *Behavioral Sciences & the Law* 25: 251–261.

Kröber, H.-L. 2007b. "Steuerungsfähigkeit und Willensfreiheit aus psychiatrischer Sicht." In *Handbuch der Forensischen Psychiatrie*, vol. 1: *Strafrechtliche Grundlagen der Forensischen Psychiatrie*, edited by H.-L. Kröber et al., pp. 159–219. Darmstadt: Steinkopff.

Kröber, H.-L. 2009a. "Concepts of intentional control." *Behavioral Sciences & Law* 27: 209–217.

Kröber, H.-L. 2009b. "Zusammenhänge zwischen psychischer Störung und Delinquenz." In *Handbuch der Forensischen Psychiatrie*, vol. **4**: *Kriminologie und Forensische Psychiatrie*, edited by Kröber et al., pp. 321–337. Darmstadt: Steinkopff.

Mezger, E. 1913. "Die Klippe des Zurechnungsproblems." In *Juristisch-psychiatrische Grenzfragen*, vol. **9**.1, pp. 35–50. Halle: Marhold.

Saß, H. 1987. *Psychopathie, Soziopathie, Dissozialität: Zur Differentialtypologie der Persönlichkeitsstörungen*. Berlin: Springer.

Saß, H. 1991. "Forensische Erheblichkeit seelischer Störungen im psychopathologischen Referenzsystem." In *Medizinrecht, Psychopathologie, Rechtsmedizin: Festschrift für Günter Schewe*, edited by H. Schütz et al., pp. 266–281. Berlin: Springer.

Schild, W. 1990. '§§ 20, 21'. In id., *Alternativkommentar zum Strafgesetzbuch*, vol. **1**, pp. 606–806. Luchterhand, Neuwied.

Schneider, K. 1948. *Die Beurteilung der Zurechnungsfähigkeit*. Stuttgart: Thieme.

Chapter 12

The American experience with the categorical ban against executing the intellectually disabled: New frontiers and unresolved questions

John H. Blume, Sheri L. Johnson, and Amelia C. Hritz

1 Introduction

More than a decade ago, in *Atkins v Virginia* [2002], the Supreme Court held that the execution of individuals with intellectual disabilities (or, in the terminology of the time, 'mental retardation') ran afoul of the cruel and unusual punishment clause of the Eighth Amendment to the US Constitution. The Court concluded that 'the evolving standards of decency that mark the progress of a maturing society' preclude the execution of persons with intellectual disabilities because of the general shift away from the practice in the years since *Penry v Lynaugh* [1989], whose ruling 13 years earlier had declined to exempt those individuals from capital punishment. When *Penry* was decided, only two states with the death penalty and the federal government prohibited the practice, but after *Penry* 16 additional states passed legislation that made persons with intellectual disabilities categorically ineligible for the death penalty (Blume and Johnson 2003). Moreover, in the remaining death penalty states, it became increasingly uncommon for juries to sentence intellectually disabled defendants to death. After citing the shift away from executing persons with intellectual disabilities, the Court applied its own moral calculus to the question and reasoned that defendants with intellectual disabilities are less culpable because they have diminished capacities to understand and process information, to communicate, to learn from mistakes and experience, to engage in logical reasoning, to control their impulses, and to understand the reactions of others. Finally, the Court noted that individuals with intellectual disabilities are at increased risk for wrongful conviction and execution because of the double-edged nature of the evidence, their reduced ability to assist counsel, and the risk that their demeanour may be inappropriate or misinterpreted.

In *Atkins* the Court did not explicitly define intellectual disability but embraced the clinical definitions accepted by the American Association on Mental Retardation (AAMR)—now the American Association on Intellectual and Developmental Disabilities (AAIDD)—and by the American Psychiatric Association (APA) (*Atkins v Virginia* [2002], 309, n. 3). Both definitions refer to substantial limitations in present functioning characterized by three requirements: significantly subaverage intellectual functioning, deficits in adaptive functioning, and manifestation of these deficits in childhood. The Supreme Court suggested that state definitions of intellectual disability for capital cases would be 'appropriate' so long as they 'generally conformed' to these clinical definitions (*Atkins v Virginia* [2002], 22).

After over ten years of litigation, some states are still reluctant to embrace varying aspects of the clinical definitions that seemed unambiguous at the time of *Atkins*.[1] Moreover, some states have interpreted *Atkins* as granting license to deviate, in some cases markedly, from the clinical definitions of intellectual disability. In so doing, these states are taking a narrow categorical ban and making it even narrower. Recently the Supreme Court has heard arguments about whether statutes requiring a defendant to show that his or her IQ falls below a strict score violates the decision in *Atkins*. This suggests that the Court is contemplating stepping in to enforce clinical definitions.

The Court explicitly left to the states the responsibility of selecting procedures for assessing who 'fall[s] within the range of [intellectually disabled] offenders about whom there is a national consensus' (*Atkins v Virginia* [2002], 317). This has created another kind of diversity in enforcement, as some states have adopted procedures that make it virtually impossible for a defendant to prove that he or she is a person with an intellectual disability.

Setting aside the disparate treatment of those who clearly fall within the clinical definition, questions remain about the fairness and morality of executing someone who falls just on the 'wrong' side of the diagnostic line but in every relevant respect is equally disabled. The Supreme Court's own judgement about factors that make a person with intellectual disabilities undeserving of the most

---

[1] The definitions seemed at least unambiguous from the Supreme Court's point of view; they were given two definitions from the AAIDD and from APA's *DSM*, and these were essentially identical. No one—neither the parties nor the Court—disputed that.

extreme punishment would seem to apply equally to individuals who are similarly disabled but, because they do not fit the clinical definition of intellectual disabilities, are not exempt from capital punishment.

The determination of whether an individual fits the intellectual disability diagnosis has life and death consequences in capital cases. This chapter first discusses how definitions and procedures used by some states have resulted in the execution of, or death sentence for, individuals who fall within the protected category of intellectually disabled people due to the level of their impairments. It then considers whether the decision in *Atkins* fails to reach defendants with similarly reduced moral culpability and increased chances of being wrongfully convicted and sentenced to death.

2 Definitional deviations

Since *Atkins*, most jurisdictions have adopted and applied clinical definitions that are similar to the definitions accepted by the AAIDD and APA. A few states, however, have interpreted *Atkins*'s statement that lower courts and state legislatures may adopt their own procedures for 'enforc[ing] the constitutional restriction' as giving license to embrace definitions of intellectual disabilities that deviate, in some cases markedly, from accepted clinical definitions and practices (*Atkins v Virginia* [2002], 317 quoting *Ford v Wainwright* [1986]). These deviations from the clinical understanding of intellectual disabilities have resulted in the exclusion of some individuals who clearly fall within the class protected by *Atkins*.

2.1 Intellectual functioning

Both the APA and the AAMR/AAIDD define the first prong of intellectual disability as 'significantly subaverage intellectual functioning' (*Atkins v Virginia* [2002], 309, citing Sadock and Sadock 2000). As a matter of definition, 'significantly subaverage intellectual functioning' requires that the measured intelligence of the individual fall at least two standard deviations below the mean.[2] Thus the first prong incorporates a statistical comparison between an individual's functioning and that of the rest of the population. The mean on the most commonly used IQ test, the Wechsler Adult Intelligence Scale (WAIS), is 100, and the standard deviations for the WAIS is 15 points (Wechsler 2008). Therefore meeting the first prong would require an IQ score of 70 or

---

[2] In this sense, significantly subaverage intellectual functioning is a statistical concept intended to capture approximately the bottom 2% of the population, which you get using a standard bell curve with a mean of 100.

below—assuming that IQ was measured perfectly. The scores in six states (Alabama, Delaware, Florida, Indiana, North Carolina, and Tennessee) created strict IQ cut-offs, which preclude the diagnosis of intellectual disability when the cut-off is exceeded (Blume, Johnson, and Seeds 2009). Such cut-offs ignore the problem of errors in the measurement of IQ. However, last term, in *Hall v Florida* (2013), the Court reaffirmed its commitment to *Atkins* when it invalidated a gloss on the definition of intellectual disability adopted by the Florida Supreme Court that had the possible effect of rendering the categorical exclusion a 'nullity' and 'risk[ed] executing a person who suffers from intellectual disability'.[3] After *Atkins*, the Florida Supreme Court had adopted a strict IQ cut-off for prong 1, which required a person claiming intellectual disability to have an IQ score of 70 or below (see *Cherry v State*, 959 So. 2d 702, 712–13 (Fla. 2007)). Because Hall had an IQ score of 71, the Florida Supreme Court ruled that, as a matter of law, his claim failed (*Hall v State*, 109 So. 3d 704, 108 (Fla. 2012)). The Supreme Court of the United States concluded that Florida's bright line test was in conflict with the unanimous clinical consensus that the standard error of measurement (SEM; + /– 5 points) in any IQ test must be taken into account; hence the US Supreme Court reversed the judgement of the Florida Supreme Court and remanded for additional proceedings where Hall's (quite strong) evidence of intellectual disability must be considered.

All psychometric measurements, including IQ scores, are subject to some variability. Potential sources of error include variations in test performance, the examiner's behaviour, and the cooperation of the test taker, as well as other personal and environmental factors. 'The term standard error of measurement . . . is used to quantify this variability and provide a stated statistical confidence interval within which the person's true score falls' (Schalock et al. 2010, 36). The SEM on the commonly used IQ tests such as the WAIS is three to five points, which means that, for a measured score of 66, there is a strong likelihood that the true score is between 61 and 71. Thus, considering the SEM, an IQ score of 75 is still within the range of significant subaverage intellectual functioning.

In addition to the variability introduced by error in measurement, IQ scores may be artificially inflated by aging norms. Aging norms, also referred to as 'the Flynn effect', are the consequence of mean IQ scores rising over time (Flynn 2006). Although an individual's IQ scores *on the same test* may rise over time, that individual is still disadvantaged when compared to the rest of the population. If the norms used in scoring the test are not recalculated so that the average value falls in the 50th percentile, the use of an older test will result

---

[3] Hall v Florida, 134 S. Ct. 1986, 2001 (2014).

in inflated scores. It has been estimated that the use of older tests can raise IQ scores by two to four points per decade, unless they are renormed (Blume, Johnson, and Seeds 2009). While the precise reasons for this phenomenon are not well understood, its existence is universally accepted. Thus, if a defendant is evaluated on the basis of outdated IQ norms, his score can be artificially and erroneously inflated above the IQ cut-off. This effect is not trivial. Research by Ceci, Scullin, and Kanaya (2003, 11–17) found that 38 percent of students who scored on the cusp of being eligible for a diagnosis of intellectual disabilities (IQ just above 70) qualified when they were retested using newer norms.

A third source of error may be introduced by repeated testing. Repetition of the same IQ test may inflate scores, depending on the interval between tests, the age of the test taker, and the number of retests (Blume, Johnson, and Seeds 2009). This phenomenon is referred to as 'the practice effect'. Unlike aging norms, the reasons for the practice effect are obvious; memory of test items leads to increased speed and more time for contemplation (Quereshi 1968, 79–85). The practice effect often is relevant to *Atkins* determinations because typically both the prosecution and the defence hire experts, each of whom administer IQ tests to the defendant. This repeated testing can cause the defendant's scores to overestimate his or her IQ, especially when the same tests are administered within a short period of time.

Failure to consider the SEM, aging norms, and practice effects can all cause IQ scores to overestimate an individual's intelligence. Some judges find these phenomena confusing and consequently refuse to take them into account, while others believe themselves to be compelled to disregard them by an applicable statute (Gresham 2009). Thus strict IQ cut-offs or the refusal to consider outdated test norms or repeated test administration can lead to the execution of individuals whose IQ should qualify them as intellectually disabled.

2.2 Adaptive functioning

The second prong of the clinical definition of intellectual disability relates to the ways in which intellectual deficits affect the individual's ability to function in life. The AAMR (2002, 1) defines this prong as 'limitations . . . in conceptual, social, and practical adaptive skills'. The APA's definition follows the same basic contours (APA 2000). This portion of the definition requires that an individual's diminished intellectual functioning involve actual impairment in the skills involved in everyday living, and is designed to ensure that the individual's IQ score reflects a real-world disability and not merely a testing anomaly. As the Supreme Court has observed, 'those who are mentally retarded have a reduced ability to cope with and function in the everyday world' (*Cleburne v Cleburne Living Center* [1985], 442). The task of courts in evaluating *Atkins* claims includes determining whether the reduced intellectual ability indicated by IQ testing had a significant impact on the individual's practical skills and functioning.

Determining deficits in 'adaptive behavior' involves the assessment of what the person with intellectual impairment cannot do, as the focus is on 'significant limitations in adaptive behavior' (e.g. AAMR 2002; APA 2000; Grossman 1983). Any person with intellectual disabilities will lack some basic skills and abilities that normal individuals typically possess. However, not every individual with intellectual disabilities will be unable to do the *same* things. The Supreme Court has long acknowledged 'wide variation in the abilities and needs' of people with intellectual disabilities (*Cleburne v Cleburne Living Center* [1985], 445). For each individual with mental retardation, there will be things that he or she cannot do, but also things that he or she *can* do. A fundamental precept in the field of intellectual disabilities is that '[a]daptive skill limitations often coexist with strengths in other adaptive skill areas' (AAMR 2002, 41). Because the mixture of skills and skill deficits varies widely among persons with intellectual disability, there is no clinically accepted list of common, ordinary skills or abilities the possession of which precludes a diagnosis of intellectual disability. Consequently, any conclusion that a defendant could not suffer from intellectual disability because he or she was able to engage in a particular common activity (such as driving a car,[4] getting married,[5] or holding a job[6]) is unsupported by, and in conflict with, the well accepted clinical understanding of intellectual disability.

Because deficits, rather than strengths, are the focus of the second prong, it becomes important to categorize the kinds of deficits that must be investigated and evaluated. According to the 1992 AAMR definition, quoted in *Atkins*, a person has intellectual disability only when significantly subaverage intellectual functioning 'exist[s] concurrently with related limitations in two or more of the [10] applicable adaptive skill areas' (Luckasson et al. 1992). Those areas are:

---

[4] Many individuals with intellectual disabilities are able to drive but may need support in obtaining a license (Lanzi 2005).

[5] Even popular culture recognizes that persons with intellectual disabilities may have romantic relationships, including marriage. For example, the documentary *Monica & David* follows the courtship and marriage of a couple in which both members have Down syndrome (Codina 2009).

[6] A significant focus of many advocacy groups today is securing more employment opportunities for persons with intellectual disabilities (Walsh 2009). At least since the 1970s, numerous public and private initiatives have been aimed at providing appropriate employment for persons with intellectual disabilities (Association for Retarded Citizens 1974).

1. *communication skills*[, which] relate to the individual's understanding and use of spoken language;

2. *self-care skills*[, which] entail an individual's capacity for feeding, dressing, and grooming himself, as well as generally maintaining personal hygiene;

3. *home-living skills*[, which] reflect housekeeping, clothing care, cooking, budgeting, safety, and property maintenance;

4. *social skills*[, which] broadly include understanding of social cues and emotions, controlling impulses, conforming to rules and laws, and understanding honesty and fairness;

5. *community-use skills*[, which] relate to the use of public transportation, shopping, or obtaining community services;

6. *self-direction skills*[, which] encompass the ability to exercise individual choice, general problem-solving, and displaying appropriate levels of assertiveness;

7. *health and safety skills*[, which] can manifest in an individual's ability to exercise caution, recognize and respond to his or her own health problems, and protect oneself from harm;

8. *functional academic skills*[, which] include reading, writing, and arithmetic skills necessary for daily living;

9. *leisure*[, which] relates to the individual's capacity to participate in community recreational activities; and

10. *work skills*[, which] relate to the person's ability to maintain employment, accept supervision, maintain punctuality and reliability on the job, cooperate with coworkers, and meet appropriate work-quality standards (Baroff and Olley 1999, 18–20).[7]

Thus, in assessing an individual's adaptive behaviour, the focus must be on *deficits* rather than strengths. If courts are to conclude that a defendant was excluded from the protection of the Supreme Court's decision in *Atkins* because of an impression or belief that people with intellectual disabilities are all incapable

---

[7] Since *Atkins*, the AAMR has revised its widely emulated formulation of adaptive functioning deficits. Instead of requiring limitations in at least two of the ten itemized 'adaptive skills areas', the new definition more concisely requires 'significant limitations . . . in adaptive behavior' in one of three broader areas: conceptual, social, or practical adaptive skills (AAMR 2002). This change is generally semantic rather than outcome determinative; AAMR (2002) notes that each of the ten skill areas of the 1992 definition is 'conceptually linked' to at least one of the broader categories of the 2002 definition (81–2). The APA's phrasing of the adaptive functioning requirement is virtually identical. The APA definition requires 'significant limitations in adaptive functioning in at least two of the following skill areas: communication, self-care, home living, social/interpersonal skills, use of community resources, self-direction, functional academic skills, work, leisure, health, and safety' (APA 2000, 41).

of a particular task or activity, this disconnects *Atkins* from its scientific mooring. Moreover, it permits the life or death decision about an individual with an intellectual disability to be based on the same type of false stereotypes that have burdened people with intellectual disabilities for generations (*Cleburne v Cleburne Living Center* [1985], 438).

2.2.1. Ex parte Briseno

In *Ex parte Briseno* [2004], the Texas Court of Criminal Appeals put Texas in the small camp of states whose substantive definitions do not comport with clinical consensus. After stating that it would follow the AAMR criteria, the court articulated a set of factors to serve as 'temporary judicial guidelines' for courts to use in assessing adaptive functioning in capital cases that strayed from accepted clinical definitions of adaptive functioning.

These factors are not consistent with the skill areas that the AAMR and APA definitions rely upon and do not comport with the governing principle that the focus must be upon deficits rather than strengths. Persons with intellectual disabilities—indeed all individuals—display 'wide variation in the[ir] abilities and needs' (*Cleburne v Cleburne Living Center* [1985], 445). In addition, as previously discussed, clinical literature explicitly warns against a focus on strengths (AAMR 2002). Instead, the *Briseno* factors seem related to lay perceptions and stereotypes of intellectual disabilities. The factors set forth by the Texas Court of Criminal Appeals are:

- Did those who knew the person best during the developmental stage ... think he was mentally retarded at that time?
- Has the person formulated plans and carried them through?
- Does his conduct show leadership or ... show that he is led around by others?
- Is his conduct in response to external stimuli rational and appropriate?
- Does he respond coherently, rationally, and on point to oral or written questions?
- Can the person hide facts or lie effectively in his own or others' interests?
- [D]id the commission of [the capital] offense require forethought, planning, and complex execution of purpose? (*Ex parte Briseno* [2004], 8–9).

According to the *Briseno* court, these guidelines were a stopgap measure, intended for use only until the Texas legislature enacted a definition of intellectual disabilities for use in capital cases. As of the publication of this book, the legislature has not heeded the call.

2.2.2. Lizcano v State

In *Lizcano v State* [2010] the Texas Court of Criminal Appeals went further than *Briseno*, explicitly supplanting the definition of adaptive functioning cited by the Supreme Court in *Atkins* with the much narrower definition from the

Texas Health and Safety Code. The *Lizcano* standard for determining adaptive functioning deficits is inconsistent with the accepted and established scientific understanding of intellectual disabilities.

The lower court's treatment of the adaptive functioning prong relies on false stereotypes about intellectual disabilities; it ignores deficits and focuses on strengths. With regard to the second prong of intellectual disabilities, without reference to the clinical definition, the lower court instructed the jury that 'adaptive behavior is defined as the effectiveness with or degree to which a person meets the standards of personal independence and social responsibility expected of the person's age and cultural group' (*Atkins v Virginia* [2002], 308, n. 3; APA 2000; *Bobby v Bies* [2009]). This definition, drawn from a pre-*Atkins* Texas Health and Safety Code provision, was approved by the *Lizcano* majority.

The lower court's treatment of the adaptive functioning prong is impermissibly narrow, as it focuses only upon personal independence and social responsibility while ignoring other skill areas. The Health and Safety Code definition is not equivalent to any currently recognized clinical characterization of adaptive skills. In contrast, at the time the Supreme Court decided *Atkins*, the clinical definition identified ten areas of adaptive functioning skills—communication, self-care, home living, social skills, community use, self-direction, health and safety, functional academics, leisure, and work—and required limitations in two (*Atkins v Virginia* [2002], 308, n. 3; APA 2000; *Bobby v Bies* [2009]). The Texas Court of Criminal Appeals has thus drastically narrowed the definition of intellectual disabilities by replacing an accepted clinical definition according to which limitations in any two of ten skill areas suffice with a requirement that an individual exhibit limitations in both of two prescribed areas. The lower court's treatment of the adaptive functioning prong also permits heavy reliance on untrained lay opinions regarding intellectual disabilities, ignoring established standards for the exercise of clinical judgement. In addition to the narrowness of the skills areas it embraces, the Texas Health and Safety Code language—'the effectiveness or degree to which a person meets the standards of personal independence and social responsibility expected of the person's age and cultural group'—focuses on strengths rather than weaknesses.[8]

Any ambiguity in the congruence between the *Lizcano* definition of adaptive behaviour and the clinical definition of adaptive functioning is resolved by examining the majority's application of their new standard to the evidence in the case. The majority found support for the jury's verdict in four facts: Lizcano's

---

[8] These deviances from the clinical understanding have not been justified other than by saying that people in Texas might have a different understanding of ID if the question is whether someone can be executed from what it would be if a different question were asked.

employment, regular car payments, romantic relationships, and money sent to assist his family. None of these, under an appropriate definition of adaptive functioning, would support the conclusion that Mr. Lizcano does not have intellectual disabilities. As discussed previously, one of the fundamental precepts in the field of intellectual disabilities is that '[a]daptive skill limitations often coexist with strengths in other adaptive skill areas' (AAMR 2002, 41).

These facts contradict only a stereotype of intellectual disabilities and have no obvious connection to the presence or absence of deficits in any of the ten skill areas. For example, 'most mentally retarded adults can work and are able to hold steady jobs—if properly trained and placed in the right job . . . Most will try hard and stay with their jobs, [and] they usually have a very good attendance record' (Best Buddies, Ursinus College 1999). In addition, having girlfriends—even getting married and having children—is not inconsistent with intellectual disabilities (AAIDD and Arc 2008). Persons with documented intellectual disabilities may marry each other and each be of the opinion that the other is 'bright', but this perception does nothing to establish that they do not suffer adaptive functioning deficits. The hard work on the job, the payments made on a car, the existence of romantic activities, and the gifts sent to his family do not call into question any of the adaptive functioning deficits testified to by lay witnesses or the consistent conclusion of experts who examined him that Mr. Lizcano is a person with intellectual disabilities.

Most state and federal courts apply *Atkins* faithfully, and their decisions reflect the clinical understanding of adaptive functioning deficits. Some have even explicitly rejected the kind of errors made by the court in *Briseno*.[9] Other lower courts, however, like the courts in *Briseno* and *Lizcano*, have ignored clinical understandings of intellectual disabilities and rejected *Atkins* claims, either relying on stereotypes about the abilities of people with intellectual disabilities or misinterpreting the presence of mental illness. A Florida court found that an intellectual disabilities diagnosis 'was contradictory to the evidence that [the applicant] was engaged in a five-year intimate relationship prior to the crime, that he had his driver's license and drove a car, and that he was employed in numerous jobs including as a mechanic' (*Brown v State* [2007], 150). Another state court cited the *Briseno* opinion and its list of 'factors' with approval

---

[9] See e.g. *State v White* [2008]: 'There [is] no evidence that "bizarre" behavior is a necessary attribute of the [intellectually disabled]'; 'Especially relevant here is Dr. Hammer's already-cited observation that retarded individuals "*may look relatively normal in some areas* and have . . . significant limitations in other areas"' (915); *Lambert v State* [2005]: 'Unless a defendant's evidence of particular limitations is specifically contradicted by evidence that he does not have those limitations, then the defendant's burden is met no matter what evidence the State might offer that he has no deficits in other skill areas' (651).

(*Van ran v State* [2006], 23–4). The dissenting judges in *Lizcano* argued, and the majority did not dispute, that the definitional deviation of adaptive behaviour permits 'some capital offenders whom every rational diagnostician would find meets the clinical definition of mental retardation to be executed simply because they demonstrate a few pronounced adaptive strengths along with their manifest deficits' (*Lizcano v State* [2010], 40).[10]

2.3 **Manifestation in childhood**

The third prong of the definition of intellectual disability requires that intellectual disabilities be present before the age of 18 (Schalock et al. 2010). This portion of the definition serves an aetiological function in the psychological community, as it distinguishes people with intellectual disabilities from people with similar impairments that are due to brain injury or drug use (Blume, Johnson, and Seeds 2008). The latter is not relevant to actual impairment and therefore bars from the protection of *Atkins* individuals in whom these similar impairments (e.g. traumatic brain injury) manifest themselves after childhood. Normally the absence of a childhood diagnosis is not challenged in *Atkins* proceedings, unless the state argues that the defendant's intellectual impairment is due to drug use or brain injury in adulthood (ibid.). This issue is further discussed in section 3.

In many *Atkins* cases the defendant did not receive an official diagnosis of intellectual disabilities as a child, or the records of that diagnosis are no longer available. The lay factfinder's immediate reaction to the absence of a juvenile diagnosis of intellectual disabilities may be that the defendant did not meet the criteria for intellectual disabilities. The clinical literature, however, recognizes that the lack of such a diagnosis may stem from various factors that do not call into question its appropriateness, such as:

◆ the individual was excluded from a full school experience;

◆ the individual's age precluded participation in special education programs;

◆ the person was not diagnosed or given another diagnosis for 'political' purposes including:

  • protection from stigma or teasing;

  • avoidance of assertions of discrimination;

  • assessment of the benefits of a particular diagnosis;

  • data reporting implications, such as school concern about the overrepresentation of diagnostic groups in the school population;

---

[10] Price J, concurring and dissenting.

- contextual school issues, such as availability of programs or funding;
- lack of entry into the referral process due to cultural, linguistic, or other reasons. (Schalock et al. 2007)

An additional complication is the reluctance to diagnose mild intellectual disabilities in school settings. In some school districts, court orders have forbidden IQ testing or classification on the basis of prior discrimination; in others, school professionals admit to substituting a diagnosis of specific learning disability for one of intellectual disabilities when the latter seems more appropriate in view of parental resistance to the former (Reschly 2009). Thus there may be a number of reasons for the absence of a diagnosis during the developmental period.

2.3.1. *Stallings v Bagley*

Michael Stallings was found guilty of murder during the commission of a burglary and sentenced to death in Ohio (*Stallings v Bagley* [2008]). After the decision in *Atkins*, Stallings sought exemption from the death penalty. The Ohio Supreme Court held after *Atkins* that an individual is intellectually disabled, and therefore ineligible for execution, if he or she has: '(1) significantly sub-average intellectual functioning[,] (2) significant limitations in two or more adaptive skills, such as communication, self-care, and self-direction, and (3) onset before the age of 18' (*State v Lott* [2002], 305).

To support his *Atkins* claim, Stallings presented evidence of two IQ scores of 76, one obtained at the age of 16 and another just before his trial. Stallings's expert, Dr Luc LeCavalier, testified that both scores were inflated because incorrect testing instruments had been used. Dr LeCavalier concluded that Stallings met the first two prongs of intellectual disability on the basis of his IQ scores and the score of an adaptive functioning test administered to Stallings in prison. Dr LeCavalier also believed that a lot of information suggested that Stallings met the third prong, yet here he was less certain, because Stallings had never been specifically evaluated for intellectual disability before the age of 18.

A second expert, Dr John Matthew Fabian, concluded that Stallings had significantly subaverage intelligence and suffered from significant deficits in adaptive functioning. He administered an IQ to Stallings that resulted in a score of 72 and stated that Stallings's previous IQ scores of 76 were inflated due to testing errors. Dr Fabian's conclusions about Stallings's adaptive functioning were based on the observations of a death row caseworker. With regard to onset, he concluded that it was more likely than not, on the basis of Stallings's school records and family reports, that this condition was present prior to the age of 18.

The trial court found that Stallings had significantly subaverage intelligence and significant limitations in adaptive functions. Nonetheless it denied Stallings' claim, reasoning that he had not established the third prong, as neither

Dr LeCavalier nor Dr Fabian were able to definitively conclude that the limitations were manifest prior to the age of 18. The Ninth District Court affirmed.

Stallings filed a habeas corpus petition. After noting that Stallings was never specifically tested for intellectual disabilities before the age of 18 and that such omissions are common among individuals of low socio-economic background, the district court expressed concern that the trial court had placed an impossible burden on Stallings. Ultimately, however, it found that the trial court's decision was not so unreasonable to meet the high standard of overturning a death sentence.[11]

3 **Procedural deviations**

Atkins v Virginia [2002] also 'le[ft] to the State[s] the task of developing appropriate ways to enforce the constitutional restriction upon [their] execution of sentences' (317). Some states have adopted procedures that make it virtually impossible for a defendant to prove that he or she is a person with an intellectual disability.

3.1 **Burden of proof**

Most dramatically, states that employ heightened standards of proof may eliminate *most* persons with intellectual disability from the sweep of *Atkins*. Typically, states require defendants to prove the presence of an intellectual disability by a preponderance of evidence. A few states impose higher burdens, however, and Georgia places upon capital defendants the burden of proving their own intellectual disabilities beyond a reasonable doubt (*Head v Hill* [2003]). The US Court of Appeals for the Eleventh Circuit held that this most stringent burden does not violate the Eighth Amendment. As explained below, the nature of clinical assessment of intellectual disabilities, combined with the special difficulties created by the context of a capital trial, will often make the burden of proof imposed by Georgia virtually impossible to meet. 'All diagnoses of mental retardation are potentially challenging', and even in ideal settings clinicians and other qualified experts ordinarily diagnose intellectual disabilities only to a reasonable degree of medical (or professional) certainty (Schalock et al. 2007, 14). Thus, the 'beyond a reasonable doubt' standard gives license to Georgia prosecutors to argue that a reasonable degree of certainty (the clinical norm) fails to satisfy the required burden of proof.

---

[11] Stallings' death sentence was ultimately commuted to life imprisonment after a finding that he received ineffective assistance of counsel during the penalty phase of his trial.

Capital cases are far from ideal diagnostic settings. Most broadly, the standards and practices for assessing intellectual disabilities evolved in large part to determine what supports are appropriate for the individual being diagnosed, a task that may easily be distorted by the adversarial process of *Atkins* determinations (Schalock et al. 2010). The clinical literature identifies four conditions that render the diagnosis of intellectual disabilities especially difficult—co-morbidity; mild (as opposed to moderate or severe) intellectual disabilities; retrospective diagnosis; and situations in which assessment is conducted under less than optimal circumstances—and virtually all *Atkins* determinations involve at least one of these conditions. In all but the most extraordinary case, the presence of one or more of these four conditions or the mere possibility of malingering, however far unsupported by the facts, will preclude proof of intellectual disabilities beyond a reasonable doubt.

3.1.1. Co-morbidity

One significant barrier to proving intellectual disabilities beyond a reasonable doubt is the prevalence of co-morbid psychiatric conditions. '[M]ental health disorders are more prevalent among individuals with MR/ID than the general population' (AAMR 2002, 15). Indeed, '[i]ndividuals with mental retardation have a prevalence of comorbid mental disorder that is estimated to be three to four times greater than in the general population' (APA 2000, 44).

Because '[t]he diagnostic criteria for Mental Retardation do not include an exclusion criterion', compliance with those criteria requires that a diagnosis of intellectual disabilities 'be made whenever the diagnostic criteria are met, regardless of and in addition to the presence of another disorder' (APA 2000).[12] In theory, then, co-morbidity should not influence the diagnosis of intellectual disabilities. However, in practice, the adversarial context of *Atkins* proceedings has often led to exclusion of an intellectual disability diagnosis on the basis of a co-morbid psychiatric condition.

With respect to the first prong of the definition of intellectual disabilities, co-morbidity makes it possible to argue that low IQ scores are not accurate measures of intellectual functioning but are artificially depressed by mental illness. In extreme cases, mental illness may preclude the administration of a standard IQ test. More commonly, mental illness, particularly depression, may diminish performance on an IQ test, even when the depression has been treated (Sackeim et al. 1992). Any ethical expert questioned about the phenomenon would have

---

12 The diagnostic criteria also do not specify the aetiology of the impairments in intellectual and adaptive functioning. In approximately half of all cases, intellectual disability has no known etiology (Schalock et al. 2007, 6).

to acknowledge the impact that depression tends to have on performance—and the possibility that a defendant with co-morbid depression and mild intellectual disabilities would, in the absence of the depression, score in the borderline range. Such questioning is obviously possible even when the burden of proof is less draconian. Satisfying an ordinary burden of proof, however, is possible by considering the consistency of earlier scores or previous academic records, or the corroborating value of limited adaptive functioning across the lifespan. In Georgia, however, such evidence would probably still not satisfy the burden of proof, because a reasonable doubt may remain as to whether the defendant was depressed at the earlier point in time.

In addition, co-morbidity makes it possible for the prosecution to argue that apparent adaptive functioning deficits are 'really' attributable to conduct and/ or personality disorders rather than to intellectual disabilities. Although the concepts of adaptive functioning deficits and the criteria for behavioural and personality disorders are distinct, there is overlap between *behaviours* that reflect adaptive functioning deficits and *behaviours* that permit an inference of criteria for other psychiatric disorders. Co-morbidity of intellectual disabilities and personality or behavioural disorders is likely to occur where intellectual disabilities have contributed to behaviours that meet one or more of the criteria for those disorders, or where adaptive functioning deficits are mistaken for attributes that satisfy those criteria (Morrissey and Hollin 2011; Moreland, Hendy, and Brown 2008; Dana 1993).

Adaptive functioning deficits have a particularly large potential to be misinterpreted as characteristics that meet the diagnostic criteria for antisocial personality disorder. Such criteria are 'failure to conform to social norms with respect to lawful behaviours as indicated by repeatedly performing acts that are grounds for arrest'; 'impulsivity or failure to plan ahead'; 'consistent irresponsibility, as indicated by repeated failure to sustain consistent work behaviour or honor financial obligations'; and 'lack of remorse, as indicated by being indifferent to or rationalizing having hurt, mistreated, or stolen from another' (APA 2000, 706). All of these factors may be wrongly inferred from adaptive functioning deficits. Psychopathy may be wrongly diagnosed in a person with intellectual disabilities because, '[f]or example, it can be difficult to differentiate between "deficient affective experience" as described by the [Psychopathy Check List-R] (shallow affect, lack of empathy and remorse) and the difficulty that people with [mental retardation] are known to have in both identifying and expressing their own emotional states and recognising them in others' (Morrissey and Hollin 2011, 135).

In *Lambert v State* [2005], the state acknowledged the existence of deficits in four skill areas, but argued that the defendant did not have intellectual disabilities because his limitations were better described by, or caused by, antisocial personality disorder, schizophrenia, conduct disorder, and/or drug abuse. The Oklahoma Court of Criminal Appeals properly dismissed this argument, finding that '[a]n alternative explanation for an agreed condition is not a negation of that condition' (*Lambert v State* [2005], 653).[13]

Less frequently, co-morbidity may preclude satisfaction of the third prong beyond a reasonable doubt. That prong requires that the intellectual and adaptive functioning deficits specified by the first two prongs originated before the age of eighteen. Drug abuse (as well as other factors, such as traumatic brain injury) may cause neurological damage that impairs both intellectual and adaptive functioning and, if that abuse occurs after the age of eighteen, may provide an alternative hypothesis for explaining current deficits in functioning. Evidence of drug abuse therefore permits the state to argue that a defendant's drug use, rather than intellectual disabilities, is the cause of his current limitations. In some instances, this argument may be well taken. However, it is not unusual for both drug abuse and intellectual disabilities to be present, in part because the genetic factors that increase the likelihood of intellectual disabilities overlap with those that increase the likelihood of substance abuse (Christian and Poling 1997). Under a 'preponderance of the evidence' standard, or even under a clear and convincing standard, the question of onset in a capital defendant with a history of substance abuse may be resolved by considering the entire picture, including, of course, evidence of pre-18 functioning. However, unless such evidence is unusually copious, attempts to create reasonable doubt as to onset from the evidence of drug abuse—even sparse evidence—will often be successful.

Not all courts faced with similar arguments have applied these principles in accordance with the *DSM-IV* mandate.[14] Over time, professionals can educate such courts. But even an educated, conscientious factfinder would be thwarted in the attempt to find *beyond a reasonable doubt* that a defendant with a co-morbid psychiatric disorder is also a person with intellectual disabilities. This is a particularly tragic result, since the personality or behavioural disorder may well be the product of intellectual disabilities and undoubtedly reflects a second

---

[13] See also *Holladay v Campbell* [2006]: faulting the prosecution's expert for 'look[ing] upon inappropriate conduct as something separate from [intellectual disabilities], rather than as indicating a lack of support which has impeded adaptation' (1344).

[14] See e.g. *Williams v Quarterman* [2008]: dismissing what Williams presented as evidence of adaptive deficits as 'bizarre and antisocial conduct' and evincing characteristics that 'could be explained by anti-social personality rather than [intellectual disabilities]' (312).

disability—a situation that renders dually diagnosed defendants even less culpable than defendants who have only intellectual disabilities.

3.1.2. Mild intellectual disabilities

The diagnosis of intellectual disabilities is more challenging when the person is in the mild range (an IQ score between 55 and 75). Almost all of the capital defendants whom *Atkins* exempts from imposition of the death penalty are persons with mild intellectual disabilities (Olley 2009; Gresham 2009). This is in large part because of the statistical fact that, of the 2.5 percent of the population whose IQ is 70 or below, approximately 75 percent fall into the 'mild' category, but also because persons who are more impaired would rarely be subject to criminal proceedings. The most impaired individuals are not likely to commit crimes at all, due to the nature of their disability. Others, who are not quite so severely disabled, commit crimes only rarely and, if they do, they might nevertheless not be competent enough to stand trial or might lack criminal responsibility.

Diagnosis of persons in the mild range is more challenging because '[t]hose individuals, while meeting the three criteria of [mental retardation], manifest subtle limitations that are frequently difficult to detect' (Schalock et al. 2007, 16). However, clinicians have noted that '[t]he concept of "mild cognitive limitations" as applied to adults with [intellectual disability] is a "gross misnomer"' (Switzky and Greespan 2006>/IBT, 30–31). Rather, mild is a relative term; those with mild mental retardation have '"mild" limitations only in comparison to those of individuals with "moderate" to "profound" mental retardation (intellectual disability)' (ibid., 31). The variability of IQ scores described in section 1 highlights the difficulty of proving that someone is intellectually disabled when his or her IQ scores are on the cusp. As described earlier, the SEM on the commonly used IQ tests is about five points, which means that, for a measured score of 66, there is a strong likelihood that the true score is between 61 and 71.

These challenges in diagnosing the mild range are a significant barrier to proving intellectual disabilities beyond a reasonable doubt. It is easy to argue that, for persons with measured IQ scores of 66 or higher, there is a 'reasonable doubt' as to their subaverage intellectual functioning, as 71 is viewed as falling outside the range of intellectual disabilities according to the substantive standard most commonly employed in litigating *Atkins* cases. Consequently, large numbers of defendants whose scores place them clearly in the range of intellectual disabilities would, because of the nature of measurement, be unable to convince a factfinder of their intellectual disabilities beyond a reasonable doubt. While more scores—all approximately the same—increase the clinician's confidence that the measurement is accurate and would permit him or her to testify to this effect, there is no formula that aggregates probabilities over the numerous scores to which a clinician could testify. Therefore even a number of such scores may lead to unpredictable results.

3.1.3. Retrospective diagnosis

Another common barrier to proving mental retardation beyond a reasonable doubt is the absence of childhood diagnoses. In many *Atkins* cases the diagnosis is wholly retrospective because the defendant did not receive an official diagnosis of intellectual disabilities as a child, or because records of that diagnosis are no longer available.[15]

As discussed in section 1, there may be ample reasons for the absence of a diagnosis during the developmental period, but the existence of such reasons is not likely to dispel the reasonable doubt created by the absence of an earlier diagnosis. Moreover, there are no obvious fixes for the difficulties of a retrospective diagnosis. Records may have disappeared, and 'the respondent's ability to correctly recall from memory the assessed individual's actual performance [is always at issue]' (Tassé 2009, 119). Should an expert be asked about the reliability of a retrospective diagnosis, he or she would have to admit that the phenomenon of '[m]emory degradation is [a] real issue, and [that] there is no solid research regarding the forgetting curve . . . regarding someone's recollection of another person's adaptive behavior' (ibid.).

Moreover, often the only people who can recall the defendant's actions at specific ages during the developmental period are family members, a fact that impairs the establishment of intellectual disabilities in two ways. First, family members may be inclined to overestimate the defendant's abilities, either because they themselves are intellectually impaired or because they are ashamed that they did not seek help for the defendant when he or she was a child. At the same time, such 'retrospective reports are frequently challenged because of the potential biases of the family member or friend who knows that their accounts will be used in determining whether the individual will be . . . protected from the death penalty due to [mild intellectual disabilities]' (Reschly 2009).

Reliance on self-ratings in retrospective diagnosis of intellectual disabilities may be tempting due to a lack of other informants, but it contains a 'high risk' of overestimating competence. Persons with intellectual disabilities have a tendency 'to attempt to look more "normal" than they actually are' and have a 'strong acquiescence bias'. What is more, intellectual disabilities can be seen as a form of social status (Schalock et al. 2007, 21–2). Incarcerated individuals may have the additional concern that a diagnosis of intellectual disabilities will make

---

[15] See e.g. *Stallings v Bagley* [2008].

them more vulnerable to predation. Although there are detailed guidelines for retrospective diagnosis (ibid., 18–22) and careful adherence to those guidelines can ameliorate some of the difficulties inherent in retrospective diagnosis, thus producing a diagnosis worthy of confidence, it is unlikely that adherence to those guidelines will overcome every reasonable doubt argued by a prosecutor arising from the lack of a diagnosis during the developmental period, every reasonable doubt arising from memory degradation, and every reasonable doubt arising from reliance on the reports of biased family members.

3.1.4. Suboptimal assessment circumstances

The fourth condition, which the clinical literature identifies as rendering assessment of intellectual disabilities particularly challenging, is something of a catch-all: 'situations that preclude formal assessment or impair its validity, reliability or utility' (Schalock et al. 2007, 22). Two of these situations that are specifically mentioned are common in *Atkins* determinations: legal restrictions (including incarceration) and cultural or linguistic factors.

Incarceration negatively affects assessment in several ways that are matters of common sense. First, it makes access to the individual himself more difficult; time may be limited, testing conditions may be less than optimal, and interviews less conducive to self-disclosure. Second, the capital charge against the defendant can make others reluctant to 'help' the defendant by providing evidence of his adaptive functioning deficits.

Perhaps more importantly, incarceration on a capital charge is likely to produce two forms of 'evidence' that the clinical literature deems unreliable. The AAIDD Users Guide instructions on the proper retrospective assessment of intellectual disabilities specifically forbid the 'use [of] past criminal behavior or verbal behavior to infer level of adaptive behavior or [the existence of mental retardation both] because there is not enough available information [and] because there is a lack of normative information' (Schalock et al. 2007, 22). Similarly, the clinical literature cautions:

> Correctional Officers and other prison personnel should probably never be sought as respondents to provide information regarding the adaptive behavior of an individual that they observed in a prison setting .... The main hesitation to involving prison personnel as respondents is related to the nature and contingencies of the prison setting. The prison setting is an artificial environment that offers limited opportunities for many activities and behaviors defining adaptive behavior (Tassé 2009, 119).

Despite the unreliability of past criminal behaviour or testimony of correctional officers, this type of evidence is frequently relied upon by courts due to the lack of alternative evidence on the current functioning of incarcerated individuals.

In addition, in *Atkins* cases, cultural or linguistic factors are common impediments to assessment. It is generally agreed that cross-cultural competence is a prerequisite for conducting valid assessments. 'Cross-cultural skills include understanding of one's own values, knowledge of the other culture(s), and the ability to interact and communicate in a sensitive fashion with members of other cultures' (Craig and Tassé 1999, 119–20). One extreme cultural barrier to assessment lies in cases involving defendants from other countries, especially from countries in which English is not the native language. With foreign nationals, logistical barriers to collecting records and informants are exacerbated by cultural barriers to communication and to the correct interpretation of information. But an examiner's lack of competence with respect to subcultures within this country can also lead to withheld, overlooked, or misinterpreted information.

Apart from the suboptimal collection and synthesis of information relevant to the determination of intellectual disabilities, persons with intellectual disabilities who are members of minority groups risk having the evidence of their disability dismissed as simply a product of their group membership. Thus some experts have testified that upward adjustments of IQ scores based on minority group membership are appropriate,[16] and others have testified that behaviour that would otherwise qualify as demonstrating adaptive functioning deficits should be disregarded because it is normal for the ethnic group of the individual concerned.[17] Although such use of a defendant's ethnicity is clearly contrary to professional norms, when proffered, it can create 'reasonable doubt' about either subaverage intellectual functioning or significant adaptive functioning deficits—if not about both (Schalock et al. 2007, 23).

Despite the heightened need for valid and reliable assessment in *Atkins* determinations, due to the difficulties of assessing incarcerated individuals and individuals from different cultures, in many cases it is unlikely that the diagnoses can satisfy the standard of being 'beyond a reasonable doubt'.

3.1.5. The possibility of malingering

In *Atkins* determinations, the defendant has an enormous incentive—his very life—to be found a person with intellectual disabilities, and no one can ignore the possibility that this would lead some defendants of normal intelligence to perform less than their best on a test of intellectual functioning or to exaggerate their adaptive functioning deficits. Thus, to any rational factfinder, the potential for malingering or for 'the intentional production of false or grossly

---

[16] See e.g. *Lizcano v State* [2010].

[17] See e.g. *Hernandez v Thaler* [2011].

exaggerated physical or psychological symptoms motivated by external incentives' (APA 2000, 739) will be salient in a capital case. A related phenomenon, suboptimal effort (also called 'incomplete effort'), is the inference drawn when maximum performance is not achieved; and may such instances have various causes (Blume, Johnson, and Seeds 2008). The possibility that the defendant is malingering or performing with suboptimal effort is another significant barrier to proving intellectual disabilities beyond a reasonable doubt.

In fact, although the available empirical evidence is limited, it suggests that, even in the *Atkins* setting, malingering intellectual disability is not particularly prevalent (Everington, Notario-Smull, and Horton 2007). This is in part because there are instruments that measure malingering and clinically recognized methods for detecting it.[18]

Malingering intellectual disability is also not particularly prevalent in part because the social barriers to feigning intellectual disabilities are substantial, rendering 'malingering well' more common than 'malingering sick' (Grossman 1968). In fact, because of the stigma attached to mental illness and developmental disabilities, affected individuals and their families take extreme measures to hide those disabilities (Ellis and Luckasson 1985, 430–31, 441).

'[T]he limited empirical research available indicates that current tests of neurocognitive and psychiatric feigning designed to detect malingering do not adequately assess feigned MR' (Musso et al. 2011, 758–9).[19] Importantly, the limitations of these tests include both false negatives and of false positives (Salekin and Doane 2009, 108). Thus, on the one hand, no responsible clinician can testify with certainty that the defendant's effort on an IQ test was optimal according to a malingering instrument. And, on the other hand, scores that appear to reflect malingering may mislead the trier of fact, because many effort tests and indicators show unacceptably high false positive rates malingering with individuals with mental retardation (Everington, Notario-Smull, and Horton 2007, 546–48). Consequently, even in cases where the evidence includes multiple scores in the range of intellectual disabilities during the developmental

---

[18] 'A diagnosis of [intellectual disabilities] must be corroborated by multiple sources of information. Defendant performance should be triangulated with scores on IQ and achievement tests, interviews with significant others, and school/psychological records .... Triangulation can be helpful in detection of malingered [intellectual disabilities] in several ways'; clinical judgment applied to multiple sources of information, with an emphasis on information obtained prior to any motive to malinger, is the most reliable method for identifying feigned intellectual disabilities (Salekin and Doane 2009).

[19] See also Salekin and Doane 2009, 107–8: 'With respect to good faith performance on tests of effort and effort indices/indicators, available literature regarding individuals with IQs below 70 has been less than adequate'.

period, a false positive on a malingering instrument may create reasonable doubt that the defendant was not putting forth optimal effort even as a child.

In part because of the weaknesses of instruments that measure malingering, the literature advises clinicians to collect 'collateral data gleaned from multiple sources . . . that, when appropriately integrated, will lead to a clinical opinion that is formulated on a constellation of relevant information, rather than gut instinct or an over-emphasis on a few variables that do not capture the full clinical presentation' (Salekin and Doane 2009, 111). However, 'successful integration of the information available . . . to tease apart areas of bona fide strength and weaknesses from those that are manufactured or purposely exaggerated is no small task' (ibid.). Nor is it a task that can be reduced to a formula. 'Clinical judgment plays a crucial role in the interpretation of this information and in the final diagnosis of malingering defendants with mental retardation' (Everington, Notario-Smull, and Horton 2007, 558). Unfortunately, while sound clinical judgement and tests for malingering may, together, provide evidence that would convince any competent professional that the defendant is indeed a person with intellectual disabilities, both can almost always be denounced by an eloquent prosecutor as insufficient for dispelling all reasonable doubt and for meeting that standard of proof.

3.1.6. *In re Hill*

Despite significant evidence of intellectual disabilities, Warren Hill was unable to meet Georgia's high standard of proof. While Hill was serving a life sentence for murdering his former girlfriend, he was charged with capital murder for the death of a fellow inmate (*Hill v State* [1993]). After his conviction was affirmed on appeal, Hill sought writ of habeas corpus, alleging that he had an intellectual disability. The habeas court found that Hill succeeded in proving beyond a reasonable doubt that he had significantly subaverage intellectual functioning, citing IQ scores ranging from 69 to 77. The court also found, however, that Hill failed to prove beyond a reasonable doubt the existence of impairments in adaptive behaviour, citing his extensive work history and 'apparent ability to function well in such employment', disciplined savings plans pursued in order to purchase cars and motorcycles, military service, active social life, writing skills, and an ability to care for himself. Consequently the court concluded that Hill had failed to prove his alleged intellectual disabilities beyond a reasonable doubt (*In re Hill* [2013]).

All mental health experts from Hill's 2000 trial agreed later on that he was a person with intellectual disabilities. Dr Thomas Sachy stated that his earlier conclusion that Hill was not intellectually disabled were unreliable because of 'lack of experience at the time' (ibid., 10). In his affidavit, Dr Sachy stated that his additional experience in practicing psychiatry and research in the field since 2000 caused him to conclude that Hill was not malingering during the 2000 evaluation and that Hill's naval records were 'not inconsistent with mild mental retardation' (ibid., 17, n. 11). Drs Donald Harris and James Gary Carter also reconsidered their 2000 opinions and stated that Hill was mildly intellectually disabled.

The court denied Hill's habeas petition, asserting that the petition was procedurally barred and the modified opinions of the prior mental health experts did not establish a miscarriage of justice that would allow him to overcome the procedural bar. Hill's application for permission to file a successive federal habeas petition based on this claim was also denied. Hill was executed on 27 January 2015, despite the fact that all of the mental health experts from his 2000 trial ultimately concluded that he was intellectually disabled.

3.2 **Decision maker**

States must determine whether a judge or a jury is the decision maker in an *Atkins* claim. In cases where judges are decision makers, the success rate is 40 percent. Defendants have much lower success rates in *Atkins* claims when the determination is made by a jury (e.g. Georgia, Texas) (Blume and Salekin 2013). In fact, in Texas no jury has ever found any defendant to have intellectual disabilities. This is probably due to jurors' more stereotypical views or misperceptions about a person with intellectual disabilities, especially mild intellectual disabilities. For example, contrary to the clinical definition described above, jurors may believe that a person who can read at all, work in any capacity, drive a car, or have a romantic relationship cannot be intellectually disabled. In addition, jurors may be more impacted by the facts of the crime than are judges, who have experience with murder trials (ibid.).

3.3 **Timing of *Atkins* hearings**

A significant procedural issue that states approach in different ways is the placement of the determination of intellectual disability in relation to the capital sentencing proceeding (Blume, Johnson, and Seeds 2009). One concern, about which there are no data to date, is that, if the hearing occurs after the jurors have heard the details of the crime, those details will cause the jury to be unwilling to exclude the defendant from death penalty eligibility. Such a biasing of the intellectual disability determination would conflict with part of the *Atkins* rationale, because characteristics of the crime that increase the jurors' perceptions of its heinousness are often due to impairments associated with intellectual disabilities such as deficits in impulse control.

4 **Impairment not due to intellectual disabilities**

The Supreme Court relied on objective evidence to the 'maximum extent' possible in deciding *Atkins*; this evidence included legislative enactments, jury verdicts, opinions of social and professional organizations with germane experience, international trends, and polling data (*Atkins v Virginia* [2002], 321). The Court, however, made its own judgement regarding the acceptability of executing offenders with intellectual disabilities, a judgement that relied on the relative culpability of intellectually disabled offenders, the relationship between intellectual disabilities and the purposes of death penalty (deterrence and retribution), and the danger that impairments lead to unacceptably high risks of wrongful execution. If a defendant is just as severely disabled, though by another condition, it would seem to be just as cruel and unusual to execute him or her. For example, a person who did not meet the diagnostic criteria for intellectual disability but had severely limited intellectual functioning would have similarly reduced culpability, would be just as unlikely to be influenced by the deterrent effect of the death penalty, would have the same difficulty on assisting his or her attorneys, and would be as easily coerced into making a false confession. Robert Moorman, who was executed in 2012, is an example of a person so impaired.

Robert Moorman was sentenced to death for the murder of Maude Moorman, his mother, in 1984 after years of sexual abuse by her. The crime occurred while he was on a 72-hour furlough from his sentence for the kidnapping and rape of an eight-year-old girl. Moorman was sharing a hotel room with his mother and killed her after they got into an argument. He dismembered her, in an attempt to hide her body.

At trial Moorman claimed that he was not guilty by reason of insanity. His psychological expert, Dr Daniel Overbeck, testified that Moorman had a history of varied diagnoses, including psychosis, cerebral palsy, intellectual disabilities, and organic brain disorder, and had been treated in the past with antipsychotic medications. Dr Overbeck diagnosed Moorman with possible organic delusional syndrome, probable persisting pedophilia, and a schizoid personality disorder. Evidence supporting his diagnosis included Moorman's dishevelled, bizarre appearance and dress after his mother's killing, his impaired social and occupational functioning, and his difficulty to cope with stressful situations. Even the prosecution's psychiatric expert stated that he 'would not give [Petitioner] a clean bill of health emotionally or mentally' and that Moorman's writings were 'bizarre' and could be indicative of a mental defect (*Moormann v Schriro* [2012], 56–8). Another expert for the state, a neurologist, testified that his exam revealed no neurological deficits, but on cross-examination acknowledged to Dr Overbeck that 'most neurologists would say somewhere around birth something probably did happen to his brain that lowered his intelligence and accounts for his behavior' (*Moormann v Schriro* [2008], 149). Thus, although he could not identify a specific deficit, he conceded that there presumably was one.

Numerous evaluations of functioning had been conducted throughout Moorman's life since he was about two years of age, and most results indicated atypical development physically, socio-emotionally, and cognitively. These findings suggest profound impairment in many adaptive areas. Moormann's varying diagnoses include:

> cerebral palsy; moderate intellectual disabilities to possibly above average intelligence; mild intellectual disabilities with behavioral reaction; chronic brain syndrome associated with birth trauma with intellectual disabilities and behavioral reaction; mild intellectual disabilities associated with pedophilia; mental deficiency (mild) with behavioral and possible psychotic reaction; no intellectual disabilities—without mental disorder/pedophilia; and, schizoid personality disorder associated with sexual deviation/pedophilia. (Ibid., 8)

Despite the variability among the diagnoses, they consistently reflect the presence of a 'marked, disabling mental disorder' (ibid.).

After Moorman's arrest, his health deteriorated and he had a stroke in 2007 that further impaired his functioning. Moorman requested a stay of execution based on his decompensation. The Ninth Circuit Court of Appeals rejected this request and did not grant permission to file a habeas petition raising an *Atkins* claim that his IQ had been diminished by his surgery and stroke (*Moormann v Schriro* 2012). The federal court held that the state court's conclusion that he was not mentally retarded—because of the requirement of a full-scale IQ 70 or lower and the failure to establish onset before 18—did not violate any clearly established federal law (ibid., 648). Moorman was executed on 29 February 2013 despite his severely limited functioning.

While we applaud the Supreme Court's holding that it is cruel and unusual to execute individuals with traits that make them less culpable—traits like youth[20] and intellectual disabilities[21]—these categorical bans leave many people with similarly reduced culpability, like Robert Moorman, unprotected. Categorical bans by definition are frequently over- and underinclusive. Currently, people with IQs of 77 who are 18 years old or are so mentally ill that they cannot control their conduct can still be executed, despite the fact that they may have the

---

[20] *Roper v Simmons* [2005].

[21] *Atkins v Virginia* [2002].

same impairments as do those protected by *Atkins* and *Roper v Simmons* [2005], or even greater ones.

5 Conclusion

In *Atkins v Virginia* [2002], the Supreme Court acknowledged that 'not all people who claim to be intellectually disabled will be so impaired as to fall within the range of intellectually disabled offenders about whom there is a national consensus' (317). In the decade since this decision, states have used this statement as a license to create their own definitions and procedures for determining who meets the national consensus for its being cruel and unusual to execute them. This has led to deviations from the clinical recommendations embraced by the Supreme Court and has resulted in the execution of people who should have been protected on the basis of the Court's determination that evolving standards of decency preclude their execution. While the Court corrected one such deviation in *Hall v Florida* [2013], it has allowed others, for example Texas' *Briseno* factors, to stand. It is too early to tell whether the *Hall* signals an intention for the Court to insist on adherence to clinical definitions or whether it is a 'one-off'. If that does happen, then the next step is to consider whether people with similar impairments ought to be included in the categorical ban. *Atkins* represents a few steps down the road towards a humanitarian recognition of the fact that many disabled people are not sufficiently culpable to receive society's most severe punishment. Ultimately this recognition may lead to the total abolition of the death penalty, because with greater understanding of individuals comes knowledge of some mitigating circumstances, be they related to mental health, family history, or circumstances of the crime.[22]

Appendix List of Court Cases

US Supreme Court Cases

Atkins v Virginia, 536 US 304 [2002].

Bobby v Bies, 556 US 825 [2009].

Cleburne v Cleburne Living Center, Inc., 473 US 432 [1985].

Ford v Wainwright, 477 US 399 [1986].

Hall v Florida, 134 S. Ct. 1986 [2014].

Penry v Lynaugh, 492 US 302 [1989].

Roper v Simmons, 543 US 551 [2005].

---

[22] See *Atkins v Virginia* [2002] (describing 'evolving standards of decency').

US Circuit Court Cases

In re Hill, 715 F.3d 284 [11th Cir. 2013].

Moormann v Schriro, 672 F.3d 644 [9th Cir. 2012].

Williams v Quarterman, 307 F. App'x 790, 792 [5th Cir. 2009].

State Court Cases

Brown v State, 959 So. 2d 146 [Fla. 2007].

Cherry v State, 959 So. 2d 702 [Fla. 2007].

Ex parte Briseno, 135 S.W.3d. 1 [Tex. Crim. App. 2004].

Hall v Florida, 614 So. 2d 473 [Fla. 1993].

Head v Hill, 587 S.E.2d. 613 [Ga. 2003].

Hernandez v Thaler, 787 F. Supp. 2d 504, 516 [W.D. Tex. 2011].

Hill v State, 207 Ga. App. 65 [Ga. Ct. App. 1993].

Holladay v Campbell, 463 F. Supp. 2d 1324 [N.D. Ala. 2006].

Lambert v State, 126 P.3d. 646 [Okla. 2005].

Lizcano v State, No. AP-75,879, 2010 WL 1817772 [Tex. Crim. App. May 5, 2010].

Moormann v Schriro, No. CV-91-1121-PHX-ROS, 2008 WL 2705146 [D. Ariz. July 8, 2008].

Stallings v Bagley, 561 F. Supp. 2d 821 [N.D. Ohio 2008].

State v Lott, 2002-Ohio-6625.

State v Stallings, 2012-Ohio-2925.

State v White, 2008-Ohio-1623.

Van Tran v State, No. W200501334CCAR3PD, 2006 WL 3327828 [Tenn. Crim. App. Nov. 9, 2006]

References

AAIDD (American Association on Intellectual and Developmental Disabilities) and Arc. 2008. 'Sexuality: Joint position statement of AAIDD and the Arc'. https://aaidd.org/news-policy/policy/position-statements/sexuality#.V2L3qZMrJE4 (accessed 16 June 2016).

AAMR (American Association on Mental Retardation). 2002. 'Mental retardation: Definition, classification and systems of support, 10th ed. American Association on Mental Retardation. Washington, DC'. *Journal of Intellectual and Developmental Disability* 28: 310–11.

APA (American Psychiatric Association). 2000. *Diagnostic and Statistical Manual of Mental Disorders, Fourth Edition, Text Revision: DSM-IV TR*. Washington, DC: American Psychiatric Association.

Association for Retarded Citizens. 1974. *Give an Opportunity—Gain an Asset.* National Association for Retarded Citizens.

Baroff, G. S., and Olley, J. G. 1999. *Mental Retardation: Nature, Cause, and Management.* Sussex: Psychology Press.

Best Buddies, Ursinus College. 1999. *Facts about Mental Retardation.* http://archive-edu-2012. com/edu/u/2012-11-21_719097_17/Facts-about-Mental-Retardation (accessed 16 June 2016).

Blume, J. H., and Johnson, S. L. 2003. 'Killing the non-willing: Atkins, the volitionally incapacitated and the death penalty'. *South Carolina Law Review* **55**: 93–143.

Blume, J. H., Johnson, S. L., and Seeds, C. 2008. 'Empirical look at *Atkins v Virginia* and its application in capital cases'. *Tennessee Law Review,* **76** (3): 625–39.

Blume, J. H., Johnson, S. L., and Seeds, C. 2009. 'Mental retardation and the death penalty five years after Atkins'. In *The Future of America's Death Penalty: An Agenda for the Next Generation of Capital Punishment Research,* edited by C. S. Lanier, W. J. Bowers, and J. R. Acker, pp. 241–60. Durham, NC: Carolina Academic Press.

Blume, J. H., and Salekin, K. L. 2015. 'Analysis of Atkins cases'. In *The Death Penalty and Intellectual Disability,* edited by E. Polloway, pp. 37–52. Washington, DC: American Association on Intellectual and Developmental Disabilities.

Ceci, S. J., Scullin, M., and Kanaya, T. 2003. 'The difficulty of basing death penalty eligibility on IQ cutoff scores for mental retardation'. *Ethics & Behavior* **13**: 11–17.

Christian, L., and Poling, A. 1997. 'Drug abuse in persons with mental retardation: A review'. *American Journal on Mental Retardation* **102**: 126–36.

Codina, A. (dir.). 2009. *Monica & David.* HBO Documentary.

Craig, E. M., and Tassé, M. J. 1999. 'Cultural and demographic group comparisons of adaptive behavior'. In *Adaptive Behavior and Its Measurement: Implications for the Field of Mental Retardation,* edited by R. L. Schalock, and D. L. Braddock, pp. 119–40. Washington, DC: American Association on Mental Retardation.

Dana, L. 1993. 'Personality disorder in persons with mental retardation: Assessment and diagnosis'. In *Mental Health Aspects of Mental Retardation: Progress in Assessment and Treatment,* edited by R. J. Fletcher, and A. Dosen, pp. 130–40. New York, NY: Lexington Books/Macmillan.

Ellis, J. W., and Luckasson, R. A. 1985. 'Mentally retarded criminal defendants'. *George Washington Law Review* **53**: 414–93.

Everington, C., Notario-Smull, H., and Horton, M. L. 2007. 'Can defendants with mental retardation successfully fake their performance on a test of competence to stand trial?' *Behavioral Sciences & the Law* **25**: 545–60.

Flynn, J. R. 2006. 'Tethering the elephant: Capital cases, IQ, and the Flynn effect'. *Psychology, Public Policy, and Law* **12** (2): 170–89.

Gresham, F. M. 2009. 'Interpretation of intelligence test scores in Atkins cases: Conceptual and psychometric issues'. *Applied Neuropsychology* **16**: 91–7.

Grossman, H. J. 1968. 'The cloak of competence: Stigma in the lives of the mentally retarded'. *Archives of General Psychiatry* **18** (4): 508–10.

Grossman, H. J., ed. 1983. *Classification in Mental Retardation.* Washington, DC: American Association on Mental Deficiency.

Lanzi, R. G. 2005. 'Supporting youth with cognitive limitations to get their learner's license: Project drive'. *Impact* **18** (3): 22–3. https://ici.umn.edu/products/impact/183/183. pdf (accessed 20 May 2016).

Luckasson, R. et al. 1992. *Mental Retardation: Definition Classification, and systems of supports.* Washington, DC: American Association on Mental Retardation.

Moreland, J., Hendy, S., and Brown, F. 2008. 'The validity of a personality disorder diagnosis for people with an intellectual disability'. *Journal of Applied Research in Intellectual Disabilities* **21**: 219–26.

Morrissey, C., and Hollin, C. 2011. 'Antisocial and psychopathic personality disorders in forensic intellectual disability populations: What do we know so far?' *Psychology, Crime & Law* **17**: 133–49.

Musso, M. W. et al. 2011. 'Development and validation of the Stanford Binet-5 Rarely Missed Items—Nonverbal index for the detection of malingered mental retardation'. *Archives of Clinical Neuropsychology* **26**: 756–67.

Olley, J. G. 2009. 'Knowledge and experience required for experts in Atkins cases'. *Applied Neuropsychology* **16**: 135–40.

Quereshi, M. Y. 1968. 'Practice effects on the WISC subtest scores and IQ estimates'. *Journal of Clinical Psychology* **24** (1): 79–85.

Reschly, D. J. 2009. 'Documenting the developmental origins of mild mental retardation'. *Applied Neuropsychology* **16**: 124–34.

Rogers, R., and Bender, S. D. 2003. 'Evaluation of malingering and deception'. In *Handbook of Psychology*, vol. **11**: *Forensic Psychology*, edited by A. M. Goldstein, pp. 109–29. Hoboken, NJ: Wiley & Sons, Inc .

Sackeim, H. A. et al. 1992. 'Effects of major depression on estimates of intelligence'. *Journal of Clinical and Experimental Neuropsychology* **14**: 268–88.

Sadock, B. J., and Sadock, V. A. 2000. *Comprehensive textbook of psychiatry*. Philadelphia, PA: Lippincott Williams & Wilkins.

Salekin, K. L., and Doane, B. M. 2009. 'Malingering intellectual disability: The value of available measures and methods'. *Applied Neuropsychology* **16**: 105–13.

Schalock, R. L. et al. 2007. *User's Guide: Mental Retardation. Definition, Classification, and Systems of Supports. Applications for Clinicians, Educators, Disability Program Managers, and Policy Makers*. Washington, DC: American Association on Intellectual and Developmental Disabilities.

Schalock, R. L. et al. 2010. *Intellectual Disability: Definition, Classification, and Systems of Supports*. Washington, DC: American Association on Intellectual and Developmental Disabilities.

Switzky, H. N., and Greenspan, S. 2006. *What Is Mental Retardation? Ideas for an Evolving Disability in the 21st Century*. Washington, DC: American Association on Mental Retardation.

Tassé, M. J. 2009. 'Adaptive behavior assessment and the diagnosis of mental retardation in capital cases'. *Applied Neuropsychology* **16**: 114–23.

Walsh, C. 2009. 'AFP launches employment initiative for citizens with intellectual & developmental disabilities'. Alliance for Full Participation. http://www.aucd.org/ecp/template/news.cfm?news_id=3720&parent=0&parent_title=Employment&url=/ecp/template/news_mgt.cfm?type%3D406%26topic%3D3 (accessed 24 May 2016).

Wechsler, D. 2008. *Wechsler Adult Intelligence Scale, Fourth Edition (WAIS–IV)*. San Antonio, TX: NCS Pearson.

Chapter 13

Typical and atypical mental disorders: Moral implications for academic–industry collaborations

Dan J. Stein

1 Introduction

The nature of medical and mental disorders turns out to be a complex issue, partly because there is a broad and diverse range of such conditions, partly because the boundaries between illness and health can be rather fuzzy, and partly because health conditions are necessarily social and evaluative constructs. This complexity is readily apparent when it comes to a number of controversial disorders, such as substance use and gambling disorders; here debate ranges around whether these conditions really are medical and mental disorders, what are the appropriate preventive and management responses from clinicians, and what is the optimal regulation of the liquor and gambling industries. To address the nature of mental disorders—including substance use and gambling disorders—and the moral implications of how clinicians should interact with the liquor and gambling industry, this chapter employs constructs drawn from the cognitive–affective sciences in order to establish a distinction between typical and atypical disorders and to examine some of the consequences of this distinction.

2 What is a mental disorder?

In this section I will draw a contrast between a classical and a critical approach to thinking through the nature of mental disorder; and I will put forward an integrative position. This conceptual framework is too coarse to capture the work of any particular author working in the philosophy of science, language, or medicine and psychiatry. Rather it is intended to provide a heuristic approach that encompasses much previous writing in the field, and that helps with thinking through important debates, particularly in the philosophy of psychiatry (Stein 1991, 2008b, 2013). In this chapter my focus is on using this conceptual framework to think through the nature of substance use and gambling disorders and the ethics of clinician–industry collaborations in research on and in services for these conditions.

A classical approach to science, language, and medicine draws on the work of many philosophers, ranging from medieval nominalism through to the early Wittgenstein and the logical positivists. In this approach, science is an objective process that uncovers the laws that govern the phenomena of the world. Language provides a means for verifying the relevant data, for example science allows operational definitions based on necessary and sufficient criteria (e.g. a square is a figure made up of four equal sides joined at right angles). In medicine and psychiatry, we can similarly adopt an objective and value-free approach to describing symptomology, relying on diagnostic criteria for operationally defining the clinical entities under scientific investigation.

It is notable that recent editions of the American Psychiatric Association (APA)'s *Diagnostic and Statistical Manual of Mental Disorders* (*DSM*), while acknowledging the fuzziness of the boundaries between disorder and normality (Stein et al. 2010), have relied on operational diagnostic criteria for making this distinction. The National Institute of Mental Health has put forward a Research Domain Criteria (RDoC) framework for psychiatric research; although emphasizing that behaviours lie on dimensions and are governed by underlying psychobiological mechanisms, the authors of the framework place hope in the idea that biomarkers will one day differentiate disorder from normality, a position that falls in line with a classical approach (Stein 2014).

A critical approach to science, language, and medicine draws on the work of a number of alternative thinkers, from Vico and Herder down to the later Wittgenstein and a range of continental philosophers. In this approach, science is a process that, like any other human activity, has subjective elements and is imbued with particular interests, agendas, and power relations. Language can be construed as a set of knowledge claims, which in turn can be conceptualized in terms of validation (establishing evidence 'beyond reasonable doubt', as in a court of law) rather than laboratory-based verification, and texts reflect the contexts from which they emerge (e.g. the definition of a weed differs from place to place and from time to time). In medicine and psychiatry, we must recognize the subjective and value-laden nature of diagnoses and should emphasize the way in which these change from time to time and from place to place.

It is notable that the World Health Organization's International Classification of Disease (ICD) (see Reed and Ayuso-Mateos 2011) and advocates of global mental health (see Jacob and Patel 2014) have been sceptical of the pseudo-precision of the *DSM* system and have focused more on ensuring that the ICD has clinical utility and directs attention to reducing the treatment gap for serious mental disorders. Some working within a cross-cultural framework have suggested that even this approach fails to address adequately key issues such as the ways in which diagnostic presentations differ across the world and the ways in which culture shapes illness, and that attention to reducing the treatment gap runs the risk of downplaying social structural determinants of health that are among the root causes of global health disparities (Kirmayer and Pedersen 2014).

An integrative framework attempts to draw on insights from both the classical and the critical approaches. According to this position, science is necessarily a social and human activity, but it is nevertheless able to provide more and more detailed depictions of the underlying mechanisms that account for the phenomena of the natural and social worlds (Bhaskar 1978). The scientific study of language reveals how categories are embedded in social contexts and embodied in human practices, how categories are often graded with both typical central exemplars and more atypical peripheral exemplars (e.g. some birds like robins are typical, some birds like ostriches are atypical), and how categories are often extended with various metaphors (Lakoff and Johnson 1999). In medicine and in psychiatry we investigate both typical diseases (e.g. bacterial pneumonia, schizophrenia) and atypical conditions (e.g. macromastia, substance use disorders); while these constructs are both theory-laden and value-laden, medical science allows us to uncover the multiple relevant underlying biological and psychobiological mechanisms (Kendler 2012).

3 Typical and atypical mental disorders

A full defence of an integrative position is beyond the confines of this paper. Nevertheless, a good deal of work in the cognitive–affective neurosciences supports this approach (Stein 2013). Cognitive psychology, for example, has documented the way in which categories are employed, noting that, when we list birds, we are quick to think of robins and slow to think of ostriches. Artificial intelligence has put forward neural network models that are able to simulate the use of such graded categories in powerful and realistic ways. From a philosophical or conceptual perspective, it is encouraging to note that a position that emphasizes that science has both transitive elements (i.e. it is a social process) and intransitive elements (i.e. it studies universal mechanisms), seems sufficiently powerful to explain how science is actually done and how it makes real progress (with the classical and critical positions providing less persuasive explanations; see Bhaskar, 1978).

A distinction between typical and atypical disorders also appears to have explanatory power. In the case of typical disorders, we conceptualize them using various metaphors of dysfunction (e.g. of an attack, a breakdown, an impediment, or an imbalance). In the case of bacterial pneumonia, for example, an external agent—the bacterium—results in a penetration of 'defences' through no fault of the patient, who is entitled to adopt the 'sick role', while a medical practitioner fights back through his antibacterial armamentarium. In contrast, in the case of a substance use disorder, the illness is a result of the patient's own actions, for which he or she must take responsibility in future choices. Advocates of a medical model argue that substance use is indeed a brain disorder—with evidence of dysfunction, breakdown or imbalance of neurocircuitry and neurochemistry—and that patients deserve treatment; but many would counterargue that the standard sick role is not appropriate here.

Put differently, whereas typical disorders are easily conceptualized in terms of a *medical metaphor*, atypical disorders are often thought about in terms of a *moral metaphor*. Thus, when clinicians and societies consider a phenomenon such as bacterial pneumonia, the idea of an underlying 'dysfunction' is non-controversial and there is unlikely to be debate about diagnostic thresholds. Furthermore, prevention and intervention are very likely to be conceptualized in purely medical terms, with an emphasis on prophylactic vaccination and antibiotic management. Exceptions do, however, arise; for example, sexually transmitted infectious diseases may be thought of through a moral metaphor, where the sufferer is blamed for contracting the illness and where prevention and intervention may focus on behaviours such as sexual abstinence. Similarly, although there is some debate about thresholds for the diagnosis of schizophrenia and about the extent to which it can be characterized by a discrete set of dysfunctions, by and large this condition is conceptualized as a medical disorder, in which various disturbances in underlying neurocircuitry and neurochemistry lead to impairment and distress.

In contrast, when clinicians and communities consider a phenomenon such as gambling disorder, there is often scepticism about whether an underlying dysfunction exists and diagnostic thresholds need to be set in a way that emphasizes the chronicity and severity of symptoms and the associated distress and disability (First and Wakefield 2013). Prevention and intervention are very likely to be conceptualized in terms of societal regulation of the relevant behaviours (e.g. laws about casino operation). Again, there may be some exceptions; there will be a group that emphasizes that gambling may reflect a brain disorder and that people with pathological gambling deserve clinical intervention just like others who suffer from medical disorders —an argument that is perhaps even harder to make in the case of so-called 'behavioural addictions' such as gambling disorder than in the case of chemical addictions such as alcohol dependence.

It is notable that *DSM-5* chose to classify gambling disorder in the same chapter as substance use disorders, on the grounds that these disorders share diagnostic validators (APA 2013). An emphasis on diagnostic validators is reminiscent of an integrative approach insofar as it focuses on underlying psychobiological mechanisms. Indeed, in determining whether a disorder belongs on any particular spectrum of conditions, it is important to address both questions of clinical utility ('Will the decision enhance clinical practice, optimizing diagnosis and treatment?') and questions of diagnostic validity (Stein 2008a). Nevertheless, there is ongoing debate about the extent of overlap between the psychobiological mechanisms underlying 'behavioural addictions' and those underlying substance use disorders (Grant et al. 2014). Further, as emphasized in the *DSM-5* introduction, a diagnosis such as gambling disorder does not provide sufficient information to allow one to make judgements on issues such as criminal responsibility; this is a disorder that, consistent with its atypical nature, does not entirely license exoneration for one's behaviour (Blaszczynski and Silove 1996; Rachlin, Halpern, and Portnow 1986).

Psychiatric disorders have been divided into those with more 'externalizing' behaviours (e.g. violent behaviour) and those with more internalizing behaviour (e.g. depression). It may be worth emphasizing that not all atypical disorders are of the externalizing type. Thus, for example, social anxiety disorder may be considered atypical in a number of respects. Social anxiety disorder, like avoidant personality disorder, has a very early age of onset, and so seems to be part of the person rather than an imposed affliction. While there is some evidence that pharmacotherapy is effective for this condition, it is notable that the cognitive behavioural therapy of social anxiety disorder requires the individual to commit to behaving in a different away (e.g. no longer avoiding social situations). Similarly, from an evolutionary perspective, a certain level of social anxiety seems to be adaptive, which, again, raises questions about whether an underlying dysfunction really is present (Stein and Nesse 2015).

4 'Good' and 'bad' industries

The medical metaphor for conceptualizing mental disorders is used not only by clinicians, but also by relevant social institutions such as academia, the pharmaceutical industry, and government agencies. Thus both universities and pharmaceutical companies are likely to be very proud of being involved in research on new drugs to fight infection, while government departments of health are likely to boast about the roll-out of preventive measures such as vaccination (i.e. addressing the factors relevant to the dysfunction seen in a more typical disorder). At the same time, conflicts of interest do arise. Thus, for example, the pharmaceutical industry not only is interested in fighting infection but also aims to make a financial profit. Much of the literature on the ethics of clinicians' collaboration with the pharmaceutical industry focuses on conflicts of interest and on how best to manage them (Appelbaum and Gold 2010; Dubovsky et al. 2010; Insel 2010). It has also been pointed out that conflicts of interest arise for clinicians who advise government institutions; for example, such institutions may also wish to cut costs, and hence they may disadvantage particular individuals (Maj 2010).

The moral metaphor for conceptualizing mental conditions may lay the blame at the door of particular individuals or relevant social actors, such as industry or government. Thus smoking, for example, is thought to reflect not only on the individual smoker's poor lifestyle choices but also on the tobacco industry as a whole, or on its governmental regulation: in the case of the more atypical disorder, tobacco addiction, there is relatively less emphasis on the notion that any underlying psychobiological dysfunction is relevant. Whereas pharmaceutical advances can be profitable for shareholders, in the case of the tobacco industry profits are inversely proportional to public health (Stein 2015). Public health clinicians have appropriately fought long and hard to ensure governmental regulation of the industry by increasing tobacco taxes and by banning smoking in public places. Furthermore, while at one point clinicians collaborated with the tobacco industry on nicotine research, most academic institutions now insist on a 'non-association' model in which no direct funding to clinician-researchers from the tobacco industry is permitted (Adams, Buetow, and Rossen 2010).

For many clinicians and other stakeholders, the liquor and gambling industries fall somewhere between these typically 'good' and 'bad' industries, perhaps in part reflecting the atypical nature of substance and gambling disorders. On the one hand, these industries may provide important benefits to individual customers, as well as significant tax money for governments (which may themselves establish lotteries for fund-raising purposes). On the other hand, these industries are also extremely risky for particular vulnerable individuals, and the sequelae of excessive alcohol use and gambling are highly costly for different societies. Partnerships with these industries entail a number of important risks, including unacceptable kinds of conflict, failure to recognize differences in power, inappropriate government–industry relationships, fragmentation of the health sector, and silencing of dissent (Adams, Buetow, and Rossen 2010). Examples of problematic outcomes abound (Babor 2009; Bakke and Endal 2010; Casswell 2013; Jernigan 2012; Miller et al. 2011; Munro 2004). Academia and governments therefore need to develop and implement appropriate models for working with such industries in order maximize harm reduction.

The argument here relies on the importance of metaphorical processes of thinking not only about categories (Lakoff and Johnson 1999), but also about moral decision-making in relation to such categories (Johnson 1994). A philosophical defence of this approach goes beyond the confines of this chapter. Nevertheless, this position, again, seems consistent with data from the cognitive–affective neurosciences. Indeed, just as a view that emphasizes that science has both transitive elements—in other words is a social process—and intransitive elements—in other words studies universal mechanisms and helps to explain how science is undertaken and progresses, so a view that the relevant metaphorical processes contribute to understanding how judgements about illness are made, evaluated, and debated appears to have useful explanatory power. In particular, in more typical disorders, social–political and legal–ethical responses are, appropriately, focused on the eradication of the factors that are viewed as causing dysfunction (e.g. tuberculosis) and on the right to receive treatment, while in more atypical disorders social–political and legal–ethical responses are, understandably, more mixed with controversy about the optimal regulation of relevant agents (e.g. alcohol), and even medical models of dysfunction and intervention emphasize that patients have key responsibilities as well.

5 Gambling versus liquor industry

It is perhaps instructive to contrast the gambling and liquor industries in particular jurisdications. In South Africa, for example, gambling has long been outlawed, but after the arrival of democracy in 1994 more liberal legislation was passed. Soon afterwards, the casino industry helped to establish a National Responsible Gambling Program, which focuses on raising awareness of responsible gambling, of doing research on gambling issues, and of providing treatment to people with gambling disorder (Collins et al. 2011). Individuals who suffer from pathological gambling are able to call a free toll line and are referred to a network of therapists. Preliminary treatment data indicate that the cognitive behavioural therapy provided by this network is efficacious (Pasche et al. 2013). It is relevant to note that I have played a role in the work done by this program at my own university.

In contrast, the liquor industry in South Africa spends a relatively small amount of funds (small by comparison to their profits) on responsible drinking and on relevant research, and takes no responsibility for the treatment of those with alcoholism. The liquor industry has funded efforts such as the Foundation for Alcohol

Related Research (FARR), which focuses on research on fetal alcohol syndrome. For some, this is an exemplar of how industry funds can be used to emphasize an important alcohol-related problem and to help with finding the best solutions. For others, however, this funding exemplifies the view that industry only provides funding for particular kinds of issue, which do not diminish profits, and fails to address many key research and policy questions that are important for harm reduction but may decrease demand (Adams 2013; Babor and Robaina 2013). There is therefore an important opportunity for the liquor industry to make larger and more robust contributions to the health of alcohol users.

Given that the liquor and gambling industries may each offer some societal good, the challenge for clinicians and other stakeholders is to interact with these industries in a way that maximizes such good and diminishes possible harms. Such an interaction may not be easy to achieve, given that these industries are driven by short-term profits rather than by concerns regarding the long-term health of the population. Such collaborations are dynamic and entail a continuum of moral jeopardy (Adams 2007). They therefore require active support from multiple parties, which hold to a vision that sustainable profits are only feasible and acceptable when societal regulations and company activities contribute to maximizing the health of the population and to reducing harms. Such an approach to industry–academic collaborations may provide all stakeholders with an important 'third way' forward.

Much further work, however, is still needed if we are to understand fully how best to facilitate academic–industry collaborations in the areas of alcohol and gambling in order to maximize public health and minimize individual harms (Adams, Raeburn, and de Silva 2009; Adams and Rossen 2012; Litten et al. 2014; Livingstone and Adams 2011; Orford 2002). Good models of such collaboration may potentially succeed in allowing profitability, but at the same time mitigate addiction-related harms. It is important to ensure, for example, that financial arrangements are transparently monitored and that other structures and processes are put in place in order to minimize potential conflicts of interest and to ensure that the goals of maximizing public health and minimizing individual harms are reached. Given that alcohol use and gambling have significant negative effects on both individuals and societies as a whole, it is important that academia, industry, and governments work to produce and to implement such models.

6 Conclusion

I have previously put forward a conceptual framework for addressing the nature of mental disorder, which attempts to integrate aspects of the classical and the critical approaches to science, language, and medicine (Stein 1991, 2008b, 2013). One defence of such a framework relies on work done in the cognitive–affective sciences on human categories; this emphasizes that categories are graded phenomena, with typical and atypical exemplars. Certainly, in the case of medical and psychiatric disorders it is notable that some conditions are more typical and can be conceptualized by using medical metaphors, while others are more atypical and may be thought through via moral metaphors. This framework can be used to address a number of key problems in the philosophy of psychiatry, including nosological issues (Stein 2008a) and questions about cognitive enhancement (Stein 2012).

In this chapter I have focused in particular on how such ways of thinking are used in considering academic relationships with industries that focus on medication, tobacco, liquor, and gambling. The liquor and gambling industries are particularly challenging for clinician-researchers and other stakeholders because they are associated with both social goods and social evils and have a spectrum of potential benefits and harms. It is notable, however, that in some jurisdictions the gambling industry has taken responsibility for assisting individuals with gambling disorder, and academic–industry collaborations may help to maximize patient and societal outcomes (Collins et al. 2011). Such a model deserves further investigation and strengthening in order to ensure sustainable positive outcomes; if attained, then it may be useful in other places too and could in principle be extended to the liquor industry.

References

Adams, P. J. 2007. 'Assessing whether to receive funding support from tobacco, alcohol, gambling and other dangerous consumption industries'. *Addiction* 102 (7): 1027–33.

Adams, P. J. 2013. 'Addiction industry studies: Understanding how proconsumption influences block effective interventions'. *American Journal of Public Health* 103 (4): e35–e38.

Adams, P. J., Buetow, S., and Rossen, F. 2010. 'Vested interests in addiction research and policy poisonous partnerships: Health sector buy-in to arrangements with government and addictive consumption industries'. *Addiction* 105 (4): 585–90.

Adams, P. J., Raeburn, J., and de Silva, K. 2009. 'A question of balance: Prioritizing public health responses to harm from gambling'. *Addiction* 104 (5): 688–91.

Adams, P. J., and Rossen, F. 2012. 'A tale of missed opportunities: Pursuit of a public health approach to gambling in New Zealand'. *Addiction* 107 (6): 1051–6.

APA (American Psychiatric Association). 2013. *Diagnostic and Statistical Manual of Mental Disorders, Fifth Edition: DSM-5*. Washington, DC: American Psychiatric Association.

Appelbaum, P. S., and Gold, A. 2010. 'Psychiatrists' relationships with industry: The principal-agent problem'. *Harvard Review of Psychiatry* 18 (5): 255–65.

Babor, T. F. 2009. 'Alcohol research and the alcoholic beverage industry: Issues, concerns and conflicts of interest'. *Addiction* 104 (Suppl. 1): 34–47.

Babor, T. F., and **Robaina, K.** 2013. 'Public health, academic medicine, and the alcohol industry's corporate social responsibility activities'. *American Journal of Public Health* **103** (2): 206–14.

Bakke, O., and **Endal, D.** 2010. 'Vested interests in addiction research and policy alcohol policies out of context: Drinks industry supplanting government role in alcohol policies in sub-Saharan Africa'. *Addiction* **105** (1): 22–8.

Bhaskar, R. 1978. *A Realist Theory of Science* (2nd edn). Sussex: Harvester Press.

Blaszczynski, A., and **Silove, D.** 1996. 'Pathological gambling: Forensic issues'. *Australian & New Zealand Journal of Psychiatry* **30** (3): 358–69.

Casswell, S. 2013. 'Vested interests in addiction research and policy: Why do we not see the corporate interests of the alcohol industry as clearly as we see those of the tobacco industry?'. *Addiction* **108** (4): 680–5.

Collins, P. et al. 2011. 'Addressing problem gambling: South Africa's National Responsible Gambling Programme' *South African Medical Journal* **101** (10): 722–3.

Dubovsky, S. L. et al. 2010. 'Can academic departments maintain industry relationships while promoting physician professionalism?'. *Academic Medicine* **85** (1): 68–73.

First, M. B., and **Wakefield, J. C.** 2013. 'Diagnostic criteria as dysfunction indicators: Bridging the chasm between the definition of mental disorder and diagnostic criteria for specific disorders'. *Canadian Journal of Psychiatry* **58** (12): 663–9.

Grant, J. E., et al. 2014. 'Impulse control disorders and "behavioural addictions" in the ICD-11'. *World Psychiatry* **13** (2): 125–7.

Insel, T. R. 2010. 'Psychiatrists' relationships with pharmaceutical companies: Part of the problem or part of the solution?'. *Journal of the American Medical Association* **303** (12): 1192–3.

Jacob, K. S. and **Patel, V.** 2014. 'Classification of mental disorders: A global mental health perspective'. *The Lancet* **383** (9926): 1433–5.

Jernigan, D. H. 2012. 'Global alcohol producers, science, and policy: The case of the International Center for Alcohol Policies'. *American Journal of Public Health* **102** (1): 80–9.

Johnson, M. 1994. *Moral Imagination: Implications of Cognitive Science for Ethics*. Chicago, IL: University of Chicago Press.

Kendler, K. S. 2012. 'The dappled nature of causes of psychiatric illness: Replacing the organic–functional/hardware-software dichotomy with empirically based pluralism'. *Molecular Psychiatry* **17** (4): 377–88.

Kirmayer, L. J. and **Pedersen, D.** 2014. 'Toward a new architecture for global mental health'. *Transcultural Psychiatry* **51** (6): 759–76.

Lakoff, G., and **Johnson, M.** 1999. *Philosophy in the Flesh: The Embodied Mind and Its Challenge to Western Thought*. New York, NY: Basic Books.

Litten, R. Z. et al. 2014. 'Alcohol medications development: Advantages and caveats of government/academia collaborating with the pharmaceutical industry'. *Alcoholism: Clinical and Experimental Research* **38** (5): 1196–9.

Livingstone, C., and **Adams, P. J.** 2011. 'Harm promotion: Observations on the symbiosis between government and private industries in Australasia for the development of highly accessible gambling markets'. *Addiction* **106** (1): 3–8.

Maj, M. 2010. 'Financial and non-financial conflicts of interests in psychiatry'. *European Archives of Psychiatry and Clinical Neuroscience* **260** (Suppl. 2): S147–S151.

Miller, P. G. et al. 2011. 'Vested interests in addiction research and policy: Alcohol industry use of social aspect public relations organizations against preventative health measures'. *Addiction* **106** (9): 1560–7.

Munro, G. 2004. 'An addiction agency's collaboration with the drinks industry: Moo Joose as a case study'. *Addiction* **99** (11): 1370–4.

Orford, J. 2002. 'Potential conflict of interest in gambling research'. *Addiction* **97** (5): 600–1.

Pasche, S. C. et al. 2013. 'The effectiveness of a cognitive–behavioral intervention for pathological gambling: A country-wide study'. *Annals of Clinical Psychiatry* **25** (4): 250–6.

Rachlin, S., Halpern, A. L., and Portnow, S. L. 1986. 'Pathological gambling and criminal responsibility'. *Journal of Forensic Sciences* **31** (1): 235–240.

Reed, G. M., and Ayuso-Mateos, J. L. 2011. 'Towards a more clinically useful International World Health Organisation classification of mental disorders'. *Revista de Psiquiatría y Salud Mental* **4** (3): 113–16.

Stein, D. J. 1991. 'Philosophy and the DSM-III'. *Comprehensive Psychiatry* **32** (5): 404–15.

Stein, D. J. 2008a. 'Is disorder X in category or spectrum Y? General considerations and application to the relationship between obsessive–compulsive disorder and anxiety disorders'. *Depression and Anxiety* **25** (4): 330–5.

Stein, D. J. 2008b. *Philosophy of Psychopharmacology*. Cambridge: Cambridge University Press.

Stein, D. J. 2012. 'Psychopharmacological enhancement: A conceptual framework'. *Philosophy, Ethics, and Humanities in Medicine* **7** (1). doi: 10.1186/1747-5341-7-5.

Stein, D. J. 2013. 'What is a mental disorder? A perspective from cognitive–affective science'. *Canadian Journal of Psychiatry* **58** (12): 656–62.

Stein, D. J. 2014. 'An integrative approach to psychiatric diagnosis and research'. *World Psychiatry* **13** (1): 51–3.

Stein, D. J. 2015. 'Academic–industry partnerships in alcohol and gambling: A continuum of benefits and harms'. *Israel Journal of Psychiatry and Related Sciences* **52** (2), 81–4.

Stein, D. J., and Nesse, R. M. 2015. 'Normal and abnormal anxiety in the age of DSM-5 and ICD-11'. *Emotion Review* **7** (3) 223–9. doi: 10.1177/1754073915575407.

Stein, D. J. et al. 2010. 'What is a mental/psychiatric disorder? From DSM-IV to DSM-V'. *Psychological Medicine* **40** (11): 1759–65.

Index